# UNIQUE
# HEALING 2 ®

# UNIQUE HEALING 2®

A Guide for Eliminating Your
"A-Z" Symptoms, Weight Problems,
Illnesses, and Addictions With This
Unique Bowel and Body Healing Program

## Donna Pessin

www.UniqueHealing.com

authorHOUSE®

*AuthorHouse*™
*1663 Liberty Drive*
*Bloomington, IN 47403*
*www.authorhouse.com*
*Phone: 1-800-839-8640*

*Published by AuthorHouse    05/02/2012*

*ISBN: 978-1-4685-8079-2 (sc)*
*ISBN: 978-1-4685-8080-8 (e)*

*Library of Congress Control Number: 2012907218*

# Warning/Disclaimer

This book is designed to provide information on how and why healing your bowel and body with the Unique Healing® program will eliminate your symptoms, illness, and future disease, addictions, and weight struggles.

The purpose of this book is to educate and inspire. It is sold with the understanding that the author is not a medical professional and that this advice has not been proven scientifically. The information in this book is based on experiential knowledge stemming from the accumulation of eighteen years of work helping clients heal their bowels and bodies. The information in this book is not intended to diagnose or treat disease, or to replace the recommendations of your medical doctor. The reader must understand that it is their constitutional right to decide how they wish to care for the health of their body. The author has not suggested that the reader cease current medical care, be it drug therapy, x-ray treatment, chemotherapy, surgery, or any other medical procedures that their medical doctor deems necessary to their health. If the reader chooses to not follow recommendations made by their medical doctor, they understand that such a decision is their responsibility and will not hold the author responsible for any consequences of such a decision. The author shall have neither liability nor responsibility to any person or entity with respect to any damage caused, or alleged to have been caused, directly or indirectly, by the information contained in this book. Every effort has been made to make this book as complete and accurate as possible. However, there may be mistakes, both typographical and in content. Therefore, this book should be used only as a general guide and not as the ultimate source for healing your bowel and body. Furthermore, this book contains information on healing the bowel and body that is current only up to the printing date.

For many people, this process has resulted in a complete elimination of their symptoms, illness, addictions, and/or weight problems.

Note: This book is an amendment to my first book *Unique Healing* (originally titled *This Works Crutches Don't*). It is to be used in conjunction with this first book, which contains the instructions you need for healing your bowel and body, as well as much other valuable information for your success.

*Unique Healing* **is a registered trademark of** *Unique Healing*® **by Donna Pessin**

# Table of Contents

# Introduction

## Summary of the Information You Learned, and Need to Know, From *Unique Healing*

### Introduction

At the age of 22, I became completely disabled with an autoimmune disease. Over twenty-two doctors told me there was no cure. I also had a history of alcoholism, an eating disorder, and drug usage. I suffered from severe food and environmental allergies, constipation, excruciating pain, depression, insomnia, Candida, and hypoglycemia.

I spent ten years trying to regain my health and get my life back. I was put on food allergy diets, fasts, and given countless herbs and supplements. I spent two years having all of my amalgam fillings removed. I spent four hours a week sitting in a doctor's office with an I.V. in my arm delivering oxygen and mega-nutrients, including very high levels of vitamin C, into my body. I had vitamin B-12 and gamma globulin shots in my behind. I did over 450 enemas and some 80 colonics. For seven months I ate nothing but millet, vegetables, and rice protein powder. I diligently followed dairy-free, wheat-free, enzyme-rich diets for years. I properly combined meals. I tried every anti-Candida diet on the market, along with all of the supplements that were recommended then, as they are today, to treat it. I practiced visualization, affirmations, meditation, biofeedback, and deep breathing. I exercised frequently, as I had been doing when I first became very ill.

I took anything and practically *everything* that was recommended then, as it is today, to eliminate my symptoms.

I was thoroughly and strictly committed to these programs, but none of them worked, so I took the matter into my own hands. I spent thousands of hours, and many years, figuring this all out.

I learned how to heal my bowel* and how to safely, but aggressively, eliminate the enormous storage of acids** in my body. This accomplished a permanent healing of my body that all of the other programs, which only treat the symptoms of an unhealthy bowel and overly acidic body, never accomplished.

The information that I presented in *Unique Healing* is "what finally worked." And it will work for you, too.

I have no more neck or chest pain, no anxiety, no depression, no constipation, no hypoglycemia, no PMS, a lot of energy, no insomnia, and no difficulty maintaining my weight. I have not drunk alcohol in twenty years and find abstaining from it is completely effortless. My eating disorder mentality is gone. Because of this program, I crave healthy foods, but I do not need to follow a strict diet or limit my carbohydrates to look and feel good. I tolerate high levels of wheat and dairy when once even the smallest amount left me crippled for days. I eat a low protein, high carbohydrate diet. I do not need extra supplements to maintain these results, either.

> My healthy bowel and body—and not a diet, exercise, or a bunch of supplements—keeps my weight down, and me feeling fabulous. My fear of becoming ill with cancer or any other disease, and of losing control of my weight, is completely gone. These outcomes are priceless.

## Chapter 1: How This Program Works

This program is *unique.* It is based on many years of personal and professional experience, schooling, and a extraordinarily high level of commitment and time. It is based on experiential knowledge stemming from the accumulation of eighteen years of work helping clients heal their bowels and bodies.

This program heals your bowel and body. I have not found either a conventional or alternative medicine program that does the same.

---

\*　　May also be loosely interpreted as colon, intestines, gut, etc.

\*\*　May also be loosely interpreted as toxins, heavy metals, pesticides, chemicals, waste, etc.

No client has ever walked into my office with health and/or weight complaints who had a healthy bowel and body.

When my clients heal their bowel and body, all symptoms, illness, disease, addictions, and weight problems go away—even the most difficult, critical, and stubborn ones. All symptoms, including those that one might think are inevitable due to mental stress, food allergies, old age, genetics, or any other cause, are eliminated. This program has helped many clients achieve this even when all else has failed. I have helped many clients eliminate conditions that modern medicine calls incurable.

In my experience, healing your bowel and body prevents the occurrence of cancer, heart disease, osteoporosis, diabetes, or any other illness. I am not aware of any other program that can deliver these results.

Vitamins, drugs, exercise, food allergy diets, low carbohydrate diets, low calorie diets, alkaline diets, fasting, organic/pesticide-free foods, detoxification programs, laxatives, enemas, chiropractic, acupuncture, alcohol, recreational drugs, nicotine and all other addictive substances, etc. are "crutches" that do *not* heal your bowel or body. When you use these crutches, you are at great risk of your symptoms, weight problems, addictions and illness returning. And they leave you vulnerable to premature death from cancer, heart disease, etc.

Relying on these crutches to look and feel great fails *you*. Stop blaming yourself.

The majority of other alternative health programs require a large intake of vitamins and herbs that help replenish the nutrients lost by an acidic body, but they do nothing to eliminate the acids/toxins that are causing the depletion in the first place. This eventually leads to failure and only short-term and minimal improvements in your health and weight, as well as a susceptibility to disease and premature death.

Vitamins do not stop the continued accumulation of acids in your body, and they do not heal your bowel and eliminate the problems associated with an unhealthy one.

I have never had an overweight client, or one with symptoms, addictions, illness, or disease, arrive at my office with a healthy bowel and body. I have never had a client improve the health of their bowel and body with this program who did not see a remarkable improvement in their health and weight.

*Unique Healing* gave you the tools needed to eventually eliminate the need for all of these crutches. When you heal your bowel and body with this program, you will look and feel great *without* diets, supplements exercise, drugs, chiropractic, acupuncture, etc.

Your body is constantly working to maintain an internal balance, or homeostasis. Daily, diet, stress, environmental toxins, heavy metals, pesticides, chemicals, drugs, and medications contribute towards an overly acidic blood pH. Acids in your blood also originate internally from the stored acids in your organs and fat cells, acids that were never eliminated from your body. Depending on what you eat, these may be released into your blood, and together with the new day-to-day acids, make up the "total acid/toxic" load in your blood.

In health, when these acids enter your blood, they move into your lymphatic system, and then into your bowel, where they are completely eliminated. Just as we generate trash in our day-to-day living that has to be thrown out, so our bodies have this acidic trash that needs to be eliminated daily, too.

For the majority of you, these acids are not completely eliminated once they reach your bowel because your bowel is not healthy enough to do so.

When you are constipated, these acids are not completely eliminated from your body. Yet, eight-five percent of my clients have daily, but poorly formed stools, and they harmfully, and mistakenly, believe that this is healthy. When you have daily stools that are not 100% well-formed, even *fewer* acids are eliminated from your body than when you are constipated.

Un-eliminated acids in your *blood* trigger symptoms, weight problems, bad blood tests, and addictions. Acids in your *organs* cause disease and death, but fewer symptoms, weight problems, bad blood tests, or addictions.

This unique program eliminates acids from *both* your organs and your blood, reducing disease/illness and numerous symptoms, including weight problems. Many programs reduce blood acidity but *increase* organ acidity, resulting in less symptoms and weight, but greater death from disease. Others simply buffer the acids in your blood, so you look and feel better, but because these acids are not eliminated, they continue to accumulate and eventually lead to disease, as well as require a strict and daily intake of numerous supplements (to buffer these acids.)

Eating fewer carbohydrates, eating fewer calories, eliminating wheat, dairy, or pesticides, exercise, yoga, chiropractic adjustments, massage, medications, vitamins and other supplements, and all of the other crutches you use to look and feel better, do little if nothing, to heal your bowel or eliminate acids from your body.

This program heals your bowel so that these acids can be safely, quickly, easily and permanently eliminated.

Healing should be safe and comfortable, and this program is!

This program heals your bowel by rebuilding the beneficial bacteria within. This process can take some time, however, so *Unique Healing* provided information on using crutches effectively, and temporarily, while healing your bowel and body. These can help you immediately look and feel better, giving you the faith and patience needed to succeed with this program. (This information has been repeated, but expanded, in Chapter 5 of this book.)

As for diet, what you eat is much more a product of the imbalances in, and ill health of, your bowel and body than your knowledge, intentions, discipline, or willpower.

You don't need me to tell you that your sugar, coffee, alcohol, meat, etc. are not good for your health. You need your body to tell you that for you. My body does that now, and yours will too as you follow this program. This program will change your internal chemical balance and in the end, you will crave a healthy diet and your fear and confusion around food will be eliminated.

When your bowel is unhealthy, it is impossible to make drastic healthy dietary changes, including the adoption of a healthy high carbohydrate diet if you are currently avoiding or limiting them, and feel good doing so. It is also unnecessary. Dietary changes in this program are gradual and extremely easy to follow. *Unique Healing* outlined a transition diet plan to follow while healing your bowel and body.

Ultimately, your healthy body will cause you to feel great and lose weight, not a strict diet.

When you heal your bowel and body and spend money doing so, you are saving up for your future, a future free from discomforts, weight struggles, bankruptcy from illness, and/or premature death. Ultimately, it is significantly more expensive and more difficult to live a life filled with fear and discomfort than it is to heal your bowel and body, which will eliminate your fears and discomforts.

There is an end to this program, unlike programs that rely on crutches, which are never-ending.

At the end of this program your stools will be daily and well-formed no matter what you eat, your weight will be effortlessly maintained, and you will be symptom-free. You will be healthier than ever before. You will crave healthy foods and not need to take extra supplements. You will look and feel great eating a high carbohydrate, healthy diet. You will realize that many of the symptoms that you put up with are not natural and are not a part of a healthy body. You will understand how excess weight, ill health, addictions, and disease develop. You will understand how you have reversed the process of disease development. You will feel utterly empowered and fear of weight gain and disease will no longer control you.

This program's difficulty lies primarily in the fact that it requires you to have a new perspective about your health and body. You have to be strong, as others will surely try to convince you to veer off the healing road. You have to let go of your possible anger about past failures to attain your ideal health and weight.

Reducing fear, skepticism, feelings of powerlessness, confusion, misunderstandings, and impatience are keys to success. *Unique Healing* aims to accomplish this.

The approaches you have been given have failed you; you, yourself are not a failure.

Healing your bowel and body takes time and you have to commit to it for a while.

Healing your bowel and body will not fail you.

## Chapter 2: How Did Everyone Get So Lost?

Most of you are zooming down the wrong road and it is not your fault. *Up until now*, these answers to your health problems, addictions, illness, and weight problems have not been available to you. Your being lost, and your failure to heal your bowel and body are not due to a lack of effort, intention, or desire. *You did your best.* If you are angry, frustrated, or in denial, replace this with a feeling of gratitude. Be grateful that an answer exists to your health and weight problems, at all.

The crutches aren't working. We are more overweight, sicker, and dying at younger ages than ever before.

Your health and weight problems are not an inevitable product of stress, genetics, age, a lack of willpower, bad luck, poor soil conditions, etc. These are under your control. If you inherited an unhealthy bowel or body, it can be healed.

You have been led down the wrong road by studies, blood tests, dangerous assumptions, misinformation, a harmful definition of health, and a lack of knowledge about how your body works and heals. You have been manipulated through fear. This program helps you take back your power and eliminate your fears. It puts you on the right road.

You have allowed success to be defined in the short-term and this has led you to choose paths that deliver short-term success but long-term failures.

There are many diet and health programs that can help you look and feel better immediately, but many of these make your body less healthy in the process, so that in the long-term you are worse off (more symptoms, susceptibility to disease, and/or weight gain) for having done so.

Relying on studies to guide you to a healthier, thinner body can be dangerous. Most of them are geared towards treating symptoms with crutches, and you will not attain a long life and weight stabilization as a result. Very little of my work has been studied. But bear in mind, the lack of a study simply means it has not been done, *not* that there is no relevant correlation.

You are stuck in a vicious cycle. Sometimes I see new clients who have spent thousands of dollars on crutches that have failed, who are then afraid to invest the necessary time and money in this program. You will not succeed if you have this mindset and fear. This is not a quick fix program. It works. But it requires time and a commitment. It requires money, although much less than you will likely spend if you don't follow this.

Dangerous definitions of health have led you down the wrong road. For example, how you look does not determine your level of health. Fit and healthy do not mean the same thing. Normal and healthy do not mean the same thing. Symptoms do not necessarily reflect your level of health. You also cannot assume you are healthy because you have relatively few symptoms, and you do not need to assume you are near death's door simply because you have many.

You need to respect, and react to, your health and weight problems *now*, before they become something deadlier.

Just as you are often wrongly and dangerously led to believe that bad genetics are your inevitable life-sentence and excuse for your health problems, there is equal danger in assuming that good genetics go on forever. This is entirely untrue.

Normal blood work does not guarantee that you are in superb health, and you should never feel safe simply because your blood tests are normal.

Muscle testing, hair analysis, live cell analysis, comprehensive metabolic and other blood tests, and pH tests done first thing in the morning and after eating also lead you to treat your symptoms and weight problems with crutches, and not heal your bowel and body. Most of these tests are unnecessary, and many are more harmful than beneficial.

An accurate definition of health that you can feel secure about, and that is created with this program, was shared in *Unique Healing,* and is as follows:

— You have a complete lack of symptoms—no acne, gas, aches and pains, fatigue, insomnia, ongoing depression, PMS, high cholesterol, constipation, diarrhea, sugar cravings, etc.
— You are slim and symptom-free, even if you are stressed or eating a lot of carbohydrates, wheat, or dairy products.
— You have an abundance of energy without drinking caffeine in any form, or taking any other stimulant.

—— You feel great, without medications, vitamins, herbs, exercise, acupuncture, massage, chiropractic adjustments, etc.

—— You have no addictions. Your body is not interested in sugar, alcohol, coffee, nicotine, or drugs.

—— Your bowel movements are twice a day and well-formed, even if you are stressed, or eat a lot of carbohydrates, spicy foods, raw vegetables, or dairy products. You do not have gas after eating beans or raw broccoli. If you are a woman, your stools do not get loose during your period.

—— You have no weight struggles. You don't have to diet or exercise to maintain it. You can eat a lot of carbohydrates and not gain weight. You do not have to constantly be vigilant about what you eat and how much you exercise. You are free of this "jail."

—— All of the medical tests that you do have—blood tests, pap smears, bone density tests, colonoscopies, etc.—show absolutely no abnormalities, not even non-cancerous polyps, cysts, ulcers, or any other conditions that you may be told are common and "nothing to worry about."

—— As a woman you do not suffer from symptoms of menopause or PMS. Your periods are every 28 days and you have no difficulty becoming pregnant and delivering your baby naturally. Your pregnancy and birth go smoothly and without complications.

—— It is effortless to maintain these results, and the results are long-term, meaning they last for decades.

—— You do not fear cancer or other diseases, because in great health, you do not feel insecure or vulnerable to them.

## Chapter 3: Why Healing Your Bowel Works

A healthy bowel eliminates acids. When they are not eliminated, they trigger reactions from your body that lead to weight gain, illness, symptoms, addictions, and eventually, disease.

There are many dangerous consequences of *not* healing your bowel.

When you heal your bowel, you create a healthy bacterial environment within it. In addition to helping your body eliminate harmful acids, these bacteria play key health and weight-regulating roles. See Chapter 1 for a detailed description of the health and weight-regulating roles of your healthy bacteria.

> This program will heal your bowel and body *all by itself.*

The most important component of your blood that needs to be kept in balance is the pH level. Your blood has an ideal pH level too, which is 7.4, or slightly alkaline. This pH needs to be maintained constantly. *Death occurs when it falls below 7.0.*

Certain foods and beverages, stress, medications, pollutants, chemicals, and heavy metals take your pH out of balance/contribute to an overly acidic bloodstream.

A description of the health and weight side-effects of un-eliminated acids due to an unhealthy bowel was given, as summarized in Chapter 1 of this book as well.

When excess acidity is eliminated, your organs become nourished and heal.

By helping your body eliminate acids, a healthy bowel improves circulation, hydration, oxygenation, and vitamin/nutrient levels in your body. (See Chapter 3 for more information on these conditions, and how they are improved by healing your bowel and body with this program.)

The variable that most affects the health of your bowel bacteria is the health of it at birth.

Studies that look at the relationship between a healthy bowel and body are not being done. A lack of scientific proof does not mean that none exists; it often means that the proof simply has not been searched for.

> Your health and weight problems are the result of a great accumulation of un-eliminated acids in your body, coupled with an unhealthy bowel bacterial environment. This program eliminates these acids, and it heals the bacterial environment in your bowel.

## Chapter 4: Why Vitamin, Drug, Exercise, and Physical Modality Crutches Don't Work

The vast majority of programs for reducing your symptoms, addictions, illness, and weight problems are crutches, and fail as a result.

These approaches (i.e. crutches) do little/mostly nothing to heal your bowel or eliminate the acids that cause your health and weight problems, and as a result, failure in the long-term is high.

Feeling good and/or looking good because you take a lot of supplements or follow a strict diet does not mean that you are healthy.

The dangers and problems of depending on programs that rely on crutches include the following: Using them gets old, so when you stop using them, your symptoms, weight, addictions, or illness returns; You may dangerously believe you are healthier, and safer from death, than you really are; Stronger ones are needed as time goes by, making it more difficult to use them, and benefit from them; You may miss an important one, like the "crutch" that could have prevented your breast cancer; The time energy and money you spend on these may mean there is not enough available for healing your bowel and body and preventing disease, etc.

You know that you are only treating your symptoms with a crutch if your weight, symptoms, or addictions return upon stopping the use of it; when there is dependence on a drug, supplement, modality, or diet; you see/feel quick results in one month or less; your elimination has not improved.

Drugs are crutches that are acidic and toxic to your body. Over the long-term they contribute to more health and weight problems.

The vast majority of vitamins, supplements, and most herbs are crutches, too. There are also no magic supplements.

Scientific studies show that people who ingest large amounts of supplements die at the same age as those who do not.

As you eliminate acids from your body with this program, your *entire* vitamin/nutrient needs plummet (calcium, B-vitamins, vitamin D, vitamin E, you name it). In other words, low levels of vitamins are not caused by many of the reasons you are given, such as soil depletion. In a healthy body, as created with this program, it is very easy to meet your entire nutrient needs, *poor soil and all*, by diet alone, because when your body is healthy, your nutrient needs are low.

Recreational drugs are also crutches. You use them to feel better. You use them to alter your brain chemistry. Like all crutches, you can easily become addicted to them and the reaction they create. With this program, recreational drugs become undesirable and no longer needed to feel good.

Exercise is a crutch too. It can help you lose weight and feel better, and it *may* make your blood tests look better, but exercise does not heal your bowel or body, and it does not prevent premature death from disease. It does not address the cause of your weight or other problems. When you heal your bowel and body with this program, you will not need to exercise to look and feel good.

If you have taken up exercise and concurrently began a high-protein diet, you are doing more harm than good.

Massage, chiropractic, acupuncture and other physical modalities are crutches too, that also do nothing to permanently heal your bowel and body or eliminate acids.

Naturopaths, acupuncturists, chiropractors, and like-minded professionals are trained to treat symptoms, just as medical doctors are. They are not trained to heal your bowel and body. The difference between them and medical doctors is that the drugs they recommend to treat symptoms are natural and non-toxic, yet many act as though they are doing much more for you. When they act as though they are helping you heal your body, they are putting you in danger. *If they recommend high-protein diets, and many of them do, you may have been safer going to a conventional doctor instead.* And if you look to them for support of the information in this book and/or "need" their "go ahead" to do this program, you are not going to succeed in healing your bowel or body.

## Chapter 5: Why Diet Crutches Don't Work

Low calorie, high protein, low carbohydrate, organic, gluten or dairy-free, food allergy, low fat, raw food, alkalinizing, macrobiotic, and cleansing or detox diets are crutches, too. They treat the symptoms of un-eliminated acids and the resultant weight and health problems. This is why they eventually fail you. You have not failed. These diet programs have failed *you*.

Worst of all, some of these are dangerous in the long-term and contribute to more difficulty losing weight in the future, and a greater occurrence of future ill health and disease, as well.

When you heal your bowel and body with this program, you will not need to eat a large amount to lose weight and/or feel great (i.e. you will look and feel great eating a lot of carbohydrates). Also, my clients always find that as their bowel becomes healthier, and they become healthier, their desire for protein goes down. It never goes up, regardless of their blood type or any other variable that is used to justify a higher intake.

Glucose and fructose are not evil. Glucose cleanses acids out of your organs and moves them into your blood and bowel. It is only when your bowel is unhealthy, or you have an excess of these acids because your body is unhealthy, that these will not be eliminated, triggering health and weigh problems. "Shoving" these acids back into your organs with a low carbohydrate diet—which may reduce health and weight problems—*increases* death and disease and is not an acceptable solution!

High protein diets cause damage to your health, whether it is immediately noticeable or not. They lead to short-term weight and symptomatic reduction; but long-term struggles and disease

If a diet calls for the restriction of carbohydrates, it is a high protein diet.

Allergy-free diets usually turn into high protein diets, and "work," but hurt, for the same reasons.

An unhealthy bowel and body cause food allergies. This program heals these so that dairy, wheat, and other food allergies do not exist.

## Chapter 6: A Healthy Bowel Explained

The form of your stools is *much* more important than the frequency of your elimination.

The health of your bowel is not simply determined by the frequency and form of your stools.

A lifetime of bad stools does not guarantee a future of them.

Frequent elimination without ideal form is the least healthy and most inefficient elimination pattern, and it leads to the greatest health and weight problems. (See this chapter in *Unique Healing* for a definition of a well-formed stool.) It is much healthier, and you are eliminating more acidity, if you go every other day and your stool is wide and hard than if you go every day and your stools are skinny or too short.

The frequency and form of your stools should meet the ideal bowel description criteria all the time, *regardless of what you eat.* If your stools are normally well formed but become looser when you eat spicy foods, or more fruit or carbohydrates, then your bowel is not as healthy as it could be. Your stools should also be well formed when you are under stress, travelling, during your period, etc.

Colonoscopies, stool analysis tests, and other colon/stool tests don't accurately measure bowel health.

Misunderstandings about bowel function are a top reason why people fail to heal their bowel and body. These were described in greater detail in this chapter.

## Chapter 7: Healing Your Bowel

Healing your bowel entails rebuilding the bacterial environment within it. In this program, *Bowel Strength,* or *Unique Healing Probiotics,* are used to accomplish this. (Note: "Probiotics" is considered synonymous with "acidophilus.")

Your bowel will not simply heal itself.

Healing your bowel is a complex process that requires a great deal of information, knowledge and understanding. Also, the *correct* amount of bowel-healing products needs to be taken in order for this to work. This chapter provided much of this information for you.

Healing your bowel takes time. There is not a magic method or product that can do this quickly. You should have 200,000,000,000,000* beneficial bacteria in your bowel, and most of you have much less than that. Building up to this number takes a while. Anyone who tries to sell you on the ability to do this quickly is "taking you for a ride." (*This number used to be stated at 10 trillion, but recent, new medical testing revealed this number to be much higher, or 20 trillion.)

Exercise, colonics, fasting, eating more healthfully, diets, acupuncture, and 99% of the supplements and modalities that you are sold do not heal your bowel. Laxatives, colon cleansers, and other programs "for the bowel" do not heal it. Products that claim a quick or inexpensive fix, or that contain probiotics or similar herbs as *Bowel Strength,* but at insufficient amounts, will not heal your bowel.

Both *Bowel Strength* and *Unique Healing Probiotics* contain ingredients that help your good bacteria grow and multiply.

*Bowel Strength* and probiotics like *Unique Healing Probiotics* do the same thing. You don't need to take both products to heal your bowel.

Instructions for using these products, and what to expect as you heal your bowel, were provided in this chapter, and questions and misunderstandings about products that heal your bowel, which are a common cause of failure, were also addressed.

Other practitioners—medical *and* alternative—*receive little to no* training or education in this bowel and body healing process. I developed this program. It is not currently taught at schools or in seminars.

It is much easier to maintain bowel health than it is to achieve it. (Personally, it has been over 18 years since I have taken a product like *Bowel Strength* or probiotics.)

For 99% of you, the bowel healing products suggested in my book will be needed, and valuable, for a *minimum* of one year or longer.

## Chapter 8: Healing Your Body

To accelerate the healing of your body and the elimination of acidity/ toxicity from it, it is very important for you to use *Body Bentonite.* This is *food grade* bentonite clay, which increases the absorption of acids in your bowel. It prevents them from being reabsorbed into your body, and therefore, it prevents the symptoms, weight problems, addictions and diseases associated with un-eliminated acids.

It helps your body eliminate the total acid load that has been stored in it. It helps heal your body. Taking it daily will immediately improve the form and frequency of your bowel movements and as a result, you will lose weight and feel better much faster than if you don't use it.

To attain your ideal health and weight, two things need to be accomplished: the elimination of old acids, and the healing of your bowel. *Body Bentonite* assists with this first one.

*Body Bentonite* is a crutch *and* a healing agent.

Like *Bowel Strength* or *Unique Healing Probiotics*, you will see greater improvements in your health, weight, symptoms, addictions, and disease *as you continue taking this product over time.* And regardless of your immediate response to it, if you stick with it for at least a year or two, you will experience significant improvements in your health, symptoms, weight, addictions, and/or disease.

*Body Bentonite* heals your body and it cannot, directly, cause you to look or feel worse. (For details on using this product, including how much to take, see Chapter 5 in this book).

If "it" doesn't result in a positive exit of acidity from your body, then "it" is not really healing you. Most diets, supplements, and alternative programs like chiropractic, acupuncture, and massage do nothing to eliminate acids from your body.

This chapter also explained what to expect as you heal your body, a vital "map" that helps you succeed as you travel down this healing road. A misunderstanding of the healing process is one of the main reasons why an individual will fail to achieve their health and weight potential.

You learned that while following this program, your symptoms/weight, etc. may be aggravated by the following: reducing your protein intake too soon; increasing your consumption of fruit and/or fruit juice; increasing your consumption of carbohydrates; exposure to more acidity; the cessation of a crutch too soon; exposure to a bacterial infection.

Ninety-nine percent of the symptoms, weight gain, loose bowels, etc. that you experience during this program will be due to the first six reasons given above, and *not* due to the use of these supplements—*Bowel Strength, Unique Healing Probiotics,* or *Body Bentonite.*

You don't need to be fearful of these products or this approach. It is the people who are *not* doing this program who should have fear, not you. Healing is not dangerous; not healing *is*.

Manipulating your blood tests to look better before you are healthier, correctly interpreting these tests, and instructions on correcting a level that is too high or too low on these tests was also covered in this chapter.

## Chapter 9: the Diet Part is Easy

It takes a very long time for dietary and other acids to negatively affect your bowel and body. You cannot reverse this quickly simply by eating healthier.

A healthier diet can help *maintain* a healthy bowel and body.

Your failure to eat "perfectly" will not prevent this program from working. In fact, the beauty of this program is that you don't have to worry about the right way to eat. It will happen naturally.

Eating healthy does not mean that *you* are healthy!

You have wrongly been led to believe that you can change your health and weight conditions by changing your diet.

If a food immediately helps you lose weight or feel better, it does not mean that that food is healthy. Some foods are healthy for you that can, in the short-term, make you feel bad or gain weight. Some foods are not healthy for you that can, in the short-term, make you feel good and lose weight.

If you have to avoid any food to look and feel better, your body is not as healthy as it could be.

The three most important variables to consider in determining if a food is *healthy* for you are its digestibility, pH value, and nutrient content.

You learned that to succeed in healing your bowel and body, you should not try to eat "perfectly" now; you should not eat foods you are allergic to or have intolerances to; you should not increase your consumption of fruit or carbohydrates, yet; and you should not eat a cleansing diet, as defined in this chapter (and a critical concept for your success).

Dietary crutches are advised while you are healing your bowel and body, and include replacing high acid foods with similar, high alkaline ones; choosing less acidic foods; choosing easier to digest proteins; eating a lot of healthy fats, including cheese; and reducing high fiber foods for *now*.

For more information on diet, review Chapter 9 of *Unique Healing*. Also, many helpful videos on diet and this program can be found at www. UniqueHealing.com and at www.YouTube.com/UniqueHealing.

## Chapter 10: Use The Right Crutch While You Heal

This chapter described how to use supplement crutches effectively so that you can look and feel better while you heal your bowel and body.

Don't attempt this program without crutches.

When your bowel and body are unhealthy, these crutches can help you look and feel better. There is no possibility of them making you look or feel worse. Never blame them for these problems.

My favorite crutches are *Body Bentonite, Unique Healing Methyl B-12, Unique Healing Colloidal Silver,* calcium citrate, melatonin, and natural progesterone cream.

On the other hand, understand they are just crutches. If they help, don't stop them just because you look or feel better; take the right amount; only use them if they work; re-try them later in the process when you are healthier; eliminate redundancy; compare apples to apples and don't stop your current crutches yet; reduce addictive crutches gradually; don't stop medication crutches.

A summary of how these crutches can help you look and feel better while you heal, and information on the dosage to take, has been updated to be more aggressive for reducing your symptoms, addictions, and weight problems more quickly. See "How to Look and Feel Better NOW" in Chapter 5. The benefits of using these crutches for your symptoms, weight problems, illness, and addictions are also covered in each individual section in Chapters 2 and 4.

For a better understanding of the important information in *Unique Healing*, watch my videos, especially "How This Program Works" and "How This Program Works 2" available at *www.UniqueHealing.com* or *www.YouTube/UniqueHealing.com*

# Chapter 1

## Why THIS Program Eliminates Your Symptoms, Weight Problems, Addictions, and Disease

When I was sick I was focused solely on trying to get rid of my current, debilitating symptoms. When I healed my bowel and body with this program, these went away, along with all of my old, pre-illness symptoms. I was angry and shocked to realize that I had bought into the idea, like most of you, that all of my symptoms and suffering were inevitable.

> This book describes how various, common conditions are eliminated with this program, but this is *not* to be interpreted as all-inclusive and representative of the only ones this program can help.

Many of these conditions are problems that I personally struggled with. The bad news is that I was so ill I had a lot of problems. The good news is that because of this, in addition to a wealth of professional experience in eliminating these, I have a lot of personal expertise in understanding and relating to them, and eliminating, them as well.

If you have a condition that is not listed here, it is simply because I thought that if I wrote a book that was thousands of pages long—the length of time it would take to discuss all possible conditions—no one would read it. Also, honestly, I have not and could not possibly have had professional experience with every possible condition and/or disease. Who has?

> However, I believe that if you focus on healing your bowel and body, the possibilities are endless. After reading about all of the conditions that follow, I hope you begin to see how a healthy bowel and body can eliminate *any* condition.

I have given you a specific description of how a healthy bowel eliminates many common conditions, and how a healthy body, as created with this program, eliminates symptoms, weight problems, addictions, and disease. I also hope to show you how the few crutches I mentioned in *Unique Healing* have widespread use and ability to help every health condition imaginable. I hope you get the tools needed to apply this to your individual condition, so if you do not have some of the conditions covered in Chapter 2, read about them anyway. This will help you better understand how this program will help yours.

At one significant point in my illness, I came to the realization that I should focus on getting healthy, and trust that my symptoms would go away. This was a turning point in my healing process. And as you know by now, it led me to the complete and permanent elimination of my current and past symptoms. Regardless of your condition, trust that if you focus on healing your bowel and body it will go away.

All health and weight problems are the result of a great accumulation of un-eliminated acids in your body, coupled with an unhealthy bowel bacterial environment.

## Heal Your Children, Too!

The conditions discussed in this book apply to children as well. I have helped many. I have worked with children from the age of 3 months to 18 years. I strongly encourage you to heal your child's bowel and body, too.

Many children inherited *less* healthy bowels than we, their parents, did. Sadly, even at a young age, many are in a state of health that is unsafe. An unhealthy bowel allows for the more rapid re-absorption of acids that eventually leads to premature death.

You have the opportunity to help your children now, and prevent much of the suffering you may have already endured (with weight problems, symptoms, illness, and/or addictions). Some of your children are already suffering more than you ever have, with autism, A.D.D., severe allergies, etc. This program will help them too.

Heal your child's bowel and body now because it is easier when they are younger. The sooner they jump on board, the less time it will take to heal. Eliminate the acids from their body now, before it accumulates to large amounts, and heal their bowels now to prevent accumulations in the future. When children are young we have some control over what they do. When they become older and independent, we lose much of this control (college-age students are perhaps my most difficult clients to work with, as a result). So the time is now.

In Chapter 5 you will find information on crutches to use for your children to help them look and feel better while they are healing their bowel and body. Many of my younger clients take large amounts of *Body Bentonite* as well. (The ideal amount to take is not a product of size and weight, as drugs are; it is a product of ill health and need.)

For information on using *Body Bentonite*, as well as *Bowel Strength* or *Unique Healing Probiotics*, refer to *Unique Healing*. In general, the amounts of these that are recommended for adults are appropriate, and needed, for children. In fact, many of my younger clients have less healthy bowels than their parents and need to use *Bowel Strength* or *Unique Healing Probiotics* at larger amounts, and for longer periods of time, than their parents.

If you have a child younger than three years old who you would like to help, I strongly advise you to contact me at ***www.UniqueHealing.com*** and schedule individual consultations with me for him/her. Under no circumstances should you use this program on a child younger than one year old without working with me personally.

## How to Use This Book

Each section is separated into the following: Why a healthy bowel eliminates the condition; Why a healthy body eliminates the condition; Why my crutches work for the condition; How long you can expect to need to use crutches for the condition; A review of additional information and misunderstandings about each condition; Success stories/testimonials about how this program has helped others with this condition.

Additionally, under the heading of some of these conditions I have recommended other conditions covered in this chapter that relate to this one, as well, and I highly recommend that you read these sections. Also, the concepts covered in Chapter 3 apply to *every* condition covered in this book, so make sure you read this chapter thoroughly as well.

# A Healthy Body Eliminates Symptoms, Weight problems, Addictions, and Disease

When you heal your body with this program, you eliminate a lifetime of stored acidity from your *organs* (toxicity, heavy metals, pesticides, etc.). You eliminate the acids that lower your oxygen and nutrient levels. With fewer acids, you have greater amounts of oxygen and nutrients available, which are needed for your organs to be healthy. Numerous symptoms, diseases, addictions, and weight problems do not and cannot exist when your organs are healthy.

When you heal your body with this program, you eliminate the acids from your *blood* that otherwise trigger numerous symptoms, diseases, addictions, and weight problems, as your body responds to protect you from these un-eliminated acids. Hence, healing your body eliminates these issues. (A healthy body, as created with this program, is not burdened by excess, stored acidity in its organs, which can at any time, become released into your blood in the first place.)

(In other words, when you have headaches, for example, you have both an unhealthy lymphatic system and excess acidity in your blood. Healing your body heals your lymphatic system and eliminates acids from your blood. In other words, in order for your kitchen to get wet, you have to have holes over the roof of your kitchen, *and* it has to be raining. Healing your body is like fixing these holes and like eliminating the rain.)

A detailed description of the sequence in which your organs/body become unhealthy, and the sequence in which they react to these un-eliminated acids, and the symptoms, diseases, addictions, and weight problems that occur in response to them, was presented in Chapter 3 of *Unique Healing*. Below is a summary of this information. At the end of this book, there is also a diagram to further help with your understanding of this. Note that while your kidneys are among your body's first line of defense against un-eliminated acids, they are among the last organs to heal. (Hence the classification of Level 4, which is meant to imply that this is the fourth area of your body to heal. This information is described in greater detail under the sections of this book titled "How long will I need crutches for" each particular condition.)

## Your first line of defense against un-eliminated acids: bowel, kidneys, lungs, skin (Level 4)

(As stated above, while this is the *first* area of your body to become unhealthy, it is the last, or fourth, to heal, hence the classification of "Level 4." This concept extends to the remaining listed below as well.)

Your organs of elimination are at the "bottom of your pipe" and they are: your bowel, kidneys, lungs, and skin. These excrete acids via your stool, urine, breath, and sweat.

These organs are your body's first line of defense against excess acidity. When you are exposed to excess acidity as a child, these are the first organs to respond to it. The bottom of your pipe "clogs up first".

As your bowel responds to un-eliminated acids, some of the symptoms you may experience are appendicitis, bloating, bulimia, Candida/yeast infections, colitis, constipation, Crohn's disease, diarrhea, diverticulitis, fissures, gas, hemorrhoids, hernias, I.B.S., nausea, polyps, stomachaches, and others. (Note: An unhealthy bowel bacterial environment causes many symptoms, diseases, addictions, and weight gain, as described below, but it too is affected by un-eliminated acids, and these can trigger the symptoms listed above, which are different from those triggered by the unhealthy bacterial environment in your bowel.)

As your kidneys respond to un-eliminated acids, some of the symptoms you may experience are acne, bedwetting, blood pressure (too high or too low), cold hands and feet, cystitis, dehydration, difficulty holding urine, dry skin or eyes, edema, gout, hot flashes, kidney stones, nephritis, night sweats, Reynaud's, sex drive (low), sweating (excessive or difficulty), swollen ankles, urination (nighttime or frequent daytime), water retention, weight gain, and others.

As your lungs respond to un-eliminated acids, some of the symptoms you may experience are allergies, asthma, coughs, cystic fibrosis, emphysema, and others.

As your skin responds to un-eliminated acids, some of the symptoms you may experience are acne, boils, dry or oily skin, eczema, hives, itchy skin, psoriasis, rashes, and others.

## Your second line of defense against un-eliminated acids: lymphatic system, nervous system/brain (Level 3)

As your lymphatic system responds to un-eliminated acids, some of the symptoms you may experience are AIDS, allergies, anemia, anxiety, appendicitis, autoimmune diseases, backache, breast pain and lumps, cataracts, chronic fatigue, colds, congestion, dizziness, earaches, fatigue, fever, fibroids, fibromyalgia, glaucoma, Grave's disease hay fever, headaches, hepatitis, herpes, hives, infertility, juvenile diabetes, laryngitis, Lou Gehrig's, lupus, macular degeneration, migraines, miscarriages, mononucleosis, multiple sclerosis, neck pain, pain and inflammation, PANDAS, prostatitis, ringing in your ears, sinusitis, snoring, sore throats, TMJ, thyroid, or TSH, imbalances, tonsillitis, tumors (benign), vaginitis, vasculitis, viral infections, vitiligo, warts, and others.

(Your lymphatic system, which includes your spleen, thymus, and lymph nodes, does not eliminate acids directly, but rather carries them to your bowel to be eliminated. I mention this because some lymphatic massage practitioners wrongly advertise that lymphatic massage eliminates toxins from your body. It does not.)

As your nervous system, including your brain, responds to un-eliminated acids, some of the symptoms you may experience are A.D.D., addictions, Alzheimer's, anxiety, autism, brain tumors (non-malignant), depression, epilepsy, insomnia, Kawasaki's, neuritis, panic attacks, Parkinson's, phobias, schizophrenia, seizures, Tourette's, and others.

## Your third line of defense against un-eliminated acids: adrenal glands, gallbladder, liver, pancreas, small intestines, stomach (Level 2)

(Many of these organs serve similar functions, hence there is great redundancy in their response to un-eliminated acids, so I have grouped these together.)

As these organs react to un-eliminated acids, some of the symptoms you may experience are Addison's disease, adrenal exhaustion, cholesterol levels (too high), cirrhosis, diabetes, fatigue, gallstones, gastritis, heartburn, hepatitis, hormonal imbalances, hypoglycemia, indigestion, infertility, irregular periods, low blood sugar (craving sweets, alcohol and/or nicotine), metabolism (lowered), pancreatitis, reflux, ulcers, weight gain, and others.

## Your fourth, and final, line of defense against un-eliminated acids: arteries, bones, cells (Level 1)

As your arteries respond to un-eliminated acids, some of the symptoms you may experience are clogged arteries, heart disease, heart attacks, blood clots, stroke, and death.

As your bones respond to un-eliminated acids, some of the symptoms you may experience are osteopenia and osteoporosis.

As your cells respond to un-eliminated acids, some of the symptoms you may experience are non-hormonal cancers, "non-curable" hormonal cancers, arthritis, and death.

## Healing Your Bowel With This Program Eliminates Symptoms, Weight Problems, Addictions, and Disease

Healing your bowel entails eliminating stored acids from it, as previously described, *as well as* creating a healthy bacterial environment within it. In addition to helping your body eliminate harmful acids, these bacteria play key health and weight-regulating roles. Some of the primary functions of your healthy intestinal bacteria are listed below.

1. Formation of acids (toxins, heavy metals, chemicals, pesticides, etc.) into stools that can be quickly and efficiently eliminated from your body.
2. Digestion of insoluble fiber in your diet, resulting in less bloating and gas.
3. Hormonal regulation, and a reduction in breast cancer, cysts, enlarged prostate, fibroids, impotence, infertility, PMS, prostate cancer, etc.
4. Manufacture of vitamin B-12, resulting in a reduction in A.D.D., addictions, alcoholism, Alzheimer's, anemia, autism, depression, drug use, Lou Gehrig's, low energy, multiple sclerosis, nerve damage, nicotine cravings, Parkinson's, seizures, sugar cravings, and Tourette's.
5. Absorption of calcium, for healthy bones/prevention of osteopenia and osteoporosis.
6. Absorption of amino acids, for healthy muscle weight gain and strength.
7. Manufacture of digestive enzymes, which reduces gas and food allergies and increases your absorption of nutrients.
8. Digestion of gluten and lactose, for the elimination of food allergies to foods containing these (especially wheat and dairy).
9. Manufacture of melatonin, for the reduction of insomnia.
10. Manufacture of vitamin K and other nutrients.

11. Improved immunity and the destruction of Candida, yeast, fungal infections, parasitic infections, and harmful bacterial infections, like E-coli, staph, pneumonia, Lyme, strep, and H-pylori.

## In summary, some of the symptoms, diseases, addictions, and weight problems directly eliminated by a healthy bowel bacterial environment, as created with this program

Acne, A.D.D., addictions, AIDS, alcoholism, Alzheimer's disease, anorexia, anxiety, athlete's foot, autism, autoimmune diseases, bacterial infections, bladder infections, bloating, breast cancer, bulimia, Candida, cavities, celiac, chronic fatigue, colitis, Crohn's disease, cystic fibrosis, dandruff, depression, diarrhea, ear infections, eating disorders, eczema, endometrial cancer, Epstein Barr Virus, fatigue, fever, flu, food allergies, fungal infections, gas, hot flashes, impotence, infertility, insomnia, itchy skin, Lyme disease, mal-absorption, malaria, memory loss, miscarriages, multiple sclerosis, nausea, nervousness, nighttime urination, osteoporosis/osteopenia, pain, parasitic infections, Parkinson's disease, pneumonia, post-partum depression, PMS, psoriasis, rashes, salmonella poisoning, schizophrenia, seizures, sinus infections, staph infections, stomachaches, strep, Tourette's syndrome, tuberculosis, underweight, uterine cancer, worms, and many more.

Additionally, because a healthy bowel eliminates acids from your body, the symptoms, diseases, addictions, and weight problems that are discussed above are also eventually eliminated.

## Additional Conditions Eliminated by Healing Your Bowel and Body With This Program

The list of conditions in 2 is not to be interpreted as all-inclusive and representative of the only ones this program can help. I have also worked with people with a number of other symptoms, as well as very complicated diseases and conditions that were called "medically incurable."

For example, athlete's foot, bad breath, boils, bone spurs, canker sores, Chlamydia, croup, cysts, dandruff, dry skin and hair, edema, fever, fibroids, fractures, gallstones, gonorrhea, gout, growth problems, Guillain-Barre Syndrome, gum disease, hair loss, hernia, herpes, hysterectomy, kidney stones, malabsorption, memory problems, polyps, Meniere's disease, ringing in the ears, syphilis, TMJ, tonsillitis, ulcers, vitiligo, warts, and worms—are just some of the many conditions that have not been covered in detail in this book, but that are eliminated by healing your bowel and body with this program.

> For now, regardless of your condition, trust that if you focus on healing your bowel and body, it will go away.

### Disease, disorder, or condition—it doesn't matter how you label it

Whether your problems are labeled as a disease, condition, or disorder, is irrelevant. They are the same thing, and if I have labeled something a disorder, like an adrenal disorder, and someone has called it adrenal disease, interpret these to be the same problems, because they are.

When a problem is called a disease, it can sound frightening, and leave you feeling as though there is no help. This label is limiting and may take away your perceived power to change this. Don't let that happen to you.

### Sorry for the redundancy

I did not go into detail with every condition possible, as I thought it would get redundant and I didn't want to offend you and your intelligence; on the other hand, after writing my first book, I was swamped with people asking me if this program could help with "x" condition, and it occurred to me that it was not so obvious how and why this program helps with *every* condition, so as a result, any redundancy you do find is a product of this experience.

## What Symptoms, Diseases, Addictions, and Weight Problems Doesn't This Program Eliminate?

I cannot think of any symptoms, diseases, addictions, or weight issues that are not caused by an unhealthy bowel and/or body.

> In my experience, an unhealthy bowel and/or body cause 100% of your symptoms, weight problems, addictions, or disease. Because this unique program heals your bowel and body, it is capable of eliminating 100% of these issues.

9

Healing your bowel and body will not make you six feet tall, if you are currently five feet tall. It will not make your brown eyes turn blue. It will not turn your black hair to blonde. While you *will* look better when you are healthier, your general physical characteristics will not change.

If your gallbladder has been removed it will not grow back. If you are missing an arm, it will not grow back. If you have a scar from a surgery, it will not go away. If you are intelligent, you will not lose this. If you are horrible at the violin, you will still be horrible, after you heal your bowel and body with this program.

So yes there are things that will not change with this program, but the ones that count, the symptoms, diseases, addictions, and weight problems that dramatically reduce the quality and quantity of your life, those will change.

## Studies

With *all* health categories covered in this book, the fact that numerous studies do not exist showing a connection between an unhealthy bowel and body does not mean that the connection does not exist; it simply means that no one has paid to have these studies done.

# Why My Crutches Work for These Conditions

Because it takes time to heal your bowel and body from a lifetime of damage, you will need to use crutches to look and feel good, as well as to have your blood tests look normal, while you are healing.

Because it will take time to fix all of the holes in your roof, you will need to drag a tarp over it everyday for a while before you can not do so and still have your house stay dry when it rains.

Under each condition, I have listed which of my favorite crutches—*Body Bentonite, Unique Healing Methyl Vitamin B-12, Unique Healing Colloidal Silver, Unique Healing Calcium Citrate,* melatonin, and natural progesterone cream—help reduce or eliminate the condition while you are healing, and why they are helpful.

For more information on using crutches for these conditions, including the amounts to use, please refer to Chapter 5.

## How long will I need to use crutches for conditions associated with an unhealthy body/un-eliminated acids?

The most effective crutch for eliminating your symptoms, weight problems, and bad blood tests while you are healing your body is *Unique Healing Body Bentonite*. If your funds are limited or your ability to take pills is limited, make this crutch your priority.

(Note that *Body Bentonite* and calcium are similar in that they both eliminate the acidity in your blood that triggers numerous health and weight reactions, but that your priority, should you be limited in ability to take or purchase these crutches, should be in taking *Body Bentonite* over calcium, as *Body Bentonite* eliminates acids from your body, while calcium citrate simply buffers them. *Body Bentonite* is a crutch that *also* heals your body, and taking it leads to a permanent elimination of the health and weight problems associated with acids, while calcium is a crutch that does not.)

How long you need to use these crutches depends on many variables, but by far, the two most relevant ones are how fast you heal (which is influenced by your desire, financial ability, fears, and misunderstandings), and which symptoms/conditions you are trying to eliminate.

Remember, healing occurs in reverse: first the bottom of your pipe, next the middle, and then the top. Symptoms/conditions associated with the organs at the top of your pipe will require crutches for far much less time than those at the bottom of your pipe.

Earlier, I reviewed the "layers of your pipe"/the process by which you accumulate acids and which organs become unhealthy and the sequence of this, and the symptoms associated with this. See also Appendix A, and the diagram "Sequence of Healing," at the end of this book.)

I have the above diagram separated into four levels: Level 1, Level 2, Level 3, and Level 4. These correspond to the different sections "of the pipe."

The organs "at the top of your pipe" heal first; the ones at the bottom heal last. The Level 1 organs, and symptoms/illnesses associated with them, heal first, and those at Level 4 heal last.

For example, if you have high cholesterol, for example, which is associated with an unhealthy liver (middle of your pipe), you will be able to stop the crutches recommended in this book and still have your blood cholesterol levels come back normal sooner than you will be able to stop your crutches and still have no water weight, for example (as this is associated with ill-health of your kidneys, or the bottom of your pipe).

In other words, going back to the house analogy, if you have holes over your living room and kitchen, both of these rooms will get wet when it rains. If you put a tarp over your roof, both of these rooms will stay dry. If the holes over your living room get fixed, but the holes over your kitchen have not been repaired yet, when it rains, your living room will stay dry, but your kitchen will get wet.

Do you have holes over your bathroom and kitchen, or do you have holes over your bathroom, kitchen, living room, family room, and bedroom? In other words, do you have an unhealthy bowel and kidneys, or do you have an unhealthy bowel, kidneys, lymphatic system, liver, adrenal glands, and heart? The more there is to heal, the longer you will need crutches. The more holes there are to fix, the longer you will need to put a tarp over your roof to keep your house dry.

Under each condition I have listed where in this level of healing it occurs, assuming that other levels are unhealthy too. In other words, if you have aches and pains, your lymphatic system is unhealthy (Level 3), and it will be the third system to heal, *if* the other levels of "your pipe:" are unhealthy too. If they are not, it may be the first area of your body to heal with this program. In general, the longer you have had a condition, the longer you will need crutches for it, but even this is not consistent, as many of you have manipulated your condition with diets, exercise, supplements, etc. and are therefore not even aware of ill health at the various levels of your body.

Some conditions are affected by more than one area of "your pipe." Some are affected by several organ systems. In these cases, you may find that as one system heals, your need for crutches are *reduced*, but that your need for crutches is not eliminated until *all* organs associated with this condition have healed.

Additionally, your organs at the "bottom of your pipe," your bowel, skin, kidneys, and lungs, are the first to become damaged when you have un-eliminated acids, and they "have more holes" and take the longest to fix. In other words, you may only need to heal your body for 12 months to heal your liver, but healing your skin may take 36 months. It takes less time to heal the organs closer to the "top of your pipe"

Under this section of each condition covered, I have indicated on which level(s) this condition occurs so as to give you an idea of how long you will need to use crutches to eliminate this condition. Consider the above concepts when you read this, and take this information as a *general* guide, but not as a *definitive* guide, as this is an understandably complex concept that is affected by numerous variables.

For many of you, you will need/find value in taking these crutches for two to four years. (Most of you have taken, and *will* take, if you do not follow this program, crutches for decades, so this is "nothing." Not to mention, the results with this program are extraordinarily superior to those you get with programs that only rely on crutches, as most do.)

Don't get too caught up with this concept. Rather, focus on the fact that you are extremely lucky that you can heal our bowels and bodies (you get a second chance at life!), and you are extremely lucky that safe and effective crutches for your conditions exist at all.

## Keep your stools well-formed

During the healing of your body, you will look and feel best, and have the best blood test results, the better you keep your stools during this process. Even though good elimination is healing, think of it as the "tarp on your roof" as well. Review Chapter 6 of *Unique Healing* for the ideal bowel description and remember, daily elimination without perfectly formed stools, or stools that are on the skinny or soft side, is worse than elimination that occurs every two days or that consists of harder stools.

## How long will I need crutches for conditions associated with an unhealthy bowel bacterial environment?

The above concepts apply to those symptoms, weight problems, and blood tests that are affected by un-eliminated acids and ill health of your body.

Remember, however, that you *also* have symptoms that are caused solely by the ill health of your bowel bacterial environment, which have nothing to do with an unhealthy body and un-eliminated acids (as reviewed earlier). The crutches you take for these symptoms, and how long you will need these, is separate from above.

> The most effective crutches for symptoms/conditions caused by an unhealthy bacterial environment in your bowel are *Unique Healing Methyl Vitamin B-12, Unique Healing Colloidal Silver, Unique Healing Calcium Citrate*, natural progesterone cream, melatonin, and a low fiber diet.

How long you will need *these* crutches depends on the health of your bowel bacterial environment, and how fast you heal it. The less healthy your bowel is on day one, and the slower you heal it, the longer you will need crutches. For many of you, you will need/find value in taking these crutches for two to four years. (Most of you have taken, and *will* take, if you do not follow this program, crutches for decades, so this is "nothing." Not to mention, the results with this program are extraordinarily superior to those you get with programs that only rely on crutches, as most do.)

For example, if your bowel bacterial environment is unhealthy and the use of *Unique Healing Methyl Vitamin B-12* increases your energy or reduces your depression, you may "need" to take this daily for two to three years before you can stop it completely and still maintain high energy levels and low levels of depression. You will need to wait until your bowel is healthy enough to make adequate amounts of vitamin B-12 on its own, in other words.

These concepts are confusing, I realize, but your understanding of them is important to your success. Re-read this section until they are clear to you. Also, watch my video titled "How Long Will I Need Crutches?" available at ***www.UniqueHealing.com*** or ***www.YouTube.com/UniqueHealing***.

## For some conditions, there are no crutches

There are *no* crutches for conditions that are degenerative or reflect damage to an organ, muscle, etc. For example, you can quickly eliminate headaches, a condition that is triggered by un-eliminated acids in your blood; you cannot quickly eliminate osteoporosis, which is a condition of damage to your bones. In other words, you can put a tarp over the holes in your roof and quickly reduce how wet your house gets; you cannot quickly fix these holes in your roof. In the conditions where an organ is involved, I have indicated this, and I have reminded you that there are no crutches for this condition.

# Dietary Crutches/Changes

The dietary crutches that are recommended in Chapter 9 of *Unique Healing* are helpful to every condition listed in this book. I have summarized these for you in the weight loss chapter, Chapter 4. I have provided a general "diet plan" you can follow that will help you look and feel better while you heal your bowel and body with this program.

Also, in some sections of Chapters 2 and 3 you will find some comments on dietary crutches that are used for specific conditions. This is done largely to clarify misunderstandings about diet as it pertains to these conditions.

Remember, however, that dietary crutches can manipulate the acids in your blood and can affect your weight, blood tests, and symptoms associated with un-eliminated acids, but that not all of your symptoms are due to un-eliminated acids. Some are the result of the unhealthy bacterial environment in your bowel and there are no dietary changes/crutches that can quickly affect these, For example, if your bowel is unhealthy and not making enough melatonin, creating insomnia, there is no dietary change you can make that will provide this needed melatonin for you.

## Why your diet won't heal you

I have created videos with dietary information and advice that support the information on diet provided in *Unique Healing*. For example, one is titled "Top 5 Diet Tips," but you will find other useful ones, as well. I also created a new video, which was not available at the time I wrote *Unique Healing*, in an attempt to address the ever-ending demand for a "quick diet fix" for your problems, which is called "Why Your Diet Won't Heal You," and I strongly encourage you to watch this, as well.

All of my videos are available at ***www.UniqueHealing.com*** or through ***www.YouTube.com/UniqueHealing***.

# Misunderstandings About These Conditions and Other Information for Your Success

My experience is that fears and misunderstandings are your greatest barrier to successfully healing your bowel and body with this program. Many exist, and I have tried my best to address the most common ones regarding each condition in Chapter 2. If I have missed yours, please email me at ***donna@UniqueHealing.com***, and I will try to incorporate these in future books/blogs/videos, etc. If you want it addressed now, contact me to schedule a consultation.

In no way can I address all of the misunderstanding that exist, so it is up to you to read what I have addressed, as well as all of my books, blogs, and videos, and determine if what I have written so far rings true. If so, then you must trust that even if your misunderstanding has not been addressed, that this program is not to be feared, and that this program has not "missed something" critical to your well being.

This section also includes some information on other widely prescribed crutches for these conditions, but for the most part, I have not spent much time on this. Crutches do not heal, and the ones that I have recommended are the ones that I have found, after 18 years of using numerous crutches, to be the most effective at reducing your symptoms, weight, and addictions while you heal your bowel and body. There are no magic supplements, and I am not missing anything if I have not recommended one. Review Chapter 4 of *Unique Healing* to better understand the limitation of crutches, and the great redundancy of the ones that are most commonly recommended.

## Success Stories/Testimonials

I warn you again, as I did in my first book, to be very careful about using testimonials to judge a program's effectiveness and/or safety.

Nevertheless, I have included some testimonials (and could have included *many* more) to appease all of you who keep asking for these.

Just as using a blood test to measure your health, measuring your health by how you look and feel, and allowing others to manipulate you through fear, produces programs that provide short-term results, and often dangerous ones, at that, you cannot use testimonials as a way to judge a program's value.

What you are left with is your intelligence and common sense. You must understand why healing your bowel and body works and why crutches don't. I have done my best to give you the information to back this up. I will keep providing this to you in future books, but ultimately, you must trust your instincts, and you cannot be afraid of failing. This program will not fail you if you commit to it with an attitude of confidence and determination and disallow others to take you off this path.

# For More Support and Information

## Watch my videos

For the majority of these conditions, I have done a video that helps you visualize the concepts I am discussing. I am a visual person, and this would be helpful to me. A great many of my clients have found these to be helpful to them, as well.

All of my videos can be accessed directly from my website at ***www.UnqiueHealing.com*** or at ***www.YouTube.com/UniqueHealing***.

(Note: The titles given in the next sections are accurate, but they will not always exactly match the ones you find on my website or on YouTube. For example, a video titled "Why THIS Program Works for Infertility" is called "Why THIS Program Eliminates Infertility" in this book. I apologize for the inconsistency, but many of these videos were done prior to my writing this book, and I neglected to keep the titles consistent. I have used a consistent title in this book in an attempt to make this easier for you, although, again, the title may vary ever so slightly once you try to locate it. I trust this will not cause any problems, and I believe you will be able to very easily find the video you are looking for.

Additionally, at the time of publication of this book, not all of the videos mentioned in here were completed. If you do not find the video you are looking for, look back in the near future. All videos will eventually be done.)

## Read every section, even if the symptom or condition does not pertain to you

Do this because there are many misunderstandings in these sections, that I have not repeated in every section, which *do* pertain to you, and which will be helpful for your success. Do this because when you are healing your bowel and body with this program, one of these conditions may arise, and it will be helpful to have read about it beforehand. Do this because, at the very least, a lot of people need your knowledge and help, and you will be better equipped to explain to your friends and family why this program can help them with their conditions, if they have ones that are different from yours, which is highly likely.

## Search for additional physiological information online or in physiology textbooks

In describing each condition, I have taken the liberty to greatly condense and summarize some of the physiology behind these conditions. There is plenty of this information for you to find on your own, such as online and in textbooks, and I encourage you to do this if desired.

I wanted this book to contain as much unique, relevant, and thought-provoking information as possible, and to focus on the information that I find is most needed for your success (because most of my clients don't care about the detailed physiology behind their conditions, so I have left much of it out of this book.)

## Do you want faster results?

Contrary to all of the approaches to health and weight loss that use crutches and fail, there is no one magic food or supplement that will help you heal your bowel and body quickly. Others will try to convince you that there are, but this is untrue. Understanding the concepts of healing is your ticket to a smooth and quick ride down the healing road.

Most, or all, of the concepts in my books will be new to you. They require you to see things from a very different perspective, and it can take time and work to change this. To fully understand the concepts and perspective of this program, re-read *Unique Healing* over and over again until you do (especially chapters 6-10), and re-read the sections in this book that pertain to you over and over again too. This is the way to get results faster. It also improves your chance of success.

Don't start this program until you read *Unique Healing* in its entirety (or schedule an appointment with me).

## 3 Steps to Success

In fact, I could quickly summarize the three steps to your success as follows:

1. **Understand the concepts and misunderstandings in my books and videos. Read and watch repeatedly until you do.**
2. **Use the right crutches, in the right amounts, to look and feel better fast.**
3. **Be prepared to commit to this program for at least one year, but three is better.**

## Schedule appointments/visit my blog/watch my videos on YouTube

If after reading this, you would like to schedule an appointment with me so that I can personally help you, as well as help you achieve faster results, contact me at *donna@UniqueHealing.com*, or 203.286.8932. If you would like to view my responses to your most common questions, my thoughts about health and healing, and current status on upcoming books/seminars/etc., please visit my blog at *www.UniqueHealing.com.* Also, from my website you can join my mailing list and receive regular e-mails with vital tips for your success, as well as specials on *Unique Healing* products.

Note: I have thousands of hours of knowledge and experience. I have done my best to address the most common concerns and questions that clients have while they heal their bowel and body with this program, but in *no way* could I address all of them in this book. It may take many more books and many years before this is done. In the meantime, if an issue/question/or concern presents itself while you are doing this, you can either trust this program and continue with it, or contact me for an appointment to address it.

# Chapter 2

## Symptoms, Illnesses, and Addictions That Are Eliminated With This Program

### Aches and Pains

This is a far-reaching symptom that includes pain from injury, headaches, neck and back pain, arthritis, infections, autoimmune diseases, and numerous other conditions that result in pain and discomfort. Pain is prevalent. For example, 40% of people have tension headaches, and 12% have migraines.

Aches and pain are one of the most common conditions that I help people eliminate.

(Note: Aches and pains are often caused by inflammation. For more information on inflammation, and why this program eliminates it, see Chapter 3.)

### A Healthy Body Eliminates Aches and Pains

The inflammatory response is an internal system of defense against acids that occur at the site of an injury and/or excess acidity in your lymphatic system that is present due to other causes (diet, stress, pollutants, drugs, etc.). It is an example of the brilliance of your body taking care of itself and doing what is best for you. Un-eliminated acids trigger the release of inflammatory chemicals by your lymphatic system to buffer these acids, and protect you from them. Thus, inflammation, rather than being an attack on your body, is a normal response of your body to deal with damaging acids.

Healing your body with this program eliminates the acids that trigger an inflammatory response. Healing your body with this program heals the organs of your lymphatic system (thymus, bone marrow, spleen, lymph nodes, appendix, tonsils, and others). Excess acidity is eventually damaging to the organs of your lymphatic system, as it reduces the oxygen and nutrients they need to be healthy, thrive, and function normally. Healing your body heals the organs of your lymphatic system so that even if there are acids, your body is strong enough to handle them without a reaction (it fixes the holes in your roof so that even if it does rain, your house does not get wet).

## A Healthy Bowel Eliminates Aches and Pains

When lactose in dairy products and gluten in grains is not completely digested, toxic by-products are created. These toxic by-products can trigger inflammatory reactions as well. A healthy bowel digests dairy and gluten and eliminates these inflammatory-stimulating toxic by-products.

Bacterial infections can also trigger aches and pains, such as sinus pain, bladder pain, vaginal pain, and others. A healthy bowel fights bacterial infections and eliminates the aches and pain associated with them.

In addition to its many other important functions, a healthy bacterial environment in your bowel is necessary for the complete elimination of acids (toxins, heavy metals, pesticides, etc.) from your body. A healthy bowel prevents the re-absorption of acids into your blood that cause an unhealthy body, and trigger the production of inflammatory chemicals.

## Why My Crutches Eliminate Aches and Pains

*Body Bentonite* binds to and eliminates acids (toxins, heavy metals, chemicals, etc.) from your body. It helps prevent them from becoming re-absorbed into your bloodstream, where they trigger a response by your body to protect you from them. It eliminates the acids that trigger the release of inflammatory chemicals, and that reduce blood flow/circulation and oxygenation.

*Unique Healing Calcium Citrate* is an alkalinizing mineral that helps neutralize the acids that your bowel does not eliminate. When these acids are neutralized, your body does not need to produce inflammatory chemicals to buffer them.

*Unique Healing Colloidal Silver* has natural anti-bacterial, anti-fungal, anti-parasitic properties. It eliminates pain that is caused by bacterial infections, such as sinus pain, bladder pain, vaginal pain, and others.

## How long will I need to use crutches for my aches and pains?

Aches and pains occur at Level 3 of your pipe. It is the second to last area of your body to heal (assuming that other areas are unhealthy too). Refer to the diagram "Sequence of Healing" in Appendix A at the end of this book to better understand this concept, as well as to Chapter 1 under this subject heading.

The bacterial environment in your bowel also affects aches and pains. To better understand how long you may need crutches for this, refer to Chapter 1 under this subject heading.

## How much do I take?/Questions about using these

See Chapter 5 for information on using these crutches, including recommendations on the amount to use, as well as a discussion of the misunderstandings about the particular crutch that may, if not understood correctly, cause you to fail to look and feel better while you heal your bowel and body with this program.

# Misunderstandings About Aches and Pains and Other Information for Your Success

## Keep your stools well-formed

Because aches and pains are caused in part by un-eliminated acids, and because well-formed stools prevent the re-absorption of acids into your blood, you will suffer from the least amount of aches and pains if you keep your stools well-formed while you are healing your bowel and body.

If you do not have a very good handle on how to define well-formed stools, review Chapter 6 of *Unique Healing* now. (And remember, when your stools are hard and slow you are eliminating more acids, and will therefore feel better, than when your stools are one or more times a day but not all extremely well-formed.)

If your stools are not well-formed, the following changes can help: increase your *Body Bentonite* intake; reduce your carbohydrate intake (pasta, breads, grains, cereals, yogurt, etc.); reduce your sugar intake (including natural healthy sugars such as agave, honey, raw sugar, cane juice, etc.); reduce your alcohol, salt, coffee, and/or soda intake; do not have a massage, chiropractic adjustment, or any other body work; drink a lot of water; rest; and keep your exercise aerobic. See Chapter 4 for more information on how to attain this, and why it is important.

If these changes do not noticeably help the form of your stools in two days, take them further (i.e. take more *Body Bentonite*, reduce your carbohydrate intake more, etc.).

Out of all of these recommendations, increasing your *Body Bentonite* intake is one of the most productive and helpful. It heals your body, unlike many of the other recommendations. It will do the most to lead you to a place where looking and feeling good is effortless, and some of the other suggestions, such as reducing sugar intake, are simply "too hard to do when your blood is too acidic."

(Note: the exception to this information is when your poorly formed stools are caused by an infection, in which case *Unique Healing Colloidal Silver* is needed to reduce your symptoms. Refer to Chapter 5 for information on when and how to use this crutch.)

## Improved circulation is healing

Anything that improves your circulation helps reduce inflammation, such as massage, Jacuzzi, heating pad, acupuncture, energy work, etc. When you increase your circulation, more blood, and therefore more oxygen and nutrients, are moved to the site of inflammation, and these help combat the toxins/acids that trigger inflammation. They are also necessary for the healing of your tissues.

An analgesic cream with menthol is a classic but often forgotten remedy that helps reduce pain and inflammation by improving circulation to the inflamed site. Ben Gay has been around for decades and natural varieties, such as "Traumeel" cream, are also available at health food stores. Apply this as often as needed.

The popular advice to apply ice to aches and pains is one I disagree with (many accepted remedies have later been proven to be wrong and/or harmful). For a more in depth discussion on this, see Chapter 3.

## Treating the symptoms with acidic drugs can make things worse

Some pain relievers, if taken more than ten days a month, can trigger "rebound headaches," which have the same dull, aching pain as tension headaches.

Excess, un-eliminated acids cause aches and pains. Drugs are acidic. So it makes sense that at some point, the acidity of the drug and its resultant ability to trigger inflammation and aches and pains, will offset the "pain-killing" drug-like aspect of it.

## There can also be a rebound effect with natural approaches, such as massage

Likewise, alternative treatments for aches and pains can also "backfire." For example, when you get a lymphatic massage, you can wrongly be led to believe that this "cleanses toxins from your body" (this statement was made in a brochure by a lymphatic massage therapist in my office suite). Massage, like lymphatic massage, does not cleanse, or eliminate, toxins/acids from your body. There are only four ways to eliminate acids/toxins and that is to poop, pee, breathe, or sweat them out!

Massage moves the toxins in your body out of one area, such as a sore muscle in your back, into another area of your body, such as your bowel. It shoves the trash from your kitchen into your bedroom. Sure it is relaxing and feels good, and for a little while your sore back may feel good, too, but when the acids/toxins that were released out of your back muscles with the massage are not eliminated by your bowel (and they won't be, because if they had been eliminated by your bowel in the first place, they never would have ended up in your back causing problems to begin with!), they eventually come right back to your back, triggering a sore back again. Or they may settle into another muscle, so that your back feels better, but you have a headache instead, for example.

## Other popular crutches

Large amounts of other alkalinizing minerals, such as sodium and magnesium, are often recommended for aches and pains, and help for the same reasons given for calcium citrate earlier. One mineral does not necessarily work better than the other. They are all equally helpful, *if taken in a strong enough/high enough dosage.*

While essential fatty acids, turmeric, and other crutches are some of the most popular ones taken for aches and pains, few of my clients experience reductions in their aches and pains with them. I am very familiar with them. I too tried them with clients many years ago. And remember, they are just crutches anyway, and are very limiting in their ability to help you as a result.

# Success With Aches and Pains

"When I came to Donna I was told that I would need surgery on my knee. I was not willing to put myself through this so I started this program.

It took some time, but eventually my knee healed and I no longer need surgery."

"For many years I had daily headaches, which became migraines several times a month. I went to doctors, neurologists, acupuncturists, and took a bunch of vitamins, but none of it helped. Soon after starting this program my headaches became much less frequent."

"When I first started this program I had neck pain, hip pain, and back pain. Immediately those became better, but I still had to be careful if I ate too much sugar or was very stressed, for example. Now, even if I eat sugar or am stressed, the pain does not come back. It just disappeared."

## My Story—severe, disabling pain that is no more

One of the most disabling symptoms that I endured on a constant basis when I was ill with an autoimmune disease was crippling neck pain. When your neck hurts, your entire head hurts, and focusing and accomplishing anything is impossible. There were many times that the pain was so bad I wanted to chop my head off. After suffering through this daily for several years, I thought that if it were gone, well, I just couldn't imagine it. It was all that I wanted in life.

During these years I tried many approaches for eliminating this pain, including massage, acupuncture, supplements, diets, and *many* chiropractic adjustments. After an adjustment I felt much better, but this lasted only a few hours before the pain returned. I worked for chiropractors for a couple of years just so that I could get these adjustments done regularly, and at no expense.

At one point I discovered the alkalinizing benefits of calcium and began taking large doses of this daily. This gave me enough relief that I could immediately go two weeks or longer without needing an adjustment. I was impressed. But I also did not know, as things are not presented this way, that calcium was a crutch and could not eliminate this pain completely, or permanently. To keep the pain down I had to take calcium daily, and as great as I felt on it, I simply knew that I was missing something. I knew I needed to find a way to eliminate the pain in a way that did not require the daily ingestion of a supplement.

I healed my bowel and body with this program and my neck pain is now gone. It has been gone for many years now. I do not need supplements, chiropractic, massage or any other crutch to do this for me. My healthier body keeps me pain-free all by itself.

## Watch my Video, "Why THIS Program Eliminates Aches and Pains"

This video, and all of my videos, can be found at *www.UniqueHealing.com* or at *www.YouTube.com/UniqueHealing*.

# Acne
See "Skin Conditions"

# ADD
See "Neurological Disorders"

# Addictions
## Alcohol, Caffeine, Drug, Exercise, Nicotine, Sugar, and Others
See also "Diabetes and Hypoglycemia"

Addiction is defined as: large amounts over a long period, unsuccessful efforts to cut down, time spent in obtaining the substance replaces social, occupational, or recreational activities, and continued use despite adverse consequences.

While we seem mostly aware and concerned about addictions to drugs and alcohol, many other addictions exist as well. Indeed, most of you are addicted to "something," whether it is sugar, high protein diets, coffee, nicotine, medications, or even exercise, for example. Yes I said exercise. Exercise is sometimes done obsessively to lose weight and keep it off. You can also get addicted to the brain-altering effects of the serotonin and endorphins produced during exercise.

Addictions can cause enormous emotional and physical pain. They can control your life, in a very unhealthy way.

Addictive substances such as alcohol, caffeine, exercise, sugar, nicotine, and pharmaceutical and recreational drugs are crutches. People who use these because they feel better—mentally and/or physically—when they do. They often use them to alter their brain chemistry. Like all crutches, one can easily become addicted to them, and the appealing reaction they create.

If you yank out the crutch and do not heal your leg you will fall down, and you will want to use that crutch again. If you yank out the addictive substance but do not heal your bowel and body, it is very likely that you will go back to the addiction.

Modern day addiction treatments do nothing to heal the underlying physical imbalances that cause addictions in the first place. They do nothing to eliminate the "need" to use a crutch to feel better. They do not heal your leg, and this is why they usually fail you in the long run.

When your bowel and body are healed, all crutches, including addictive ones, become undesirable and are no longer needed to feel good. Your brain chemistry will be altered naturally and you will be "high on life."

(My focus in the following sections is largely on alcohol addictions, but you can substitute *any* addictive substance into this information, as the concepts explained regarding alcohol addictions apply to *all* addictive substances.)

## Healing Your Body With This Program Eliminates Addictions

When your blood sugar levels are too low, you feel weak, tired, irritable, and depressed, because blood sugar is needed to fuel your muscles and brain. Low blood sugar levels reduce your brain's levels of serotonin and endorphins, chemicals that combat depression. (Scientists have found that using medications to reduce the release of the neurotransmitter serotonin after drinking, takes away the pleasure of drinking, resulting in a significant reduction in the consumption of alcohol.)

Alcohol, caffeine, some drugs, sugar, and nicotine are some of the substances that can quickly increase your blood sugar levels and improve your brain chemicals, if they are too low, quickly reducing the undesirable symptoms mentioned above. When your blood sugar is low, you will crave one or some of these substances. When your blood sugar levels are normal, you won't. Before I altered my brain chemistry naturally by healing my bowel and body, I was in love with recreational drugs. Also, when I was an alcoholic I had a serious sweet tooth. When I healed my body and balanced my blood sugar, the desire for *both* alcohol *and* sugar were eliminated.

Un-eliminated acids reduce blood sugar levels, and healing your body eliminates these acids, stabilizing blood sugar levels, and eliminating the desire for theses addictive substances.

Un-eliminated acids aggravate your nervous system. When acids are eliminated, your nervous system is relaxed. There is less anxiety and depression. Since many addictive substances are used to treat the symptoms of these psychological issues as well, eliminating acids eliminates the need to use these substances in order to feel good (mentally), as well.

Healing your body with this program eliminates the acids that trigger low blood sugar and nervous system irritation. Healing your body with this program heals your liver, pancreas, and adrenal glands, which play key roles in regulating your blood sugar levels. Excess acidity is eventually damaging to these organs, as it reduces the oxygen and nutrients they need to be healthy, thrive, and function normally. Healing your body heals these organs so that even if there are acids, your body is strong enough to handle them without a reaction (it fixes the holes on your roof so that even if it does rain, your house does not get wet).

## Healing Your Bowel With This Program Eliminates Addictions

Scientists have called your bowel "your second brain," as it is responsible for the production of a large number of brain chemicals, such as serotonin, that help "keep you happy."

When your brain chemistry is out of balance you can feel anxious, irritable, and/or depressed. Addictive substances stimulate neurotransmitter production, or brain chemicals that make you feel good. We like to feel good—naturally! For me, alcohol and marijuana made me feel more relaxed and less anxious. When I stopped these, I suffered severe, debilitating anxiety attacks. The addictions had eliminated these symptoms. For most people, if given a choice between debilitating anxiety or drug use, they're going to pick the drug.

Vitamin B-12, manufactured adequately when your bowel is healthy, is needed for the production of the brain chemicals, such as serotonin and benzodiazepines. (Valium and Xanax are pharmaceutical benzodiazepines.) Low levels of B-12 have been scientifically implicated in cases of depression, sugar cravings, nicotine cravings, alcoholism, and drug use.

In addition to its many other important functions, a healthy bacterial environment in your bowel is a necessity for the complete elimination of acids (toxins, heavy metals, pesticides, etc.) from your body. A healthy bowel prevents the re-absorption of acids into your blood that cause low blood sugar levels, nervous system irritation, and depression, which therefore reduces your desire for addictive substances to feel better.

# Why My Crutches Eliminate Addictions

*Body Bentonite* binds to and eliminates acids (toxins, heavy metals, chemicals, etc.) from your body. It eliminates the acids that interfere with blood sugar regulation, and helps create normal blood sugar levels. This increases your brain's levels of serotonin and endorphins, chemicals that reduce depression and the "desire" for alcohol, nicotine, caffeine, and other "drugs" that otherwise stimulate these same enjoyable levels of chemicals. It eliminates the acids that irritate your nervous system, helping to keep you calm and relaxed without the need for a drug to do this for you.

*Unique Healing Calcium Citrate* is an alkalinizing mineral that helps neutralize the acids that your bowel does not eliminate. When these acids are neutralized, your blood sugar stabilizes, and nervous system irritation is reduced, which reduces anxiety and depression.

*Unique Healing Methyl Vitamin B-12* provides your body with easy to assimilate levels of this nutrient, which can reduce anxiety, depression, sugar cravings, irritability, and other conditions that are otherwise remedied by the ingestion of an addictive substance.

Until your bowel is healthy enough to produce adequate amounts of vitamin B-12, use this crutch. I have seen significant reductions in clients' pharmaceutical and recreational drug, alcohol, coffee, and sugar cravings and usage with the addition of sufficient amounts of vitamin B-12.

## How much do I take?/Questions about using these

See Chapter 5 for information on using these crutches, including recommendations on the amount to use, as well as a discussion of the misunderstandings about the particular crutch that may, if not understood correctly, cause you to fail to look and feel better while you heal your bowel and body with this program.

## How long will I need to use crutches for my addictions?

Addictions occur at Levels 2 and 3 of your pipe. They are the second, and second to last, areas of your body to heal (assuming that other areas are unhealthy too). Refer to the diagram "Sequence of Healing" in Appendix A at the end of this book to better understand this concept, as well as to Chapter 1 under this subject heading.

The bacterial environment in your bowel also affects addictions. To better understand how long you may need crutches for this, refer to Chapter 1 under this subject heading.

# Misunderstandings About Addictions and Other Information for Your Success

## Keep your stools well-formed

Because addictions are caused in part by un-eliminated acids, and because well-formed stools prevent the re-absorption of acids into your blood, you will be most successful in conquering your addictions if you keep your stools well-formed while you are healing your bowel and body.

If you do not have a very good handle on how to define well-formed stools, review Chapter 6 of *Unique Healing* now. (And remember, when your stools are hard and slow you are eliminating more acids, and will therefore feel better, than when your stools are one or more times a day but not all extremely well-formed.)

If your stools are not well-formed, the following changes can help: increase your *Body Bentonite* intake; reduce your carbohydrate intake (pasta, breads, grains, cereals, yogurt, etc.); reduce your sugar intake (including natural healthy sugars such as agave, honey, raw sugar, cane juice, etc.); reduce your alcohol, salt, coffee, and/or soda intake; do not have a massage, chiropractic adjustment, or any other body work; drink a lot of water; rest; and keep your exercise aerobic (see Chapter 4 for more information on how to attain this, and why it is important.)

If these changes do not noticeably help the form of your stools in two days, take them further (i.e. take more *Body Bentonite*, reduce your carbohydrate intake more, etc.)

Out of all of these recommendations, increasing your *Body Bentonite* intake is one of the most productive and helpful. It heals your body, unlike many of the other recommendations. It will do the most to lead you to a place where looking and feeling good is effortless, and some of the other suggestions, such as reducing sugar intake, are simply "too hard to do when your blood is too acidic."

(Note: the exception to this information is when your poorly formed stools are caused by an infection, in which case *Unique Healing Colloidal Silver* is needed to reduce your symptoms. Refer to Chapter 5 for information on when and how to use this crutch.)

## Blame the program for your failure, not yourself

Only 25% of people remain substance-free one year following a treatment program for their alcohol or drug addiction, and the typical person entering treatment is doing so for the third time. Since the "war on drugs" was launched thirty-five years ago, our government has spent over $500 billion on this, yet today the number of Americans using drugs remains virtually unchanged.

Treatments for alcohol and other addictions are ineffective, yet many of you have accepted this as the best you can get. Do you think you are worthless and don't deserve better? Many of you have also bought into the idea that these addictions are forever; they are demons waiting to surface at any moment, that you must spend a lifetime fighting. Many people and institutions profit handsomely from these accepted beliefs. It is you who suffers, needlessly.

It's sad and very unfortunate that we blame the person with the addiction for their failure, as if it is their fault and they are bad people. Traditional programs can't lose because nobody blames them! It is an easy excuse to blame the person, as many of us have some emotional issues that negatively affect us. It is easier to blame the person than to take responsibility for the fact that you, the therapist or recovery center, do not have the answer, and cannot honestly help cure them of these addictions.

The most common approach to controlling addictions is much like our typical approach to weight loss. And they have both failed you miserably. You may believe you are on the right road because in the short-term there is often success with these programs. For a little while, you lose weight, or stop drinking alcohol or using your drugs. Then when you fail to stick with it in the long-term, you blame yourself. The ability to go cold turkey for a short bit of time does not make the advice you followed desirable, or successful, in the long run.

If your leg is broken and you yank out your crutches, you will fall down, and you will want to use those crutches again. If you yank out an addictive substance, but do not heal your bowel and body, you will eventually go back to the addiction.

Modern day addiction treatments do nothing to heal the underlying physical imbalances that cause addictions in the first place. They do nothing to eliminate the "need" to use a crutch to feel better, and this is why they frequently fail in the long run. This program eliminates your need for *all* crutches, addictive ones included.

If you follow an addiction program and you are not able to stay off your "drug," your addictive substance, in the long-term, blame the program, not yourself!

## A high tolerance to alcohol is unhealthy

As you heal your bowel and body, you will find that it takes less alcohol to get drunk than it did before. Your tolerance level will go down. Wrongly, a low tolerance is usually perceived as bad, unhealthy, and/or a sign of weakness. On the contrary, the less healthy your bowel and body are, the stronger the crutch is that is needed to make you feel good; the more alcohol it takes to make you feel good.

When I first drank too much, I become very ill the next day. As I continued to drink and I became less healthy, I could drink all night, black out, wake up the next morning feeling fine, and go to school and get "As."

Feeling fine after drinking, and tolerating a large amount of alcohol, are signs of a very unhealthy bowel and body.

When you liver is healthy, it transports the toxins (acids) of alcohol into your organs of elimination, where, if not completely eliminated by your bowel, they will trigger symptoms. Even when your bowel is healthy, it can only handle so many toxins at once, and excessive drinking will overwhelm your bowel with acids and trigger reactions. The reaction of your other organs of elimination to these un-eliminated toxins/acids can cause vomiting, headaches, fatigue, dehydration, and other hangover symptoms.

As your liver becomes less healthy, it no longer has the strength to "send" alcohol toxins into your organs of elimination. This means that in the short-term you feel better, but there is a serious price being paid. The toxins deplete and harm your liver instead, for example. When your liver cells die, this produces no discomfort, and you can easily and wrongly think you are not being harmed.

Feeling bad after drinking a lot of alcohol is a strong deterrent, and a reason why alcohol treatments have included drugs to induce vomiting if an alcoholic drinks. It is easy to become addicted when you don't feel bad. When I felt fine the day after drinking in excess, it was very easy to repeat the behavior again. I also thought, "Gee, I'm getting away with this. I guess I must not be hurting myself." Deep down I knew it was harmful, but when you are led to believe that a lack of symptoms equates with health, it is easy to think, "Maybe I'm the exception."

I no longer "crave" alcohol; I no longer need alcohol, sugar, cigarettes, or any of the other drugs I used to take to feel happy and calm; but I am further kept away from drinking by the knowledge that if I did, I would feel horrible the next day.

33

## Alcohol can damage *every* organ in your body

When I went back to school to study nutrition, my final thesis was titled, "Alcoholism: A Nutritional Approach." It received rave reviews from my university's administration. In writing this, I spent many hours at the University of California Irvine medical library. I was shocked to find thousands of studies that showed the negative effects of alcohol on *all* of the body's organs, not just the highly publicized liver. And there were hundreds of studies that showed a positive effect when alcoholics improved their nutrition. I wondered, "Wow, there is a lot of helpful and useful information here, so why haven't we heard of it? And why do so many of us generally believe that only our liver is harmed by alcohol?" (People who smoke have been equally led to wrongly believe that only their lungs are damaged by this addiction, etc.)

Of course alcohol can damage every organ in your body, because alcohol is highly acidic, and a highly acidic diet, as you have learned, leads to organ damage.

Two misunderstandings are at the core of the belief that alcohol is less harmful than it really is: First, blood tests are used to measure liver health and the affect of alcohol on it, and second, you have been led to believe that when you stop drinking alcohol, or any other addictive substance, any damage it has caused is miraculously fixed.

## A normal blood test result does not mean that your liver is healthy and that your drinking is not harming you.

Your blood test results can look normal even if your organs are very unhealthy. Review Chapter 2 of *Unique Healing* to understand why blood tests are a dangerous way to measure the health of your body, your liver included. Unfortunately, many of you have been harmfully led to believe that you are "getting away" with your drinking because of a normal blood test result. A liver biopsy, or at the very least a scan of your liver, are the only reliable tests that can detect serious damage to it. But these are extraordinarily more expensive than blood tests, and your insurance company usually doesn't want to pay for a bunch of tests. And hey, your doctor is probably ok with this anyway, because he is better liked if he can tell you that your liver is healthy, amidst all of your abuse to it, than if he has to tell you to stop drinking. And really, all of you are not much different than I was in wanting to believe that you are "getting away with it." You want to and need to believe this because no one has given you a way to stop your addiction and not feel horrible, and fail, when you do so.

## If you stop drinking alcohol, your liver, or any other organ that is unhealthy, does not automatically heal itself

If you throw rocks at your windows and they break, they do not fix themselves once you stop throwing the rocks. Stopping reduces the *future* damage to your house and is invaluable from that perspective, but it does not fix the damage already done.

Likewise, when you stop drinking, the damage already done to your health remains when you stop. You have merely reduced any future damage, although given the approach most take to stop drinking, which usually involves replacing one acidic, damaging substance such as alcohol with another, such as a drug, smoking, extra protein, or more sugar, the future damage is often not lessened after all.

Lung cancer is much more prevalent than liver disease, as your lungs become unhealthy before your liver does, per the description in Chapter One. Therefore, we have many more stories of people who have stopped smoking who many years later develop lung cancer "anyway" than we do of alcoholics who later developed liver cancer "anyway," but the analogy is the same. We are shocked when we hear of the person who stopped smoking decades ago only to suffer from lung cancer later. But we shouldn't be shocked.

Unless specific action is taken to heal your body, the damage done from your addictions—alcohol, drugs, sugar, nicotine, etc—*will* one day catch up with you.

## Your liver can be very unhealthy even if you have never drunk alcohol

People who have not been heavy drinkers often wrongly believe that they therefore cannot have an unhealthy liver, because of the highly publicized comment that "drinking alcohol is bad for your liver." Non-smokers often wrongly think they are immune from lung cancer, as well.

If you never drank alcohol or smoked a cigarette, but ate a lot of acidic foods like chicken, salt, sugar, and coffee, and/or were exposed to numerous chemicals/heavy metals, for example, and your bowel was too unhealthy to eliminate the acids from these, your lungs and liver would eventually be harmed.

A recent study titled "Long term nutritional intake and the risk for non-alcoholic fatty liver disease (NAFLD): A population based study," found a higher rate of non-alcoholic fatty liver disease in participants who ate 27% more meat and twice as many soft drinks (soda) than non-users.

Meat and soft drinks, like alcohol, are acidic, and a highly acidic diet is harmful to the health of your liver.

## Replacing one addiction with another is *not* success

If you avoid the rain and never fix the holes in your roof, you will always have to avoid the rain to keep your house dry. And the reality is, you won't be able to.

Likewise, you won't always be able to manipulate circumstances so that you aren't vulnerable to your addiction. If you do not heal your bowel and body, you will always be vulnerable. Since accepted treatments for addictions do not heal your bowel and body, when you do follow them, you are left vulnerable to the addiction returning, and you are told, correctly, to "fear" the "ever-present demons" lurking that cause you to become addicted again. The treatments do not eradicate these demons.

Modern day approaches to addictions define success as the stopping of an addiction. Because they do not heal your bowel and balance your blood and brain chemistry, you will find another substance to fill in for the one that was abandoned. This new substance often comes in the form of medication, coffee, recreational drugs, high protein diets, sugar, intense exercise, and/or cigarettes. (If you go to an A.A. meeting or talk to a "recovering" alcoholic, you will find heavy coffee, cigarette and/or sugar use.)

(Even scientists, who are looking for a treatment for alcoholism based on specific alcohol-related genes, acknowledge that alcohol genes can overlap with genes for nicotine, cocaine, and other addictions. This is one way to explain it; mine is another.)

These substitute substances replace the action that the eliminated one had on your body's blood and brain chemistry. You may no longer drink alcohol to feel better, you now eat large quantities of sugar, or exercise religiously, to feel good, for example. One crutch has been replaced with another. One addiction is replaced with another. And this is called success? Are you healthier or happier for having done this? More importantly, it sets you up for failure. Many of these crutches contribute to further ill health and worsening of your blood and brain chemistry that triggered the addiction in the first place. This means that you have a greater probability of returning to your addiction in the future.

Also, if you are an alcoholic and stop drinking and use a medication to satisfy your unbalanced brain chemistry, for example, there will be a high likelihood of your drinking again if you are ever around alcohol at a time when your crutch (the drug) has been forgotten. Maybe you forgot to take your medication and you are at a party with alcohol and well, since the drug is not in your body balancing your brain chemistry, that alcohol sure looks good to you, and you dive right in!

Using a new crutch to satisfy your blood and brain leaves you very vulnerable to returning to your old crutch if the new one is ever not available to you. This is another reason why modern day treatments, which depend on crutches, usually fail.

A couple of years ago an ex-Division 1 college basketball player came into my office. He was there to sell me something, but somehow we got onto the subject of marijuana and addictions and crutches. He was interested in my viewpoint and it made sense to him. He related a story to me of a friend who was addicted to crack, who had been able to quit. I know that you cannot simply quit using a crutch without replacing it with another, and sure enough, as I dug for more information, he revealed to me that his friend was smoking pot all day, and it was because of this that he was able to quit the crack. He traded one addiction for another.

When you heal your bowel and body, then, and only then, will you be able to get off *all* your crutches. Then and only then will you be able to eliminate *all* addictions.

## The high protein approach to addictions—another doomed crutch

A high protein diet is often recommended for addicts. Eating more protein than is needed and healthy for your body is another approach that contributes to the short-term gain, long-term pain syndrome, and ultimate failure to heal the addiction. It treats the symptoms of the addiction and not the cause, and it makes the addiction harder to break in the future.

A high protein diet stops your body's internal cleansing process, causing acids to remain in your cells, where they do serious harm. The appeal, however, is that these acids are prevented from moving into your blood, where they can trigger low blood sugar and depression when they are not eliminated from your body. Again, these two situations make you vulnerable to craving alcohol or other addictive substances in order to relieve these discomforts.

A high protein diet makes you feel better in the short run and can, in the short run, help you stop your addictions. But because this diet is very acidic and damaging to your body, in the long run, it makes the underlying cause even worse. Your bowel becomes less healthy, for example, and less able to eliminate acids and keep your blood and brain chemistry healthy, making you even *more* vulnerable to an addiction and making it more difficult to conquer it (unless you are able to constantly maintain a strict high protein diet forever, a feat that, ironically, may kill you sooner than the original addiction!). This same scenario holds true when you use drugs, nicotine, sugar or any other acidic substance to replace your current one.

## Other programs that claim to address the cause of an addiction, but don't

Alternative approaches to addictions also replace one crutch, the addiction, with another, such as massive supplementation or restrictive diets that need to be followed on a daily basis, forever.

These approaches also describe the brain chemistry and blood sugar imbalances as the cause, but they fail in their ability to heal your bowel and body, which when unhealthy, cause your brain and blood sugar imbalances.

In addition to a high protein diet, these approaches often recommend wheat-free and dairy-free diets and the use of numerous supplements to take the place of other crutches such as alcohol, coffee, drugs, and sugar. Herbs and vitamins that help balance your blood sugar and help your body produce beneficial brain chemicals are often prescribed. In the long run, this is preferable to using an acidic drug or nicotine, as supplements are not acidic and do not contribute to the further breakdown of body organs. They fail however because they are still only crutches, and all crutches usually fail eventually. They fail because they require the strict adherence to a diet and daily handfuls of supplements. It becomes much easier to simply take a little pill (drug) to feel better.

When you heal your body and bowel and stabilize the chemistry of your body, the appeal of *all* of these addictive crutches is eliminated.

A successful alcohol addiction program, therefore, is defined as one where an individual loses their desire, not only for alcohol, but for drugs, sugar, meat protein, coffee, and cigarettes as well. A successful addiction program does not require a lifetime of avoiding wheat and dairy and the ingestion of a handful of supplements daily. A successful addiction program delivers effortless, long-term results, as this one does!

## It takes time to eliminate addictions: the necessity of gradual reductions in alcohol, pharmaceutical and recreational drugs, cigarettes, coffee, etc.

It takes time to heal an unhealthy bowel and body. As a result, in the short-term, you will need to depend on *some* crutches or else risk failing to stop your addiction. Wrongly, many people think they won't succeed at stopping their addiction unless they exert total control over it immediately, only to find that eventually they lose all control over it!

You can't heal your body and bowel overnight, so do not expect to be able to stop your addictions overnight either. But at least it will happen one day. One day, with this program, you will be taken to a place where you do not need any crutches to look and feel good; where addictions do not exist.

Likewise, if you are healing your body and you use your "drug," this should not be interpreted as a failure on your part. It is impossible to function without any crutches immediately, and the sooner you accept that, the more successful you will be.

For example, if you are healing your bowel and body and you drink, after having stopped for two weeks, you have not failed. This has also not prevented you from healing your bowel and body. The fact that you drank is simply a reflection of the fact that your bowel and body are not strong enough yet to function without a crutch; your leg has not healed yet. You have not failed. It is only when you rely on crutches alone, and do not heal, that your risk of failure is extremely high.

To successfully conquer your addictions, you must be committed to this healing program and look at your results one year or more, not one week, from starting it. Take the crutches listed earlier to support your blood and brain chemistry, and take them daily until your bowel and body are healed.

In a study published in the *International Journal of Biosocial and Medical Research,* more than 70% of patients who received nutritional support during withdrawal remained abstinent for several years after treatment.

## In other words, do not go cold turkey

While many programs for addictions rely on a "cold turkey" approach, most people who have followed this advice have failed to remain addiction-free. The approach is wrong, not you.

I find little value in going cold turkey with a substance, because the only way to succeed with this is to replace it with *another* harmful substance, so what is the point?

Many who claim to have quit their addictions cold turkey really have not done this at all. Often an addict will be given pharmaceutical medications, which means that they have simply traded one crutch—the addictive one with a bad name, such as cocaine—for another crutch—a pharmaceutical one, such as an anti-depressant, that is viewed as acceptable.

On the other hand, because driving drunk can kill you and innocent people, if you have an alcohol addiction, it is advisable that you replace the alcohol with a drug or other crutch that does not impair your driving.

Time and again clients reduce their drinking and other addictions on their own during this program, and they don't miss it. But if you are forced to stop cold turkey, you will miss it. You will miss the feel-good feeling the substance gave you.

## Symptoms of withdrawal are not detox and can go on "forever"

When I became ill and quit alcohol and drugs cold turkey, I felt horrendous. I expected this to only last a short time, as I was wrongly led to believe that "detox" symptoms were a reaction to the elimination of harmful alcohol and drug poisons that had accumulated in my body and would shortly be gone.

When you stop alcohol, drugs, coffee, marijuana, or any other toxic substance, the horrible feelings you experience are caused not primarily by the action of your body eliminating the substance, but rather from the elimination of the "crutch like" effect the substance provided to you.

In my case, when I stopped using drugs I experienced years of debilitating panic attacks. These were not caused by "detox." Rather, my unhealthy body created them. The drugs were simply crutches I had used to eliminate them. When the crutches were taken away, the symptoms reappeared.

There are two serious problems created by the mistaken belief that when you stop putting a toxic chemical into your body it will be eliminated in a short period of time. First, it contributes to the wrong and harmful thinking that you can abuse your body for many years and quickly reverse the ill effects of this. It contributes to the harmful "quick-fix" mentality. Is this why people wrongly think they can do a "spring cleanse" for four days and eliminate all of the toxins that have accumulated in their body over the year? It may make it difficult for someone who is trying to heal his or her bowel and body with this program to understand why it takes as long as it does.

Second, if you do not understand that the symptoms of withdrawal are symptoms that can persist indefinitely, as they did for me, you will likely find another "drug" to take its place and pollute your body another way, or you can suffer, as I did, thinking that the symptoms would eventually disappear. My symptoms of "detox" went on for many years and did not disappear until I healed my bowel and body with this program.

## Psychotherapy and addictions

Psychotherapy does not heal your bowel or body, or eliminate the physiological basis of addictions, but it is invaluable for an addictive person. Many people with addictions harbor a great deal of anger, hurt, feelings of worthlessness, and other forms of emotional problems, and these can not, and will not, be changed when you heal your bowel and body with this program. This requires a good therapist. Additionally, when these issues are worked on, you are more likely to succeed in healing your bowel and body and the physiological basis of your addictions.

A vicious cycle can occur when an addict, who already has self-esteem issues, refuses therapy, as this can make them feel even more worthless, which is something they just can't handle. This is very unfortunate. I like to have clients think of therapy as a treat, like a massage. It is a luxury to have someone to talk to who will not judge, criticize, or manipulate you, as perhaps too many others, such as parents and friends, have already done to you in your past. It would be wonderful if we all had close family members and friends who could provide this to us. That is how it should be, but for many, it simply is not the case. Don't get frustrated over the lack of power to change "the family you were born into." Instead, realize that you can "buy" the emotional support you need by seeing a therapist. I don't view therapists as people who help others with problems. I view them as people who can help those who don't have a strong, healthy emotional support system. In a sense, they can be the healthy family you may not have ever had.

Even if you do not have an addiction, for many of you, an occasional visit to a therapist will help you succeed in healing your bowel and body faster. When I have a client who is struggling with this process, it always stems from an emotional issue.

Ultimately, however, the main cause of your addiction is a physical one, and I want to scream, and cry, when I watch shows that denigrate individuals for not having the "strength" to stop their addictions.

When you heal your bowel and body with this program your addictions will go away, even if you never get one day of psychological counseling (although you will likely be much happier and fulfilled, if you do.).

## A.A.

I attended two A.A. meetings when I was ill. I was an alcoholic, but I was also very sick, and my focus was both on stopping my alcohol addiction and becoming healthier. The environment I found at A.A. meetings was not at all conducive to the physical healing I needed (as the people I met were alcoholics who had now become nicotine, drug, sugar, and other "addicts"). So I never went back.

A.A. is a crutch for your addictions. I do not criticize this entirely; however when used alone, as is often the case, and your underlying blood and brain chemistry imbalances that are at the core of your addiction are not corrected by healing your bowel and body, the statistics for your success are slim.

## Medication crutches may be helpful temporarily

If other crutches don't help, or you are especially vulnerable, a drug may be in order. Anti-depressants can be helpful in these cases, and I support their short-term use. In the short-term it won't harm you, and if it "keeps you from jumping off a bridge" it will help you. I always say, "I can't help someone if they are no longer alive." Of course, this is something you must discuss with your doctor.

## It's NOT about willpower

Recently a friend had someone she knew die from complications related to her alcoholism. My friend's sentiment about it was one you hear all the time, which goes something like this: "Well, the doctors told her she needed to stop drinking or else she would die, and she just wouldn't do it."

This sentiment has to stop—immediately!

People who have addictions don't want to have addictions. They don't want to die. They just can't stop.

Threatening someone to stop an addiction but not giving them the tools to do so successfully (which means healing their bowel and body and changing their blood and brain chemistry so that the addiction is no longer needed to function/feel good), is unfair, and doomed for a lot of heartache and failure.

And don't ever take it personally when a loved one has an addiction and won't "stop for you" It has nothing to do with you. They simply can't stop. If someone you love is addicted, help them heal their bowel and body and do not criticize or judge them for their addictions. Be compassionate, and know that all of the love in the world won't "cure" them. Healing their bowel and body will.

Stopping your addiction is not about willpower or strength; it is about a healthy bowel and body. If they are not healthy, your unbalanced physiology will win out over your willpower.

## Your environment influences your addiction

The majority of you have an unhealthy bowel and body and are susceptible to some sort of "addiction"—sugar, caffeine, nicotine, medications, exercise, etc. The addiction you choose to satisfy your unbalanced blood and brain chemistry is often one that you are exposed to by your family members. If you have an unhealthy bowel and body and your parents exercise seven days a week, that may be the way you learn to cope with your imbalances; if your parents takes medications to cope, that may be how you learn to manage your imbalances; if they eat vast quantities of sugar, that may be what you are exposed to, to large amounts of candy and cookies in the pantry, for example, and therefore, what you use to satisfy your imbalances.

## Genetics, Hollywood, and other excuses given by failed programs

The failure to quit drinking or stop any other addiction occurs because of the approach that is taken. Addictions are not a lifetime sentence caused by genetics. If you have family members that have struggled with alcoholism and other addictions, then they have an unhealthy bowel and body. You may have inherited this, making you more susceptible to following in their footsteps *unless you take action to change this* inherited weakness. If your house was built with cheap windows you can actively buy new ones and replace them. When you heal your bowel and body with this program, your family and genetic tendencies towards addictions are eliminated. Bad genes mean an unhealthy bowel and body, and these can be altered/healed.

Likewise, do not blame Hollywood, the death of your dog, or anything or anyone else for your addictions. These may be triggers—the rain hitting your roof—but when your health (or your roof), is strong, you will not react to them.

## If your child eats a lot of sugar now, he/she may drink a lot of alcohol later

There is a lot you can do to help prevent addictions, such as alcoholism, from developing in your children.

Because sugar increases your blood sugar in the same way that alcohol does, and because this reaction makes you "feel good" when your blood sugar levels are low (which happens when you have excess un-eliminated acids in your blood), someone who eats a lot of sugar (i.e. likes to eat a lot of sugar) can very easily become someone who drinks a lot of alcohol (i.e. likes to drink a lot of alcohol).

Before my alcoholic days, I ate *a lot* of sugar. Once I was older and exposed to alcohol, I found that just as appealing as the sugar I used to eat as a kid (in other words, had I been offered alcohol as a kid, I would have probably liked it then too!).

So what is "a lot of sugar," and don't all kids eat a lot? In answer to the second question, "no they do not." In answer to the first, "a lot of sugar" is more than two pieces of candy, or more than two cookies, more than one soda, or more than three pieces of fruit/day, for example.

If your child has a sweet tooth, heal his or her bowel and body now. When you do and he or she reduces their sugar intake, you will very likely find that he or she drinks very little alcohol as a teenager or young adult.

# Success With Addictions

"I went to addiction centers all over the country to stop using drugs. They never worked. Since doing this program, I have been drug-free for 2 years—the longest I have stayed away from drugs in 25 years!"

"It is amazing that I no longer crave sugar all the time."

"I stopped smoking one pack of cigarettes a day, which had been a fourteen year addiction. One and a half years later I still don't smoke."

"When I came to Donna I drank 2-3 glasses of wine most nights after work. I drank to relax. I never thought I would or could give this up. I did, however, and now I am relaxed without wine, and I also have more energy, fewer headaches, and have lost weight."

"The last time I tried to stop drinking, I ended up eating a lot of sugar, and gained weight as a result. I was depressed and satisfied this with sweets. I did not want to go back there again. So I really didn't believe Donna when she said I would want less alcohol AND sugar when I healed my bowel and body, but it really happened. I feel great. I feel more confident. I can't believe I can stay away from these things and not miss them. All I can say is "wow."

## My story

At the age of fourteen I began drinking regularly and smoking pot. By the time I was eighteen I was a raging alcoholic. I was also using many other drugs as well, such as cocaine, speed, and acid. Four years later I was completely disabled with an autoimmune disease.

Since healing my bowel and body with this program, I have cured myself of my alcoholism. I am not an alcoholic any more than I am a person with an immune disorder, or someone who loves steak and sugar, as I used to. I have been around drinking people for the last twenty-five years and I have never once felt vulnerable to drinking again. I have had numerous triggers in the last twenty years. They have never set off my alcoholism.

The desire to drink is 1,000% gone. Alcohol looks and smells unappealing to me. There is no struggle or fear of relapse. There are not many recovering addicts who can honestly say this. This program can give you these results too.

You may say, hey, if you stopped drinking, you probably weren't really that much of an alcoholic to begin with, because after all, we all know that alcoholism can't be cured! Or, you may judge me by the way I look. I am not the "scruffy, dirty, and uneducated" alcoholic that is stereotyped. If so, you are wrong. By the time I was eighteen I was blacking out after drinking excessively, which happened all the time. I could not control how much I drank; it had complete control over me. I used alcohol to make me happy and feel good, and when I stopped drinking, I felt horrible and had to drink again to stop the discomfort. Eventually, it led to the complete collapse of my job and relationships. I was a hard-core alcoholic.

This program alone cured me of my addictions. I did not join AA, take medications, or use any other traditional alcoholism treatment approach.

## My dream

My heart goes out to everyone who is struggling with alcoholism and other addictions and failing, needlessly. When I first began working as a nutritionist in southern California I dreamed of devoting myself to helping alcoholics. I contacted all of the local alcohol treatment facilities in the area and only a couple responded to me. I was shocked. Didn't they want to hear about how I cured myself of alcoholism? Surely this is not a story they often hear. Weren't they discouraged by the futile results of accepted treatment approaches, and wouldn't they do anything to try to find a better approach? Nope. The same thing happened when I moved to Boulder. Only in Boulder, not a single person or organization responded to my calls and letters. Frustrated and incredulous, I gave up (and have no intention of making similar attempts here in my new hometown of Fairfield, CT). But I have not given up my dream, and never will.

One day, I would love to open a center for treating alcoholics and people with other addictions, including eating disorders, with this program.

## Watch my Video, "Why THIS Program Eliminates Addictions"

This video, and all of my videos, can be found at *www. UniqueHealing. com* or at *www. YouTube.com/UniqueHealing*.

## Addison's Disease

See "Adrenal Disorders"

## Adrenal Disorders
### Adrenal Exhaustion, Adrenal Fatigue, Addison's Disease, and Others
See also, "Diabetes and Hypoglycemia"

Adrenal problems are a very popular diagnosis given by alternative health care practitioners (seemingly just as popular as the thyroid problems that are diagnosed among the conventional healthcare profession). Both of these professions have been well trained to search for these problems, and more relevantly, they have been trained how to offer a remedy, a crutch, to treat them. You may be led to believe that the "answer" to your problems has been discovered when you get one of these diagnoses. But in truth, the majority of the population could be diagnosed similarly, and adrenal supplements, or thyroid medications, are not a magic cure-all (as *many* of you have already experienced, and many more of you may soon find out.). Unfortunately, the months, or years, you spend chasing down the promise of "fixing" these problems with these crutches means wasted time not healing your bowel and body, which is the only way to eliminate these conditions and the symptoms associated with them—effortlessly, completely, and permanently.

## Healing Your Body Eliminates Adrenal Disorders

Excess acidity disturbs the secretion of adrenaline, and interferes with cortisol production. Healing your body with this program eliminates the acids that interfere with adrenaline and cortisol regulation.

Healing your body with this program heals your adrenal glands. Healing your body heals your adrenal glands so that even if there are acids, your body is strong enough to handle them without a reaction (it fixes the holes on your roof so that even if it does rain, your house does not get wet).

## Healing Your Bowel With This Program Eliminates Adrenal Disorders

In addition to its many other important functions, a healthy bacterial environment in your bowel is a necessity for the complete elimination of acids (toxins, heavy metals, pesticides, etc.) from your body. A healthy bowel prevents the re-absorption of acids into your blood that cause unhealthy adrenal glands, and that trigger a disruption in your adrenalin and cortisol levels.

## Why My Crutches Eliminate Adrenal Disorders

***Body Bentonite*** binds to and eliminates acids (toxins, heavy metals, chemicals, etc.) from your body. It helps prevent them from becoming re-absorbed into your bloodstream, where they trigger a response by your body to protect you from them. It eliminates the acids that interfere with the proper balance of adrenaline and cortisol in your body.

***Unique Healing Calcium Citrate*** is an alkalinizing mineral that helps neutralize the acids that your bowel does not eliminate. When these acids are neutralized, your body's levels of adrenalin and cortisol are not disrupted.

## How much do I take?/Questions about using these

See Chapter 5 for information on using these crutches, including recommendations on the amount to use, as well as a discussion of the misunderstandings about the particular crutch that may, if not understood correctly, cause you to fail to look and feel better while you heal your bowel and body with this program.

## How long will I need to use crutches for my adrenal disorders?

Adrenal disorders occur at Level 2 of your pipe. It is the second area of your body to heal (assuming that other areas are unhealthy too). Refer to the diagram "Sequence of Healing" in Appendix A at the end of this book to better understand this concept, as well as to Chapter 1 under this subject heading.

# Misunderstandings About Adrenal Disorders and Other Information for Your Success

## Keep your stools well-formed

Because adrenal disorders caused by un-eliminated acids, and because well-formed stools prevent the re-absorption of acids into your blood that trigger this condition, you will feel best and have fewer adrenal problems if you keep your stools well-formed while you are healing your bowel and body.

If you do not have a very good handle on how to define well-formed stools, review Chapter 6 of *Unique Healing* now. (And remember, when your stools are hard and slow you are eliminating more acids, and will therefore feel better, than when your stools are one or more times a day but are not all extremely well-formed.)

If your stools are not well-formed, the following changes can help: increase your *Body Bentonite* intake; reduce your carbohydrate intake (pasta, breads, grains, cereals, yogurt, etc.); reduce your sugar intake (including natural healthy sugars such as agave, honey, raw sugar, cane juice, etc.); reduce your alcohol, salt, coffee, and/or soda intake; do not have a massage, chiropractic adjustment, or any other body work; and keep your exercise aerobic (see Chapter 4 for more information on how to attain this, and why it is important.)

If these changes do not noticeably help the form of your stools in two days, take them further (i.e. take more *Body Bentonite*, reduce your carbohydrate intake more, etc.)

Finally, of all of these recommendations, increasing your *Body Bentonite* intake is the most productive and helpful. It heals your body, unlike the other recommendations. It will do the most to lead you to a place where looking and feeling good is effortless, and some of the other suggestions, such as reducing sugar intake, are simply "too hard to do when your blood is too acidic."

(Note: the exception to this information is when your poorly formed stools are caused by an infection, in which case *Unique Healing Colloidal Silver* is needed to reduce your symptoms. Refer to Chapter 5 for information on when and how to use this crutch.)

## Cortisol levels that are too high or too low are corrected with this program

Just as levels of calcium in your blood that are too high or too low, or levels of iron in your blood that are too high or too low, are balanced and corrected by healing your bowel and body with this program, so too are cortisol levels that are too high or too low.

When your blood is overly acidic due to many un-eliminated acids, your adrenal glands may at some point respond to these with the secretion of cortisol. This can raise your blood cortisol levels. Over time, as your adrenal glands become unhealthy and exhausted, they may not be able to properly regulate these levels; in a sense, they may "run out of" cortisol to excrete, causing blood cortisol levels to plummet.

In both cases, acids in your blood have triggered cortisol levels that are too high or too low, and eliminating them with this program corrects this.

## Not caused "just by stress"

Many of you have been told that your adrenal problems are caused by stress, but that is not entirely true.

Stress can make your body more acidic, but your adrenal glands, like all of your organs, are damaged from *all* sources of acidity, not just stress. If you were never stressed, but ate a highly acidic diet, or were exposed to many acidic chemicals, and your bowel was not healthy enough to eliminate these acids, your adrenal glands, like all of your organs, would eventually become unhealthy.

Just as there is danger in promoting the idea that alcohol only damages your liver, leaving you to wrongly believe that alcohol cannot damage your other organs, it is dangerous to be told that your adrenal glands are damaged by stress. If you are not stressed, you may wrongly believe that your adrenal glands are safe from becoming unhealthy.

## Nor are they an inevitable product of stress

Most of us have stress in our lives. But if you are led to believe that stress invariably causes adrenal damage, then you can easily accept the idea that your adrenal glands will inevitably become damaged as a result, and that there is no chance of healing them. This is not true.

When your bowel and body are healthy, stress does not harm any of your organs, your adrenal glands included. When you have no holes in the roof of your house, it does not get wet when it rains.

## Adrenal supplements are not a magic cure-all

Millions of dollars of adrenal supplements have been sold with the promise that they will cure you of many of your problems. I purchased many hundreds of dollars worth of these myself when I was sick. They did not turn out to be the magic cure-all I was led to believe they would be, because they are crutches and crutches cannot cure you.

My clients eliminate their adrenal disorders without ingesting any adrenal supplements. They eliminate these disorders because when they heal their bowel and body with this program, their adrenal glands heal, *and they stay healed*. These are results that "magic adrenal supplements" cannot deliver.

# Success With Adrenal Disorders

"I came to Donna with a diagnosis of extreme adrenal exhaustion. My cortisol levels were completely out of whack. I took dozens of supplements every day for this and yet I still felt horrible most of the day. Since doing this program, I have been able to stop all of the adrenal supplements I was taking, which is shocking, and I feel better than I did when I was taking all of them."

## My story

"I too was diagnosed with adrenal fatigue over twenty-five years ago when I was very ill. The symptoms that I had associated with this—extreme anxiety, exhaustion, and very unstable blood sugar levels—are now completely gone. I do not take any supplements, as I did back then, for this condition. I spent a lot of money treating these symptoms, and now I spend nothing."

### Watch my Video, "Why THIS Program Eliminates Adrenal Disorders"

This video, and all of my videos, can be found at *www. UniqueHealing. com* or at *www.YouTube.com/UniqueHealing*.

# AIDS

See "Autoimmune Diseases" and "Viral Infections"

# Alcoholism

See "Addictions"

# Allergies (Environmental)
## Chemicals, Mold, Pesticides, Pollutants, and Others

When I was ill, I "lived in a bubble." I was told that environmental toxins were causing my problems, and I avoided as many as I could. I threw out books that were more than a few years old (due to the mold), stopped reading the newspaper (due to the toxic ink), moved out of a new house (due to the toxic fumes from the new carpeting and paint), stopped wearing perfume, bought diodes (to combat the negative electrical charges from computers, televisions, etc.), used only natural products for cleaning, washing, etc., and even became paranoid about pumping gas, as my nutritionist told me the fumes from it might set off my symptoms! (See my full story under "Success with Environmental Allergies.")

This was twenty-five years ago, long before most of you became aware of environmental toxins/acids. Now, the awareness of these problems has increased significantly, but there is also a significantly larger number of you who are sensitive to environmental toxins, as well. Is this purely due to awareness, or is it due to ever-worsening health? I believe it is due to both, with health decline being the greatest contributing factor.

I am grateful for my knowledge, and for knowing that avoiding these toxins is good for my health, but simply avoiding them is not the solution to your problems (as it wasn't for me, either). Avoiding the rains that hit your roof so your house doesn't get wet is good, but your roof will last longer if it has no holes in it, and avoiding rain does not fix these holes. Healing your bowel and body with this program creates strength against environmental toxins that leads to a much longer life, with fewer symptoms and disease.

## Healing Your Body With This Program Eliminates Environmental Allergies

Your immune/lymphatic system may respond to un-eliminated acids (irritants, chemicals, etc.) by secreting histamines and mucus. These substances entrap these acids in an attempt to prevent them from harming your body, but they are also largely responsible for the symptoms associated with allergies, such as a runny nose, watery eyes, sneezing, etc.

Healing your body with this program eliminates the acids that trigger immune system reactions, such as inflammation and the secretion of histamines. Healing your body with this program heals your lymphatic/immune system organs. Healing your body heals these organs so that even if there are acids, your body is strong enough to handle them without a reaction (it fixes the holes on your roof so that even if it does rain, your house does not get wet).

## Healing Your Bowel With This Program Eliminates Environmental Allergies

In addition to its many other important functions, a healthy bacterial environment in your bowel is a necessity for the complete elimination of acids (toxins, heavy metals, pesticides, etc.) from your body. A healthy bowel prevents the re-absorption of acids into your blood that cause allergies.

# Why My Crutches Work for Environmental Allergies

**Body Bentonite** binds to and eliminates acids (toxins, heavy metals, chemicals, etc.) from your body. It helps prevent them from becoming re-absorbed into your bloodstream, where they trigger a response by your immune system to protect you from them. It eliminates the acids that trigger the release of histamines and mucus.

**Unique Healing Calcium Citrate** is an alkalinizing mineral that helps neutralize the acids that your bowel does not eliminate. When these acids are neutralized, your body does not need to produce histamines and mucus to buffer them.

### How much do I take?/Questions about using these

See Chapter 5 for information on using these crutches, including recommendations on the amount to use, as well as a discussion of the misunderstandings about the particular crutch which, if not understood correctly, may cause you to fail to look and feel better while you heal your bowel and body with this program.

### How long will I need to use crutches for environmental allergies?

Environmental allergies occur at Level 3 of your pipe. It is the second to last area of your body to heal (assuming that other areas are unhealthy too). Refer to the diagram "Sequence of Healing" in Appendix A at the end of this book to better understand this concept, as well as to Chapter 1 under this subject heading.

## Misunderstandings About Environmental Allergies and Other Information for Your Success

### Keep your stools well-formed

Because un-eliminated acids cause allergies, and because well-formed stools prevent the re-absorption of acids into your blood, you will suffer least from allergies if you keep your stools well-formed while you are healing your bowel and body.

If you do not have a very good handle on how to define well-formed stools, review Chapter 6 of *Unique Healing* now. (And remember, when your stools are hard and slow you are eliminating more acids, and will

therefore feel better, than when your stools are one or more times a day but not all extremely well-formed.)

If your stools are not well-formed, the following changes can help: increase your *Body Bentonite* intake; reduce your carbohydrate intake (pasta, breads, grains, cereals, yogurt, etc.); reduce your sugar intake (including natural healthy sugars such as agave, honey, raw sugar, cane juice, etc.); reduce your alcohol, salt, coffee, and/or soda intake; do not have a massage, chiropractic adjustment, or any other body work; drink a lot of water; rest; and keep your exercise aerobic (see Chapter 4 for more information on how to attain this, and why it is important.)

If these changes do not noticeably help the form of your stools in two days, take them further (i.e. take more *Body Bentonite*, reduce your carbohydrate intake more, etc.)

Out of all of these recommendations, increasing your *Body Bentonite* intake is one of the most productive and helpful. It heals your body, unlike many of the other recommendations. It will do the most to lead you to a place where looking and feeling good is effortless, and some of the other suggestions, such as reducing sugar intake, are simply "too hard to do when your blood is too acidic."

(Note: the exception to this information is when your poorly formed stools are caused by an infection, in which case *Unique Healing Colloidal Silver* is needed to reduce your symptoms. Refer to Chapter 5 for information on when and how to use this crutch.)

## Allergy shots

Allergy shots are crutches that may be helpful for reducing the discomfort of allergies, but be careful that you do not rely on these alone. If you do, you are ignoring the "cry" from your lymphatic (immune) system that it is being attacked, and becoming unhealthy.

Allergy shots do not heal your lymphatic/immune system; they only serve to make you comfortable, which can make you believe that you are healthier than you really are. If you do not heal your lymphatic system, as this program does, then one day you may "outgrow your allergies" only to find greater immune system symptoms and ill health in its place. For example, your allergies may "turn into" arthritis, instead.

Just as it is dangerous to assume that outgrowing asthma (see the later section on asthma) is a sign that you have miraculously become healthier, it is dangerous to assume that you have miraculously become healthier if you outgrow your allergies, too.

# Success With Environmental Allergies

"I used to have allergies all spring long. This past spring, I had none. None!"

"I had chemical allergies and allergies to cats. I took a million vitamins to treat these but I still suffered. Nothing really helped. After a couple of years of healing my bowel and body, these allergies are gone, and I can even be around cats now and not start wheezing."

## My story

"I was plagued with horrible hay fever as a young child. The hay fever disappeared later on, "replaced" by a crippling autoimmune disease instead. At this time I suffered from severe chemical allergies as well. I even had to move out of a newly built rental home after only two weeks, as I had a severe reaction to the toxins emitted from the fresh paint and carpeting. I lived in a bubble of sorts, or so it felt. The smell of gasoline, moldy books, perfume, and many other irritants made me feel miserable. I was afraid to go out. How could I survive this way?

Now, while I am sensitive to the smell of toxins—a blessing that reminds me to remove myself from them as much as possible—I do not react to them. They do not cripple me as they did before I did this program. In fact, just last month I had my house re-carpeted and while it smelled very toxic, and it was cold outside so I could not open my windows or escape the fumes, I was fine. This was a completely different experience from the one I had many years ago. The fear of exposure to these, and the dire consequences of the exposure to them, is gone. It is a much better way to live. My hay fever no longer exists either (although it did "re-appear" temporarily while I has healing my bowel and body, which occurred when I was much healthier and felt much better overall, so that all in all, the experience was a positive, not a negative, one.)

## Watch My Video, "Why THIS Program Works for Environmental Allergies"

This video, and all of my videos, can be found at *www.UniqueHealing. com* or at *www.YouTube.com/UniqueHealing.*

# Allergies (Food)

Thirty to fifty million Americans produce insufficient amounts of lactase to digest the lactose, or sugar, in milk products. Between 1997 and 2002, there was a 100% increase in the incidence of peanut allergies in children. Gluten allergies are soaring. Twenty years ago when I was diagnosed with a gluten allergy I was considered odd. Nowadays, it's a common discussion. A client came in the other day and said that at her son's soccer game it is all the mothers talk about. The number, and sales, of gluten-free products, has increased dramatically in the last few years. Someone is cashing in.

Food allergies have skyrocketed in the last five years, and as with environmental allergies, one must ask, are we merely more aware of these allergies, or is it due to our ever-worsening health? Again, I say the latter.

In this section I have focused mainly on dairy and gluten allergies, as these are the most common, however the concepts mentioned here apply to any food you may be allergic to—nuts, egg, citrus, soy, shellfish, peanuts, milk, wheat, etc.

If you have symptoms after eating dairy or gluten-containing products, these products are the trigger of your symptoms, not the cause. Many of my clients have been able to eat dairy and wheat again without any problems after following this healing program.

## Healing Your Body With This Program Eliminates Food Allergies

Many of the symptoms of food allergies reflect the reactions of your organs to the acidic/toxic irritants in some foods, such as molds, chemicals, pesticides, etc. This is especially true of foods such as peanuts and other nuts, shellfish, and highly processed foods. For example, hives result from the release of histamine, which itself is a protective response from your immune/lymphatic system in reaction to irritants in foods, and asthma occurs when your body releases inflammatory chemicals and oxygen in order to buffer acidity in your lungs.

Healing your body with this program eliminates immune system responses such as inflammation and the secretion of histamines. Healing your body with this program heals your organs. Excess acidity is eventually damaging to them, as it reduces the oxygen and nutrients they need to be healthy, thrive, and function normally. Healing your body heals your organs so that even if there are acids, your body is strong enough to handle them without a reaction (it fixes the holes on your roof so that even if it does rain, your house does not get wet).

# Healing Your Bowel With This Program Eliminates Food Allergies

Your beneficial bowel bacteria are involved in the manufacture of digestive enzymes, and the breakdown of gluten and lactose. When these are digested properly it eliminates the negative reaction to undigested particles of gluten and lactose that otherwise can trigger symptoms.

Studies have found that mice with poor bowel bacteria were more susceptible to allergies than healthier mice. Also, a study of 29 Estonian and 33 Swedish two-year old children found that 36 were non allergenic and 27 had a confirmed diagnosis of allergy, with at least one skin prick test positive to egg or cow's milk. The allergic children were less often colonized with lactobacilli (a beneficial bacteria), than the non-allergic children in both countries. Allergic children had higher counts of aerobic microorganisms, specifically coliforms and *Staphylococcus aureus,* but lower proportions of anaerobic microorganisms such as *Bacteriodes.* ("The Intestinal Microflora in Allergic Estonian and Swedish 2-Year-Old Children," Bjorksten B, et al, ***Clin Exp Allergy***, 1999; 29:342-346.

From ABC News online, 2/24/04: "Treatment may reduce child allergy development." "Researcher's believe 'good bacteria' may be the key to preventing children developing allergies. In the first of its kind in Australia, a trial has begun at Perth's Princess Margaret Hospital that involves administering dietary supplements known as probiotics, to babies twice a day for their first six months. An estimated 40 percent of children have some kind of allergy."

In addition to its many other important functions, a healthy bacterial environment in your bowel is a necessity for the complete elimination of acids (toxins, heavy metals, pesticides, etc.) from your body. A healthy bowel prevents the re-absorption into your blood of acids from irritating foods that cause an unhealthy body, and trigger the symptoms associated with food allergies.

# Why My Crutches Work for Food Allergies

***Body Bentonite*** binds to and eliminates acids (toxins, heavy metals, chemicals, etc.) from your body. It helps prevent them from becoming re-absorbed into your bloodstream, where they trigger allergic responses by your body to protect you from them.

***Unique Healing Calcium Citrate*** is an alkalinizing mineral that helps neutralize the acids that your bowel does not eliminate. When these acids are neutralized, your body does not need to produce inflammatory chemicals and other responses to buffer them.

As for additional crutches for food allergies, one of the best is to avoid the food until your bowel is healthier. If a food creates a serious reaction, that is an appropriate time to resort to medications intended for this purpose.

## How much do I take?/Questions about using these

See Chapter 5 for information on using these crutches, including recommendations on the amount to use, as well as a discussion of the misunderstandings about the particular crutch that may, if not understood correctly, cause you to fail to look and feel better while you heal your bowel and body with this program.

## How long will I need to use crutches for my food allergies?

Food allergies occur at Levels 3 and 4 of your pipe. These are the second to last, and the last, areas of your body to heal (assuming that other areas are unhealthy too). Refer to the diagram "Sequence of Healing" in Appendix A at the end of this book to better understand this concept, as well as to Chapter 1 under this subject heading.

The bacterial environment in your bowel also affects food allergies. To better understand how long you may need crutches for this, refer to Chapter 1 under this subject heading.

# Misunderstandings About Food Allergies and Other Information for Your Success

## Keep your stools well-formed

Because allergic reactions are caused in part by un-eliminated acids, and because well-formed stools prevent the re-absorption of acids into your blood, you will suffer from the least amount of food allergies if you keep your stools well-formed while you are healing your bowel and body.

If you do not have a very good handle on how to define well-formed stools, review Chapter 6 of *Unique Healing* now. (And remember, when your stools are hard and slow you are eliminating more acids, and will therefore feel better, than when your stools are one or more times a day but not all extremely well-formed.)

If your stools are not well-formed, the following changes can help: increase your *Body Bentonite* intake; reduce your carbohydrate intake (pasta, breads, grains, cereals, yogurt, etc.); reduce your sugar intake (including natural healthy sugars such as agave, honey, raw sugar, cane juice, etc.); reduce your alcohol, salt, coffee, and/or soda intake; do not have a massage, chiropractic adjustment, or any other body work; drink a lot of water; rest; and keep your exercise aerobic (see Chapter 4 for more information on how to attain this, and why it is important.)

If these changes do not noticeably help the form of your stools in two days, take them further (i.e. take more *Body Bentonite*, reduce your carbohydrate intake more, etc.)

Out of all of these recommendations, increasing your *Body Bentonite* intake is one of the most productive and helpful. It heals your body, unlike many of the other recommendations. It will do the most to lead you to a place where looking and feeling good is effortless, and some of the other suggestions, such as reducing sugar intake, are simply "too hard to do when your blood is too acidic."

(Note: the exception to this information is when your poorly formed stools are caused by an infection, in which case *Unique Healing Colloidal Silver* is needed to reduce your symptoms. Refer to Chapter 5 for information on when and how to use this crutch.)

## Many symptoms are due to cleansing reactions, and not due to food allergies

Many of your weight problems and symptoms that are currently being blamed on food allergies are not caused by food allergies at all.

In fact, according to the Wall Street Journal (12/7/10—"New Rules for Food Allergies"), the percentage of people allergic to the following foods are listed as: fish: 0.3%-0.6%, soy 0.2%-0.7%, peanuts 0.6%-0.75%, tree nuts.1%-0.45%, milk 0.9%-3%, wheat 0.2%-2%, eggs 0.3% to 1%. (An allergy to a food is defined roughly as the occurrence of wheezing, turning red, and/or breaking out in a rash suddenly after eating one of these foods.)

These are very small numbers. Yet very large numbers of you have been told that your symptoms/weight/etc. are being caused by food allergies, which means something doesn't add up.

On a similar note, when discussing gluten allergies and celiac disease (Wall Street Journal 8/24/10), the author Melinda Beck notes that ". . . . as many as 20 million Americans appear to be sensitive to gluten without having full-blown celiac disease. For them, symptoms may be less typical, including depression, mental fogginess, mood swings and behavior changes. *Much less is known about this group.*" These "non food allergy" symptoms baffle experts, but they are not really baffling at all.

My knowledge and experience is that most of you who are being told you have food allergies don't have these at all, but rather, you are reacting to the cleansing effect of the food that is eaten.

You may also find these cleansing reactions referred to as "food intolerances." They mean the same thing. However, I have used the term "cleansing reactions" as I feel it more accurately describes the condition and is more helpful for your success in eliminating it.

While true allergic reactions to a food occur immediately after its consumption, cleansing reactions to foods eaten are delayed. They can occur within hours or even days after a cleansing food has been consumed and the un-eliminated acids created by its consumption show up as symptoms.

The most common foods that cause cleansing symptoms are *all* fruit, *all* grains/carbohydrates such as rice, bread, pasta, etc. (non-gluten grains included!), yogurt, kefir, agave, honey, and other natural sweeteners.

When I was extremely ill, I spent one and a half years writing down everything I ate, looking for allergic reactions to foods. I followed food allergy and food elimination diets to try to determine which foods were aggravating my symptoms. I never found a correlation (and clearly remember tossing this notebook across my bedroom in frustration at some point).

As with most of you, my symptoms were aggravated by the cleansing reactions of certain foods I ate, and because no one understood this concept, and because these reactions were delayed, I never found the direct cause and effect relationship I was looking for. Most of you won't either.

For more information on cleansing diets, and reactions to them, see Chapter 9 of *Unique Healing*, and watch my videos, "Avoid Cleansing Diets" and "Blame the *Right* Food," available at ***www.UniqueHealing. com*** under my videos, or at ***www.YouTube.com/UniqueHealing***.

## . . . . or from a highly acidic diet

In addition to symptoms caused by cleansing reactions as stated above, many other symptoms, weight problems, etc. are triggered by the acidity of the food consumed. Again, this is a much more common cause of your problems than food allergies themselves. And your negative reactions to these foods is, once again, often delayed (rather than immediate, as with a true food allergy.)

The acidic foods that are likely to trigger the most symptoms for you are: alcohol, salt, coffee, soda, vinegar, and sugar. (While chicken, beef, turkey and other animal proteins are also acidic, remember, they acidify your organs, not your *blood*, and it is only the acids in your blood that trigger symptoms.) So if you eat ice cream, which is acidic *and* cleansing, you may react to the powerful increase in blood acidity triggered by these two variables, and this should be called an "acidic" reaction, not a food allergy.

## Food allergy diets do not heal your bowel or body

When you avoid a food that you are allergic to but do not heal your bowel and body, you may see a quick improvement in your symptoms, but you rarely see a complete elimination of them. In this program, your symptoms will be completely eliminated.

When you avoid food allergens you create a stressful eating environment, with fear around food, and fear when eating out when the ingredients of a dish are not always known. When you are done with this program, you will be able to eat *any* food and not react poorly to it, and your fear around food will be eliminated.

When you avoid foods you are allergic to, you are overlooking the fact that your bowel and body are unhealthy. They will *continue* to become less healthy even as you avoid these foods, leading to *more* debilitating conditions down the road, including a higher possibility of early death. When you follow most food allergy diets, you are lulled into a false sense of security about your health.

Food allergy diets are more widely known about today, but this is *not* a "new" magical dietary program. Like all of the other crutches, they are back in print because there is a whole new population of people who haven't tried, and ultimately failed, following them. Again, I got on this bandwagon twenty-five years ago. These diets existed back then and failed to heal me, and they are failing to heal millions of you too. I have worked with many people who have ultimately failed to permanently eliminate their symptoms, excess weight, and/or avoid disease with this approach, and some of my most seriously ill clients have followed food allergy diets and still remained highly symptomatic.

A healthy bowel digests gluten and lactose without producing discomfort. When you focus on a strict diet and do not heal your unhealthy bowel, your symptoms may improve, but as soon as you stray from the diet, they will return. And straying from this diet is very easy to do. Unfortunately, at this point, most of you think you have failed, rather than blaming the approach. Many practitioners blame the person when they stray from a ridiculously strict diet and their symptoms return, when the real blame lies in the approach that the practitioner recommended. As in so many other cases, you have been led to believe that if something gives you immediate, short-term benefits, you are on the right track, and that the approach is not the ultimate reason for your failure.

A naturopath writes of treating a child with eczema and how the elimination of dairy produced formed stools for the first time in the child's life, and that as soon as dairy was re-introduced the symptoms returned. If a symptom returns, you have not healed your bowel or body. If you eliminate a food group and your stools improve, it does not mean you have healed your bowel. You have not.

The long-term consequences of following these diets have not shown up, yet. But they will. If you do not heal your bowel and body and only avoid foods that you are allergic, or sensitive to, you are at risk of other serious health problems down the road. Problems such as breast cancer and prostate cancer, that are directly associated with an unhealthy bowel.

True food allergies can be deadly in the immediate term, so respect them. But in the long-term, if you avoid a food you are allergic or sensitive to and do not address the cause of the problem, especially if you incorporate a high protein diet, as most people do (see the discussion below), you will likely end up with more serious problems down the road as a result of a continually worsening of your bowel and body health.

### They are dangerous when they turn into high protein diets

Gluten (wheat) and dairy are very common ingredients in the foods we eat. When these are eliminated, the majority of people replace them with high protein foods such as chicken, fish, and eggs.

In other words, allergy-free diets usually turn into high protein diets, and "work," but hurt, for the same reasons. Review Chapter Five of *Unique Healing* for a complete understanding of the dangers of these diets.

### Genetics can be altered

Some people blame food allergies and intolerances on genetics. What you are not told is that yes, you can inherit an unhealthy bowel from your parents, and this will manifest as allergies *unless you actively work to heal it.*

## Success With Food Allergies

"My daughter had allergic reactions to dairy when we started this program, and now she can eat it without any problems."

"I was diagnosed with gluten allergies by my naturopath. I avoided gluten for many years but I still was overweight, had horrible headaches, joint pain, and gas and bloating after eating gluten-containing foods. After I followed this program for a while I added these back in—probably faster and in greater quantities than I should have!—but I felt fine doing so, and I was so tired of avoiding these for so long, I just did it."

"This program was the first to explain why I was reacting to the foods that I ate the way that I did. I am no longer confused about what to eat, and I understand how and why certain foods affect me the way they do. Often I will take extra *Body Bentonite* if I eat something I shouldn't yet, and it prevents me from reacting badly to it."

"Dairy products used to trigger bad diarrhea. I now eat dairy and I haven't had diarrhea in many months."

### My story

"When I was very ill, I ate a strict wheat-free, dairy-free, sugar-free diet. I followed this for approximately five years. I even went to the emergency room twice after consuming pizza (and remember the "looks" given to me by the emergency room staff when I claimed the pizza had caused my problems—I'm lucky they didn't try to lock me away!). Eventually, I just couldn't keep this strict diet up. My symptoms improved slightly on this diet, but were still significantly worse than when I healed my bowel and body and added wheat and dairy, including pizza, back into my daily diet. I now consume wheat and dairy daily, with zero ill effects."

### Watch My Video, "Why THIS Program Eliminates Food Allergies," and My Videos "Important Information on Wheat/Gluten-Free Diets," and "Avoid Cleansing Diets"

These videos, and all of my videos, can be found at *www. UniqueHealing.com* or at *www.YouTube.com/UniqueHealing*.

## Aluminum Toxicity
See "Heavy Metal Toxicity"

## Alzheimer's Disease
See "Neurological Conditions"

## Anemia
See also "Fatigue"

Common symptoms of anemia include fatigue, dizziness, and depression.

You may be anemic, even if your blood test shows normal iron levels. Blood tests are a very unreliable way to test the health of your body/organs, and an unhealthy body can be anemic. So if you have the above symptoms, even if your blood tests for iron levels are normal, read the following section and consider the possibility that you are suffering from anemia, anyway.

## Healing Your Body With This Program Eliminates Anemia

Iron oxygenates your blood. When you have excess un-eliminated acids in your blood, your body may "use up" iron to buffer these, causing low iron levels, resulting in anemia.

Your spleen, one of the main organs of your lymphatic system, stores iron. It is the responsibility of your spleen to regulate iron levels in your blood, and when your spleen is healthy, this is done effectively.

Healing your body with this program eliminates the acids that trigger the symptoms associated with anemia. Healing your body with this program heals your lymphatic organs so that even if there are acids, they are strong enough to handle them without a reaction (it fixes the holes on your roof so that even if it does rain, your house does not get wet).

## Healing Your Bowel With This Program Eliminates Anemia

In addition to its many other important functions, a healthy bacterial environment in your bowel is a necessity for the complete elimination of acids (toxins, heavy metals, pesticides, etc.) from your body. A healthy bowel prevents the re-absorption of acids into your blood that cause an unhealthy body, and trigger anemia.

## Why My Crutches Work for Anemia

***Body Bentonite*** binds to and eliminates acids (toxins, heavy metals, chemicals, etc.) from your body. It helps to prevent them from becoming re-absorbed into your bloodstream, where they trigger a response by your immune system to protect you from them. It eliminates the acids that reduce oxygen levels in your blood and reduce iron levels as a result.

***Unique Healing Calcium Citrate*** is an alkalinizing mineral that helps neutralize the acids that your bowel does not eliminate. When these acids are neutralized, your body does not need to "use up iron" to buffer them.

***Unique Healing Methyl Vitamin B-12*** Technically, vitamin B-12 is not a helpful crutch for anemia. However, I mention it here because low levels of this nutrient are very common, and they can cause fatigue and other symptoms that are associated with, and similar to, anemia.

### How much do I take?/Questions about using these

See Chapter 5 for information on using these crutches, including recommendations on the amount to use, as well as a discussion of the misunderstandings about the particular crutch that may, if not understood correctly, cause you to fail to look and feel better while you heal your bowel and body with this program.

## How long will I need to use crutches for my anemia?

Anemia occurs at Level 3 of your pipe. It is the second to last area of your body to heal (assuming that other areas are unhealthy too). Refer to the diagram "Sequence of Healing" in Appendix A at the end of this book to better understand this concept, as well as to Chapter 1 under this subject heading.

# Misunderstandings About Anemia and Other Information for Your Success

## Keep your stools well-formed

Because un-eliminated acids cause anemia, and because well-formed stools prevent the re-absorption of acids into your blood, you will suffer from the least amount of anemic symptoms if you keep your stools well-formed while you are healing your bowel and body.

If you do not have a very good handle on how to define well-formed stools, review Chapter 6 of *Unique Healing* now. (And remember, when your stools are hard and slow you are eliminating more acids, and will therefore feel better, than when your stools are one or more times a day but not all extremely well-formed.)

If your stools are not well-formed, the following changes can help: increase your *Body Bentonite* intake; reduce your carbohydrate intake (pasta, breads, grains, cereals, yogurt, etc.); reduce your sugar intake (including natural healthy sugars such as agave, honey, raw sugar, cane juice, etc.); reduce your alcohol, salt, coffee, and/or soda intake; do not have a massage, chiropractic adjustment, or any other body work; drink a lot of water; rest; and keep your exercise aerobic (see Chapter 4 for more information on how to attain this, and why it is important.)

If these changes do not noticeably help the form of your stools in two days, take them further (i.e. take more *Body Bentonite*, reduce your carbohydrate intake more, etc.)

Out of all of these recommendations, increasing your *Body Bentonite* intake is one of the most productive and helpful. It heals your body, unlike many of the other recommendations. It will do the most to lead you to a place where looking and feeling good is effortless, and some of the other suggestions, such as reducing sugar intake, are simply "too hard to do when your blood is too acidic."

(Note: the exception to this information is when your poorly formed stools are caused by an infection, in which case *Unique Healing Colloidal Silver* is needed to reduce your symptoms. Refer to Chapter 5 for information on when and how to use this crutch.)

## High blood iron levels

In optimum health, your iron levels will be neither too high nor too low. In health, your blood pressure will be neither too high or too low, your blood sugar will be neither too high or too low, etc. When a health variable is too high or too low, the situation and cause of this is much more similar than you may know. Perhaps surprisingly, health variables that are too high (high blood sugar or high iron levels, for example) may result from the same situation or cause as when they are too low (a variable that is too high is usually a sign of a much less healthy body than when it is too low.)

High blood iron levels occur when you have severely low levels of oxygen in your blood, which is caused by a lot of un-eliminated acids in your blood, coupled with an unhealthy lymphatic system. To protect you from these acids, your lymphatic system (spleen) may respond by "dumping" a lot of iron into your blood in an attempt to oxygenate it.

If you have high blood iron levels, this is corrected by taking *more* iron, not less (just as other blood nutrient variables that are high are corrected by taking more of that nutrient, not less). You will likely be given contrary advice, but I have seen high iron levels lowered to normal with the ingestion of large quantities of iron in 100% of the clients that I have given, and who have followed, this advice.

## No harm from taking iron

Likewise, iron intake does not harm your heart, cause cancer, or harm your body whatsoever. It has been observed that in cases of heart disease and cancer there may be high blood iron levels, and some people have wrongly assumed that one caused the other.

When two variables co-exist, it does not automatically mean that one caused the other. When you have a non-hormonal cancer or heart disease, you are in a state of great ill health; there has been a large accumulation of acidity in your body and a great decline in the health of your lymphatic system as well (which regulates iron levels in your blood and prevents them from becoming too low or too high). So when you see high iron levels in cases of serious disease, it is a symptom of the ill health of your body; it is *not the cause* of your ill health.

Iron intake does not cause cancer, heart disease, or any other diseases or problems. Excess acids cause high iron levels, and excess acids cause many diseases, too.

I have also read that bad bacteria feed off of iron, which again, can wrongly alarm you about taking this mineral. Has this correlation been proven, or is it simply another one of those "cause and effect guesses" that are so immensely prevalent in the medical and health field? I have seen no evidence that it has been proven. Maybe high iron levels simply *coexist* with high levels of bad bacteria, because an unhealthy bowel causes poor elimination of acids, and once again, high acids levels can cause your body to dump a lot of iron into your blood to oxygenate, and therefore protect you, from these acids.

## Using an iron crutch

Iron is not a crutch that I routinely recommend, because my knowledge and experience is that the use of *Body Bentonite* and *Unique Healing Calcium Citrate* are sufficient to correct blood iron levels, for the reasons explained earlier (except where one is not willing to take the amount necessary to create well-formed stools, which helps to keep your iron levels normalized). However, if you have this condition and would like to take iron, make sure you buy a "chelated" iron supplement (likely only found at the health food store or online). Try 150 mg/day and if you do not feel better/have more energy in 2-3 days, consider that you are taking the wrong crutch, and stop (or, if you have high blood iron levels, consider taking 300 mg/day daily *up until the day* that you have these tests re-done).

# Success With Anemia

"I did not think I was anemic or that iron could help me feel better because my blood tests showed normal levels, however when I started it, immediately I had more energy and less depression. After healing my bowel and body for the last 1 ½ years, I have stopped it and still feel great."

"I was diagnosed with an autoimmune disease when I came to Donna. For two years, my blood iron levels were too high and I was told to avoid it. She convinced me to take larger amounts and by my next blood test a couple months later, my levels were back to normal!"

## My story

"There was a moment in my illness when my lymphatic system was still healing, and I found that the addition of just 100 mg of iron/day increased my energy levels from a '2' to a '9.' The difference was remarkable."

### Watch My Video, "Why THIS Program Eliminates Anemia"

This video, and all of my videos, can be found at *www.UniqueHealing.com* or at *www.YouTube.com/UniqueHealing*.

# Anorexia
See "Eating Disorders"

# Anxiety
See "Mental Health"

# Apnea
See "Sleep Disorders"

# Arsenic Poisoning
See "Heavy Metal Toxicity"

# Arteriosclerosis
See "Cholesterol/Heart Disease"

# Arthritis

Arthritis is more than just inflammation and aches and pain (for more information on these conditions, see "Aches and Pains"). With arthritis, there is inflammation and aches and pain, but there is also degeneration. It is a more serious condition, and represents a much less healthy body.

# Healing Your Body With This Program Eliminates Arthritis

Your body's first line of defense against excess un-eliminated acids in your blood are your four elimination channels—lungs, kidneys, skin, and especially, your bowel. After they become unhealthy, your liver, adrenal glands, stomach, pancreas, and small intestine are stimulated to protect you against these acids. It is after *they* become unhealthy that your body turns to its alkaline reserves—calcium, magnesium, sodium, and potassium—to neutralize this acidity.

Your joints contain a lot of these alkaline minerals, and when they are leached out of your bones to buffer these un-eliminated acids, they degenerate, and eventually create the condition of arthritis. (Review Chapter 3 of *Unique Healing* for a description of this degenerative process in response to un-eliminated acids.)

Healing your body with this program eliminates the acids that cause your body to leach calcium and other minerals from your joints.

# Healing Your Bowel With This Program Eliminates Arthritis

In addition to its many other important functions, a healthy bacterial environment in your bowel is a necessity for the complete elimination of acids (toxins, heavy metals, pesticides, etc.) from your body. A healthy bowel prevents the re-absorption of acids into your blood that cause damage to your organs and body, including your joints.

# Why My Crutches Work for Arthritis

There are no crutches for degenerative conditions. Crutches can offset the effects of acids in your blood, or the effects of poor function of your bowel bacterial environment (as these can be quickly altered), but degeneration is caused by depletion and damage to your organs, and organs take time to heal.

You can put a tarp on your roof and quickly stop your house from becoming wet, but you cannot quickly repair the holes in your roof. Your house getting wet causes many conditions, but degenerative conditions are the "holes in your roof" and there are no quick fixes for these.

(Nevertheless, I do highly recommend that you use *Body Bentonite* and *Unique Healing Calcium Citrate,* as these crutches can reduce the pain and inflammation that make arthritis uncomfortable.)

### How long will I need to use crutches for my arthritis?

Again, there are no crutches for degenerative conditions like arthritis; however, degenerative conditions are the first to be eliminated as you heal your bowel and body with this program.

## Misunderstandings About Arthritis and Other Information for Your Success

### Arthritis does not only affect old people

Degenerative conditions, like arthritis, are occurring at younger and younger ages. As our bowels become less healthy, we are faced with a quickening accumulation of acidity and ever-quickening damage, or degeneration, in our bodies.

Be careful that you do not wrongly believe that just because you are young you are safe from this condition.

### Nor is it an inevitable product of old age

On the other hand, degeneration, like arthritis, is not an inevitable product of aging. You can get younger as you age. You can prevent the accumulation of acidity that eventually leads to degeneration, and you will, when you follow this program.

### Surgery can be helpful, but heed the warning signs of this condition

Knee and hip replacement surgery, for example, is a wonderful tool of modern medicine, and it can, relatively quickly, improve the quality of your life. While there is a risk with every surgery, and that is true here too, there is also a risk involved with having surgery and avoiding the physiological cause of your degeneration in the first place.

Degeneration is a very strong warning sign that your body, and bowel, need a lot of healing; that you are getting a "bit too close to the top of your pipe" for comfort.

## Take *Unique Healing Calcium Citrate*

If you are diagnosed with arthritis, I strongly advise you to take extra calcium, in a very easy-to-assimilate form, like *Unique Healing Calcium Citrate*, until you get a "clean bill of health." Extra calcium can help you build a stronger skeletal system. (For information on using *Unique Healing Calcium Citrate*, see Chapter 5).

# Success With Arthritis

"An MRI showed degeneration of the femur of my hip bone. Two years after doing this program I had another MRI done and the degeneration is gone."

"I was diagnosed with arthritis and suffered from daily discomfort as a result. The pain went away quickly when I started this program, but more amazingly, the arthritis went away too!"

## Watch My Video, Why THIS Program Works for Arthritis."

This video, and all of my videos, can be found at *www.UniqueHealing. com* or at *www.YouTube.com/UniqueHealing.*

# Asthma

Asthma affected 8.2% of all U.S. residents in 2009, up from 7.3% in 2001, an increase of 12.3% (according to the Centers for Disease Control and Prevention). Children are more prone to asthma than adults, and women are more prone than men. The incidence has risen, as has the use of toxic medications to treat it, but the death rate is down (due to early detection and better treatments), but what about the long-term affects of these treatments? And what is the death rate from *other* conditions of people who have treated their asthma with medications?

The increase in asthma has brought with it an increased interest and awareness about the conditions that trigger this condition. The environment, additives in food, or food allergies, like dairy and wheat, are commonly blamed for asthma. While it is true that all of these have the potential to *trigger* asthma, the real culprit is an unhealthy bowel and body.

Why has asthma increased in the last decade? I suggest that this correlates to the ever-worsening health of the bowel bacterial environments of children born today.

# A Healthy Body Eliminates Asthma

A low level of oxygen, and inflammation in your lungs, are the primary contributors to the symptoms of asthma.

Oxygen is taken into your lungs, and carbon dioxide is excreted, with every breath in and out. If your lungs do not get enough oxygen, they tend to "gasp" for air.

Excess acids in your blood may be buffered with oxygen to protect you from the danger of them. As oxygen levels are "used up" to buffer these acids, less is available for your lungs (and rest of your body) to function healthfully.

Low oxygen levels and asthma are at the core of this condition. Surely you have heard of "exercise-induced asthma"? (I have never heard of exercise-induced cancer, high cholesterol, or diabetes.) During strenuous exercise, an excess production of lactic acid, coupled with shallow breathing due to exertion, can lead to low levels of oxygen in your blood, triggering asthma.

Haven't you seen ill people with more serious lung problems, like emphysema and lung disease, who walk around with oxygen tanks? I wonder if asthma symptoms and deaths would decrease if asthmatics were given an oxygen tank, too. It seems very likely that it would, although I understand that it would be impractical and costly.

Another condition that contributes to asthma is inflammation. When your lungs become inflamed, they constrict, making it more difficult to get needed oxygen to them. Many traditional treatments for asthma, including inhalers and steroids, reduce inflammation in your body.

Inflammatory chemicals are secreted by your lymphatic system in response to un-eliminated acids in your blood. By eliminating acids from your body, you eliminate inflammation.

Healing your body with this program eliminates the acids that trigger the symptoms associated with asthma. Healing your body heals your lungs and lymphatic system so that even if there are acids, your body is strong enough to handle them without a reaction (it fixes the holes on your roof so that even if it does rain, your house does not get wet).

(For more information on how this program increases oxygenation and reduces inflammation, see Chapter 3).

# A Healthy Bowel Eliminates Asthma

Food allergies have been linked to asthma because undigested food particles are irritants/toxins that can trigger inflammation. A healthy bowel digests *all* of the components of your food, including lactose and gluten (dairy and wheat), so that undigested particles are not created to trigger inflammatory reactions.

Children living on farms who are exposed to bacteria and other microbes have a lower risk (30% or more) of developing asthma than children who don't, according to a large published study on this matter. (*Wall Street Journal*—2/24/11)

In addition to its many other important functions, a healthy bacterial environment in your bowel is a necessity for the complete elimination of acids (toxins, heavy metals, pesticides, etc.) from your body. A healthy bowel prevents the re-absorption of acids into your blood that cause an unhealthy body, and trigger low oxygen and increased inflammation, and the symptoms associated with asthma.

# Why My Crutches Eliminate Asthma

***Body Bentonite*** binds to and eliminates acids (toxins, heavy metals, chemicals, etc.) from your body. It helps prevent them from becoming re-absorbed into your bloodstream, where they trigger a response by your body to protect you from them. It eliminates the acids that trigger the release of inflammatory chemicals, and that reduce oxygenation.

***Unique Healing Calcium Citrate*** is an alkalinizing mineral that helps neutralize the acids that your bowel does not eliminate. When these acids are neutralized, your body does not need to produce inflammatory chemicals, or "use up" oxygen, to buffer them.

### How much do I take?/Questions about using these

See Chapter 5 for information on using these crutches, including recommendations on the amount to use, as well as a discussion of the misunderstandings about the particular crutch that may, if not understood correctly, cause you to fail to look and feel better while you heal your bowel and body with this program.

### How long will I need to use crutches for my asthma?

Asthma occurs at Level 4 of your pipe. It is the last area of your body to heal (assuming that other areas are unhealthy too). Refer to the diagram "Sequence of Healing" in Appendix A at the end of this book to better understand this concept, as well as to Chapter 1 under this subject heading.

The bacterial environment in your bowel also affects asthma. To better understand how long you may need crutches for this, refer to Chapter 1 under this subject heading.

## Misunderstandings About Asthma and Other Information for Your Success

### Keep your stools well-formed

Because asthma is caused in part by un-eliminated acids, and because well-formed stools prevent the re-absorption of acids into your blood, you will suffer from the least amount of asthma if you keep your stools well-formed while you are healing your bowel and body.

If you do not have a very good handle on how to define well-formed stools, review Chapter 6 of *Unique Healing* now. (And remember, when your stools are hard and slow you are eliminating more acids, and will therefore feel better, than when your stools are one or more times a day but not all extremely well-formed.)

If your stools are not well-formed, the following changes can help: increase your *Body Bentonite* intake; reduce your carbohydrate intake (pasta, breads, grains, cereals, yogurt, etc.); reduce your sugar intake (including natural healthy sugars such as agave, honey, raw sugar, cane juice, etc.); reduce your alcohol, salt, coffee, and/or soda intake; do not have a massage, chiropractic adjustment, or any other body work; drink a lot of water; rest; and keep your exercise aerobic (see Chapter 4 for more information on how to attain this, and why it is important.)

If these changes do not noticeably help the form of your stools in two days, take them further (i.e. take more *Body Bentonite*, reduce your carbohydrate intake more, etc.)

Out of all of these recommendations, increasing your *Body Bentonite* intake is one of the most productive and helpful. It heals your body, unlike many of the other recommendations. It will do the most to lead you to a place where looking and feeling good is effortless, and some of the other suggestions, such as reducing sugar intake, are simply "too hard to do when your blood is too acidic."

(Note: the exception to this information is when your poorly formed stools are caused by an infection, in which case *Unique Healing Colloidal Silver* is needed to reduce your symptoms. Refer to Chapter 5 for information on when and how to use this crutch.)

## Avoid allergic foods

As is true in all cases where I make dietary suggestions, if you are allergic to a food, do not consume it until your bowel and body are healed, and you can consume it without harm or symptoms. In the case of asthma, this is especially important, given the potential danger of this condition.

I do not conduct food allergy tests because the majority of the clients I see (and you) do not have them; the majority of the clients I work with who do have them have already had these tested and determined; and because the most common allergens like dairy, wheat, shellfish, nuts, and eggs can be tested on your own by avoiding these and/or observing your reaction to them.

If desired, you can very likely find a local allergist or practitioner who will do extensive food allergy testing for you.

And re-read the section on "Food Allergies" in this chapter for a better understanding of this concept, including an explanation of why many of your "food allergies" are not true allergies at all.

## Take this seriously, and use crutches daily

Minimizing the occurrence of asthma is important because at any time an attack can be deadly. The above crutches are non-toxic and best used on a daily basis to help *prevent* an asthma attack. During a bad attack, however, use a reliable and strong drug, like an inhaler. Go to the hospital if needed. This is not the time to try to treat this symptom with a natural crutch.

Because of the potential danger of this condition, it is especially important that an aggressive approach be taken to heal your bowel and body and eliminate your susceptibility to this condition altogether.

## Buffer the acids that trigger inflammation and low oxygenation with additional crutches

A study of 2,633 adults assessed them for magnesium intake and it was found that those who ingested the most had a lower incidence of wheezing, less incidence of bronchi spasms, and more efficient flow of air through the bronchial passages than did those with lower magnesium intakes. (Britton J. et al. *Dietary magnesium, lung function, wheezing, and airway hyperactivity in a random adult population sample.* Lancet, 1994;344:357-362.)

Alkalinizing minerals like magnesium (and calcium, sodium, and potassium) can buffer the acids that lead to this condition, as described earlier under the recommendation for *Unique Healing Calcium Citrate*.

If you or your child has difficulty breathing, but it is not serious, in addition to *Body Bentonite*, take 3,000 mg of *Unique Healing Calcium Citrate*.

Antioxidants like vitamin A, E, and selenium, and essential fatty acids like fish oils and flaxseed oil, can also reduce inflammation. A recent (2007) Dutch study found that kids who eat the most fish and whole grains are two to three times less likely to have asthma. Antioxidants in whole grains and fatty acids in fish both have anti-inflammatory properties. Antioxidants can buffer acids and reduce asthma symptoms, but it is far more effective to use *Body Bentonite* to eliminate these, as this has a cumulative, permanent, healing effect on the health of your lungs, while antioxidants, fish oils and alkalinizing minerals do not.

Buffering the acids that trigger low oxygen levels and inflammation is valuable; healing your lungs so they don't react badly to these acids is even better. *Body Bentonite* heals your lungs.

## Deep breathing, heart rate monitors, and oxygen therapy

To improve the oxygenation to your lungs, learn how to breathe deeply (this entails breathing with your diaphragm (or belly) *and* lungs, not just with your lungs). You can learn this on your own, or in yoga, Pilates, meditation, and other classes.

If you are an adult and exercise, buy a heart rate monitor from a sport, cycling, or running store and use it when exercising. It will help keep you from overexerting yourself and getting into an oxygen-depleted (i.e. asthma-inducing) state.

## Low carbohydrate/high protein diets cause more harm than good

A high protein diet can reduce the symptoms of asthma, because it prevents acids that are stored in your organs from moving into your blood, where symptoms are triggered when they are not eliminated from your body/bowel. This can lead to less asthma, but an increase in cellular degeneration (due to the accumulation of acidity in your organs that occurs as a result of these diets). Sure, asthma, which is triggered by un-eliminated acids in your blood, is bad, but cancer, which is triggered by un-eliminated acids in your organs, is worse. Don't let anyone sell you on this diet as a "cure" for asthma. It is a dangerous "treat the symptom" approach.

## You do not simply outgrow asthma

Your lungs are part of your body's first line of defense against excess un-eliminated acidity in your blood. Asthma is more prevalent when you are younger because you are usually healthier than when you age, when acids are more likely handled by your second, third, or fourth lines of defense, which create symptoms other than asthma. As an adult, asthma is less prevalent, but diabetes, cancer, and heart disease, which are problems associated with damage "further up your pipe" are much more prevalent, for example.

In other words, if you had asthma as a youngster and it disappeared, you are not as healthy as you may think. When you have a health condition like asthma and it "goes away" it is not because health problems magically disappear. True, asthma can disappear if you heal your bowel and body, but that is not the case with the vast majority of you who have had this experience. When nothing has been done to heal your bowel and body and your asthma "disappears," it is not because your lungs are healthier; it is because your other organs are less healthy. If you ask around you will find plenty of people who "outgrew" their asthma only to be stricken at an early age with cancer or heart disease.

Asthma is a very strong warning sign that your bowel and body are very unhealthy and if not fixed, something more serious will likely develop later on.

# Success With Asthma

"Prior to this program I was very allergic to nuts and can now eat them without my symptoms of asthma flaring up."

"I used to need my inhaler all the time. Now I rarely do."

"I had bad asthma and outgrew it, only to be diagnosed in my early 50's with breast cancer. I now get that my asthma "grew into" something more dangerous, and I am now healing my bowel and body with this program and have never felt better."

## Watch my Video, "Why THIS Program Eliminates Asthma"

This video, and all of my videos, can be found at *www.UniqueHealing. com* or at *www.YouTube.com/UniqueHealing*.

# Atherosclerosis
### See "Cholesterol/Heart Disease"

# Athlete's Foot
### See "Fungal Infections"

# Autism
### See "Neurological Disorders"

# Autoimmune Diseases

(See also "Aches and Pains," "Adrenal Disorders," "Allergies," "Anemia," "Bacterial Infections," "Fatigue," "Fungal Infections," "Thyroid Problems," and "Viral Infections")

There are over 100 named autoimmune diseases, and they are prevalent. Regarding just Chronic Fatigue alone, the Centers for Disease estimates 1-4 million Americans have it, and they are spending an average of $3286 annually on medical treatments for it; a lot more than this program costs, and with results that are significantly inferior.

The autoimmune diseases that you may be most familiar with are listed below, however, do not interpret this list as all-inclusive, and if you have been given a diagnosis of one, know that this program can help (even if you do not see your condition's name on the list).

Additionally, there are numerous conditions that contribute to autoimmune diseases, and you will find many of these conditions covered in earlier, and later, sections in this book, under other headings (for example, colitis is an autoimmune disease but you will also find it under "Bowel Conditions," so look for more specific information on these conditions in the index of this book as well.)

Some of the more common autoimmune diseases are: Addison's, ankylosing spondylitis (Lou Gehrig's disease), arthritis, cardiomyopathy, celiac, chronic fatigue, Crohn's, Cushing's syndrome, cystitis, diabetes mellitus type 1, eczema, Guillain-Barre, Grave's, Hashimoto's, interstitial cystis, juvenile arthritis, Kawasaki's, meniere's, multiple sclerosis, myasthenia gravis, PANDAS, pernicious anemia, psoriasis, pulmonary fibrosis, Reynaud's, rheumatoid arthritis, Sjogrns, ulcerative colitis, vasculitis, and vitiligo.

## Healing Your Body With This Program Eliminates Autoimmune Diseases

Your lymphatic system may respond to un-eliminated acids by secreting inflammatory chemicals to protect you from them. Pain and inflammation are very common complaints of people with these diseases, as was very true in my case as well. So is fatigue, and your lymphatic system is also responsible for making sure there is an adequate flow of iron into your blood, which is needed to oxygenate your brain and blood, and which gives you physical and mental energy. High levels of un-eliminated acids reduce oxygen, and iron, levels, as they are "used up" to buffer these acids and protect you from them. Your brain may also be considered a "giant lymph node" on top of your shoulders. You have numerous lymph nodes in your neck, head, and sinuses. Mine were in a constant state of inflammation due to a large amount of un-eliminated acidity in my body, and this caused my brain to be unclear, foggy, fuzzy, and irritable—again, common complaints of those of you who have these conditions.

Your lymphatic system is also responsible for fighting viral infections. When I was first diagnosed with my autoimmune disease, Epstein Barr Virus and cytomegalovirus were found, and the mindset was that this condition was caused by a viral infection. (And while this relationship is controversial, as discussed later on, the concept that an unhealthy immune system is at the core of these problems is not. This program heals your lymphatic, or immune, system.)

Un-eliminated acids can also cause your blood sugar levels to drop. A healthy liver, adrenal glands, pancreas, etc. (middle of your pipe) are needed to regulate energy and blood sugar levels. Many of you suffer from low blood sugar problems and must eat constantly to feel better.

Healing your body with this program eliminates the acids that trigger the symptoms associated with autoimmune diseases. Healing your body with this program heals your organs so that even if there are acids, your body is strong enough to handle them without a reaction (it fixes the holes on your roof so that even if it does rain, your house does not get wet).

(Dizziness, low blood pressure, skin and lung conditions, thyroid problems, hormonal problems, food allergies, environmental allergies, constipation, diarrhea, and many other symptoms and conditions that are the result of an unhealthy bowel and body/un-eliminated acids, are common among those of you who have these diseases, and you can find information in this chapter that specifically addresses each of these conditions and explains why this program eliminates them, as well as information on the best crutches to use to eliminate your symptoms while you are healing your bowel and body with this program.)

## Healing Your Bowel With This Program Eliminates Autoimmune Diseases

Your bowel bacteria are responsible for the production of vitamin B-12, and low levels of this vitamin have been linked to fatigue, depression, anxiety, sugar cravings, and neurological problems—all conditions that are common with autoimmune diseases.

Your bowel bacteria are also involved in the manufacture and regulation of melatonin, a hormone needed for deep, uninterrupted sleep. Insomnia, and the resultant fatigue that accompanies it, are also common in these conditions.

Your bowel bacteria are also responsible for fighting fungal, bacterial, and parasitic infections. When present in your body, these infections can trigger fatigue, insomnia, irritability, mental disorientation, and other symptoms associated with autoimmune diseases.

In addition to its many other important functions, a healthy bacterial environment in your bowel is a necessity for the complete elimination of acids (toxins, heavy metals, pesticides, etc.) from your body. A healthy bowel prevents the re-absorption of acids into your blood that cause an unhealthy body, and trigger some of the symptoms associated with autoimmune diseases.

# Why My Crutches Work for Autoimmune Diseases

*Body Bentonite* binds to and eliminates acids (toxins, heavy metals, chemicals, etc.) from your body. It helps prevent them from becoming re-absorbed into your bloodstream, where they trigger a response by your body to protect you from them. It eliminates the acids that trigger the release of inflammatory chemicals, and that reduce blood flow/circulation and oxygenation and blood sugar levels.

*Unique Healing Calcium Citrate* is an alkalinizing mineral that helps neutralize the acids that your bowel does not eliminate. When these acids are neutralized, your body does not need to produce inflammatory chemicals or "use up" oxygen to buffer them. The presence of fewer acids also results in more stable blood sugar levels, and more energy as a result as well.

*Unique Healing Methyl Vitamin B-12* provides your body with easy to assimilate levels of this nutrient, which can reduce fatigue, depression, anxiety, sugar cravings, and the neurological conditions that are associated with these diseases.

*Unique Healing Colloidal Silver* has natural anti-bacterial, anti-fungal, anti-parasitic properties, and helps to eliminate the fatigue, insomnia, irritability, mental disorientation, and other symptoms associated with these infections.

## How much do I take?/Questions about using these

See Chapter 5 for information on using these crutches, including recommendations on the amount to use, as well as a discussion of the misunderstandings about the particular crutch that may, if not understood correctly, cause you to fail to look and feel better while you heal your bowel and body with this program.

## How long will I need to use crutches for my autoimmune disease?

Autoimmune diseases occur at Levels 2 and 3 of your pipe. They are the second, and the second to last, areas of your body to heal (assuming that other areas are unhealthy too). Refer to the diagram "Sequence of Healing" in Appendix A at the end of this book to better understand this concept, as well as to Chapter 1 under this subject heading.

The bacterial environment in your bowel also affects autoimmune diseases. To better understand how long you may need crutches for this, refer to Chapter 1 under this subject heading.

## Misunderstandings About Autoimmune Diseases and Other Information for Your Success

### Keep your stools well-formed

Because autoimmune diseases are caused in part by un-eliminated acids, and because well-formed stools prevent the re-absorption of acids into your blood, you will suffer from the least amount of symptoms if you keep your stools well-formed while you are healing your bowel and body.

If you do not have a very good handle on how to define well-formed stools, review Chapter 6 of *Unique Healing* now. (And remember, when your stools are hard and slow you are eliminating more acids, and will therefore feel better, than when your stools are one or more times a day but not all extremely well-formed.)

If your stools are not well-formed, the following changes can help: increase your *Body Bentonite* intake; reduce your carbohydrate intake (pasta, breads, grains, cereals, yogurt, etc.); reduce your sugar intake (including natural healthy sugars such as agave, honey, raw sugar, cane juice, etc.); reduce your alcohol, salt, coffee, and/or soda intake; do not have a massage, chiropractic adjustment, or any other body work; drink a lot of water; rest; and keep your exercise aerobic (see Chapter 4 for more information on how to attain this, and why it is important.)

If these changes do not noticeably help the form of your stools in two days, take them further (i.e. take more *Body Bentonite*, reduce your carbohydrate intake more, etc.)

Out of all of these recommendations, increasing your *Body Bentonite* intake is one of the most productive and helpful. It heals your body, unlike many of the other recommendations. It will do the most to lead you to a place where looking and feeling good is effortless, and some of the other suggestions, such as reducing sugar intake, are simply "too hard to do when your blood is too acidic."

(Note: the exception to this information is when your poorly formed stools are caused by an infection, in which case *Unique Healing Colloidal Silver* is needed to reduce your symptoms. Refer to Chapter 5 for information on when and how to this crutch.)

## If you recover with other programs, what is your mortality rate?

Some of you have been led to believe that your autoimmune disease will simply, and magically, disappear on it's own after a number of years. There is a 31% recovery rate in the first five years of Chronic Fatigue, and 48% after 10 years. But hold on, it is unfortunately not this simple.

When you have an autoimmune disease, initially your immune system and liver, adrenal glands, etc. are very fragile, but often your cellular system is not, so these conditions come with disabling symptoms, but are often not present (at least not initially) with conditions related to cellular damage, like cancer or heart attack.

In other words, my experience is that people in these shoes have very unhealthy middle and bottoms of their pipe, but the top is still okay. They have very unhealthy livers, adrenals, pancreases, lymphatic systems, kidneys, skin, bowels, etc, but the acidity has not damaged the top of their pipe yet, where deadly cancers and heart disease occur.

Similar to the discussion on "outgrowing asthma" discussed under this section of the book, in many cases, when someone is said to recover from an autoimmune disease, we must look at his or her longevity after this recovery. Does the acidity move to the "top of the pipe," reducing some of the horrible autoimmune symptoms, only to be replaced with more deadly symptoms, like cancer or heart disease? If so, then in this case, "recovery" is not as great as it seems.

## Which came first, the illness or the virus?

As mentioned earlier, some of these conditions have been linked to a virus (a retrovirus), but this is controversial. A strong cause and effect relationship has failed to be proven.

Does a virus *cause* these conditions, or does it simply *co-exist* with them? I suggest that it is the latter (and hence, the failure of this theory to be proven.) My experience is that an unhealthy bowel and body cause these conditions, not by a virus.

## Complicated, and often requires additional support

Due to the complexity of these diseases, the many organs involved and the severity of damage to these organs that occurs with them, if you have one, you may need to consult with me directly for 6-12 months at the start of this program so I can give you more aggressive, and individualized, recommendations for healing your bowel and body and feeling better while you heal. These diseases occur when your bowel and body are extremely unhealthy, requiring very strong crutches, stronger than routinely recommended. Also, the more complicated the condition, and the sicker you are, the greater your fears and misunderstandings may be, and I can help you overcome these so you can find the success that is possible with this program, and that you deserve.

## Review the misunderstandings in other sections, too

Again, there are numerous conditions within this diagnosis that exist that have been covered in detail in other sections of this chapter. When you read these, read the misunderstandings that apply to them as well.

# Success With Autoimmune Diseases

"When I came to Donna I had been ill with an autoimmune disease for over 15 years. Many of these years were spent trapped inside my home, too ill to leave. One chore was a struggle, which resulted in my needing to come home and rest the remainder of the day afterwards. A lot of time was spent going to doctors, having tests done, seeing specialists, naturopaths, etc. I spent a lot of money on this. I was told many times from the people I saw that they had the answer and I would get better, but I never did. When I started this program I was very skeptical. It made sense, but after so many failures, I didn't believe anyone anymore. But here I am over two years later, and even though I am not done with healing my bowel and body yet, my fatigue, pain, dizziness, mental fogginess, insomnia, and anxiety are remarkably better. I am able to do things that I haven't done in over 15 years. I am riding this thing out to the end and I am excited to see where it takes me. For the first time ever, I know that this really is the answer."

## My story

After a year and a half of one doctor visit after another, looking for the answer to my extreme, disabling ill health twenty-five years ago, including

85

waiting three months to get into a well-known immunologist affiliated with UC Irvine, I was given the vague diagnosis of "autoimmune disease." It was the first official diagnosis that I was given during all that time, and it left me with nothing to hold on to. There were no treatments, and there was no hope. I was told I would have to learn to live with my symptoms (I was only 22 years old, so that seemed completely unrealistic, living this way for decades. I am extremely strong, but this I could not do.)

In the introduction of *Unique Healing* I summarized my horrendous ordeal battling an autoimmune disease (as well as briefly at the beginning of this book), and I also described my amazing recovery. So I will not repeat the story again here, but will emphasize that as a result of this program, my autoimmune disease is completely, 100%, gone. And by gone, I mean not only are my disabling symptoms gone, but I do not need to avoid wheat, dairy or any other foods to feel great, take supplements, or use medications, acupuncture, or any other crutch to feel good.

Nineteen years into this work and thousands of clients later, I rarely see someone who is as ill as I was, and so as unfortunate as that was for me, I hope you take comfort in knowing that if this program helped me recuperate from the enormous depths of ill health that I was in, it can help you can beat your autoimmune disease too.

## Watch My Video, "Why THIS Program Works for Autoimmune Diseases"
This video, and all of my videos, can be found at *www.UniqueHealing. com* or at *www.YouTube.com/UniqueHealing*.

## Backache
See "Aches and Pains"

## Bacterial Infections
### Bronchitis, Fever, Lyme's, Pneumonia, Sinus Infections, Strep, Staph, Tuberculosis, and others
(See also "Diarrhea/Loose Stools")

Infections are either viral or bacterial. To generalize, viral infections are prevented by your lymphatic, or immune system, and the beneficial bacteria in your bowel prevent bacterial infections. (Learn more about viral infections later in this chapter.)

Sinus infections, some cases of the flu, staph, pneumonia, bronchitis, Strep, fungal infections, bladder infections, some cases of acne, parasitic infections, some yeast infections, Lyme's disease, most cases of diarrhea that last more than three days, tuberculosis, many cases of food poisoning, and e-coli are examples of infections than can loosely be classified as "bacterial."

You are *very* likely to get a bacterial infection(s) during this program, and these will cause many uncomfortable symptoms for you.

Therefore, read the following section carefully, and frequently.

## Healing Your Body With This Program Eliminates Bacterial Infections

A healthy body does not prevent bacterial infections. An unhealthy bowel bacterial environment is the sole cause of bacterial infections. Even if you have a very healthy body, if your bowel is not healthy, you are vulnerable to these infections.

## Healing Your Bowel With This Program Eliminates Bacterial Infections

The good bacteria in your bowel are your "army" that kills these invaders. When your bowel bacterial environment is healthy, it fights bacterial infections, preventing them from thriving and causing symptoms and distress.

However, it takes time to heal your bowel and create natural immunity against bacterial infections, even with this extraordinarily aggressive healing program. Therefore, it is very likely that at some point during this program, as stated above, you will suffer from a bacterial infection, or infections.

## Why My Crutches Work for Bacterial Infections

**Unique Healing Colloidal Silver** has natural anti-bacterial, anti-fungal, anti-parasitic properties.

## How much do I take?/Questions about using these

See Chapter 5 for information on using these crutches, including recommendations on the amount to use, as well as a discussion of the misunderstandings about the particular crutch that may, if not understood correctly, cause you to fail to look and feel better while you heal your bowel and body with this program.

## How long will I need to use crutches for my bacterial infections?

The bacterial environment in your bowel affects bacterial infections. To better understand how long you may need crutches for this, refer to Chapter 1 under this subject heading.

# Misunderstandings About Bacterial Infections and Other Information for Your Success

### Signs that you likely have a bacterial infection

If you have very well-formed stools, very few acids will be re-absorbed into your blood, and this prevents many symptoms, addictions, and weight problems. But very well-formed stools do *not* prevent bacterial infections. If your stools are well-formed during this program and you are fatigued, have bladder discomfort, difficulty sleeping, sinus congestion, a skin rash, or acne, for example, it is likely that a bacterial infection is causing these symptoms, and treating this with a anti-bacterial crutch, like *Unique Healing Colloidal Silver*, is likely to help these problems go away.

Also, if your stools are green, yellow, more than 2x/day, and/or loose "for no reason" (i.e. you have not recently consumed larger than normal quantities of alcohol, sugar, fruit, had a massage, or any thing else that can increase the acidity of your blood and bowel, as defined in Chapter 8 of *Unique Healing*), you likely have a bacterial-type infection and taking *Unique Healing Colloidal Silver* is highly recommended in these situations.

I have also had a number of clients complain that *Body Bentonite* causes them nausea or stomach discomfort. This is usually a sign of a bacterial infection which, once eliminated with colloidal silver, allows the client to take advantage of *Body Bentonite* without discomfort.

It is very important that you try *Unique Healing Colloidal Silver* during this program if you do not feel well and/or your stools are loose, as a number of the symptoms you experience while you heal will be caused by a bacterial infection.

Sometimes a client will wrongly blame *Bowel Strength* or *Body Bentonite* for their symptoms, when the true culprit is a bacterial infection. Don't make that mistake.

## Get your family (and pets) on board too

It can be hard, if not impossible, to eliminate your bacterial infection with *Unique Healing Colloidal Silver* if you are constantly being re-infected by a family member who also has one. Ideally, you will do your best to determine if your spouse, partner, children, or even pets (yes, they can carry many infections that affect you) have an infection, as defined above, before you start the colloidal silver. If they do, have them take the *Unique Healing Colloidal Silver* at the same time that you do too. (See Chapter 5 for information on the amount to take, including working with your pets). Not only should they appreciate feeling better as a result of this, but you will save money with this approach, as two or more people taking silver for a very short time is less expensive than having just yourself take it repeatedly, for days or weeks on end (as may be your experience if they do not get on board with you).

## *Bowel Strength* contains some anti-bacterial crutches, probiotics do not

*Bowel Strength* contains goldenseal, black walnut, garlic, and other herbs that have mild antibacterial properties, and its use can help prevent these infections, but it is likely that you will need additional anti-bacterial crutches at times. *Unique Healing Colloidal Silver* is generally stronger than goldenseal, etc., and is preferable to use if you have symptoms of a bacterial infection. (Note: *Unique Healing Probiotics*, and all other probiotics, do not contain antibacterial crutches as *Bowel Strength* does. Therefore, if you are using these to heal your bowel, add 1-2 tsp/day of *Unique Healing Colloidal Silver* to your *daily* regimen as well.)

## Do not use *Unique Healing Probiotics* as crutches to fight bacterial infections

Contrary to some much-heeded advice, probiotics cannot immediately eliminate a bacterial infection. They are not crutches, and they cannot help you get better right away, as *Unique Healing Colloidal Silver* can. Time and again I see this mistake made. Probiotics, and *Bowel Strength*, are products that heal your bowel and *eventually* prevent bacterial infections from occurring, but they are not crutches that can immediately fight an infection when it occurs.

If you are sick, you can continue taking *Bowel Strength* or *Unique Healing Probiotics*, or you can stop them for a few days as well. You will not feel worse if you stop them. If you just don't feel well enough to take them, and need a break from swallowing supplements, stop these until you feel better. The supplements that you want to focus on at these times are the ones that can help you feel better right away—the "crutches," like *Unique Healing Colloidal Silver*.

## Crutches that help viral infections do not fight bacterial ones

Taking zinc or vitamin C, for example, for a bacterial infection, will not help you get better. These are crutches that help fight viral infections, not bacterial ones.

If you are uncertain if your infection is a viral or bacterial one, use crutches for both (see "Viral Infections" for more information on this). It will not hurt you to take one that you don't need. More commonly, I see clients who are taking a crutch for a viral infection when they have a bacterial infection, and not getting better because of it.

## Changing your diet will not eliminate bacterial infections

Bacterial infections occur when your bowel is unhealthy, and you are exposed to a harmful bacterium. Your diet, stress, exercise habits, etc. have no impact on whether or not you get a bacterial infection, only the first two variables listed trigger them.

It confuses and frustrates many of my clients when they get one, even as they are trying hard to take care of their body with diet, reducing stress, etc. Likewise, it causes a lot of unnecessary suffering, as you may get one of these infections and wrongly think that "being good" with your diet will make it go away.

A healthy diet, reducing stress, etc. are valuable for reducing acids in your blood and organs, and for increasing your health, but these do not prevent bacterial infections.

## Likewise, *Body Bentonite* will not eliminate a bacterial infection

*Body Bentonite* will not help you if you have a bacterial infection, either. It eliminates acids that trigger many of your symptoms, weight problems, addictions, illnesses, and bad blood tests, but it does *not* fight bacterial infections. You need a healthy bowel, or *Unique Healing Colloidal Silver* until your bowel is healthy, to fight a bacterial infection.

If you are getting bacterial infections often, or are very bothered by them, consider healing your bowel faster. I can personally assist you with this process, if desired.

## Take an antibiotic if necessary

Bacterial infections can be much more serious than viral ones, and can be much more difficult to treat naturally. If *Unique Healing Colloidal Silver* does not work for you soon, or you are very ill, especially of you have diarrhea more than three times a day for more than two days, go to your doctor (and get antibiotics, if he deems them appropriate). While antibiotics are toxic and inflict some damage to your bowel bacteria, one round of antibiotics did not cause your bowel to be unhealthy. One round of antibiotics is not going to prevent you from healing it, either.

## . . . but not too often

The current trend to treat kids with Lyme, PANDA's, and other bacterial and neurological problems with large and long-term amounts of antibiotics is horrifying.

In the short-term, there is potential to see some progress, but these drugs make the bacterial environment in their bowel less healthy over time, and since the ill health of their bowel *is a major causative factor* of these problems in the first place, it only stands to reason that the long-term affects of this treatment will be devastating, and life-threatening (and yet this treatment is being followed all over the country with no data to back up its long-term effectiveness, or safety, to your child, and it is especially dangerous when it is coupled with high protein diet recommendations).

## . . . and increase your *Body Bentonite* during this time

*Body Bentonite* will help offset some of the possible adverse side effects of using antibiotics, as these drugs can be highly toxic, and excess toxins/acids can trigger numerous symptoms. *Body Bentonite* can help eliminate these aggravating symptoms, but it does not and will not offset the effectiveness of the antibiotic itself. It is necessary, however, that you take your antibiotics at least one hour away from your taking of *Body Bentonite*.

Take extra *Body Bentonite* if you take antibiotics because you will feel better if you do, and because if you do not, you might be tempted to blame your side effects of these antibiotics on the wrong thing, like your ingestion of *Bowel Strength*, for example. Also, antibiotics may help you feel much better, and *Body Bentonite*, by offsetting the possible discomforts of using these drugs, may help you "continue taking them as directed" so you get the help you need.

## Food borne outbreaks have increased in recent years

According to an article in the *Wall Street Journal* (12/1/10) titled "Food Borne Illnesses:"

"There are about 76 million cases of food-borne illnesses every year in the U.S. that result in 325,000 hospitalizations and 5,000 deaths, according to the Centers for Disease Control and Prevention."

Also, between 2009-2010, there were 72 reported illnesses from cookie dough; 272 from red/black pepper, 1,442 from jalapenos and tomatoes, 3 dead and 199 ill from spinach, 1,600 ill from eggs, and 9 dead and 714 ill from peanut butter and related products.

And, not too long ago, it was reported that approximately 25% of the turkey and chicken that was tested contained staph bacterium.

In other words, you should be concerned about the quality of your food, and you should understand that you are likely to eat contaminated food during this program, while you are healing your bowel, that is likely to cause problems/infections. You can easily ascertain when your stools are loose or you feel unwell due to drinking too many margaritas; you cannot easily ascertain when the eggs you just ate contained salmonella. You can more easily avoid toxic, acidic, cleansing foods that aggravate your bowels and symptoms; you cannot easily avoid foods that are contaminated with bacterium that do the same.

## Other sources of bacterial infections

Contaminated food, and contaminated people, will trigger most of your bacterial infections; yet there are many ways you may come in contact with bacteria that cause you problems. For example, old sponges, toothbrushes, cutting boards, food that has expired, food purchased from a "buffet" bar, including that sold in health food stores, hospitals, and airplanes can be infested with germs.

Fecal matter is often highly contaminated with germs, so if you have a dog with an infection and his behind is not clean when he sits on your coach, you could pick this up. The other day a client found that mice had invaded her basement and left a huge pile of infected waste. The possibilities are somewhat endless.

I recently heard a report on the radio in which the level of bacterium was measured in various places, and the results were shocking, and very interesting. Unfortunately, I tuned in when it was halfway done, but here is what I heard. It was discovered that some of the highest sources of germs were soap dispensers in public bathrooms, soda dispensers in fast food restaurants, and new clothes. The explanation for the latter is that when people try on new clothes, they can leave fecal matter from their underwear on the inside of the pants. Crazy, huh?!

Finally, travelling to a foreign country often increases your risk of coming in contact with bacterial infections, and I strongly encourage you to take *Unique Healing Colloidal Silver* while you are travelling, as well. A large number of my clients who have, have reported that they were the "only one" in their family, or group, who did not get diarrhea, or sick.

(I am not trying to make you germ-phobic. I am very "non germ-phobic" myself. Rather, I am trying to make you aware of the great possibly that you will get a bacterial infection while you are healing your bowel, and I am trying once again to emphasize the need to understand the information and advice in this chapter, as it is very important for your success.)

## Organic does not mean, "free of bad bacteria"

Eating organic foods is a great way to reduce your ingestion of pesticides, chemicals, food colorings, and other toxins/acids. But eating organic foods does *not* eliminate your risk of food borne contaminants and subsequent bacterial infections, as a result.

## Scientists warn of a "superbug"

Scientists warned that a "superbug" that gives bacteria the power to resist virtually all known antibiotics may be spreading, and poses a global health risk (*Wall Street Journal*, 4/8/11). "So much of modern medicine . . . depends on our ability to treat infection. If resistance destroys that ability then the whole edifice of modern medicine crumbles," says David Livermore, director of antibiotic resistance monitoring at the U.K.'s Health Protection Agency.

In this country, we are lucky that we are not exposed to as many dangerous bacteria, like tuberculosis, or even parasites, like malaria, as many poorer countries are. But many predict that one day a strain of deadly bacteria *will* make its way to our country with devastating effects, and millions will be killed. Your chance of surviving is significantly higher if you have a healthy bowel bacterial environment.

## "Silver Lining to Fighting Germs"
## (Wall Street Journal, 7/19/11)

The use of *Unique Healing Colloidal Silver* is not as "strange" as it may sound. Consider the article headline above. According to this, silver is making a comeback as a germ-fighting agent (in part because of new technology that allows it to be woven into fabrics), and it has been known for its "anti-microbial powers *for more than a century* (italics mine)."

Silver is showing up in bandages and gels for treating wounds and burns (long used in hospitals, by the way!), and for $3,599 you can buy a queen-size mattress with silver woven into its cover (which the company who sells these, Magniflex USA Ltd., claims inhibits bacteria, dust mites, and allergens). Several years ago, plastic food containers with silver bottoms were marketed on television to fight bacterium and keep food fresh longer.

In other words, the use of silver to fight bad bacterium is known by many others, and many others have tried to help others from this knowledge, as well as to profit from it (for the cost of that mattress, you could buy over 100 bottles of *Bowel Strength* and heal your bowel and prevent infections, as well as disease, weight problems, other symptoms, etc., which would be a much more productive use of your hard earned money).

# Success With Bacterial Infections

"Before starting this program I was getting sick all the time. It has now been one year since my last infection. I feel great."

"Prior to this program I experienced diarrhea pretty often, but it was a trip to India, and diarrhea afterwards, that left me in a very bad place. I spent many months seeing doctors about this, had a stool analysis test done, took a lot of probiotics, avoided wheat and dairy, and still nothing helped, and no one could figure out what was wrong or how to help me. I always knew my bowel was unhealthy so it made sense to heal it with this program. It has been two years and I have not had diarrhea in over a year now. My bowel is the healthiest it has been in a very long time."

"My daughter's very bad acne cleared up right away after we started giving her a large amount of colloidal silver."

"I rarely get sinus infections now, but if I do, it is much less severe, and lasts much less time, than it used to. As soon as I feel one coming I take *Unique Healing Colloidal Silver* and I am fine by the next day."

"My son was diagnosed with PANDAS and strep. As his strep has improved with this program, so have his symptoms."

"My son was on a constant treatment of antibiotics for Lyme's and he felt better, but never great, and later he developed juvenile arthritis. I knew I had to change our path, and luckily someone told me about Donna's program. He is now off the antibiotics and his pain and inflammation is significantly better, and I feel better now that we are healing his bowel and he is no longer taking antibiotics, which always concerned me."

## My story

My children, ages thirteen and sixteen, have never had a bacterial infection in their life. As for myself, it has been 20 years since my last one. None of us ever use colloidal silver, as we don't need to.

### Watch My Video, "Why THIS Program Works for Bacterial Infections."

This video, and all of my videos, can be found at *www.UniqueHealing. com* or at *www.YouTube.com/UniqueHealing*.

# Bedwetting
See "Urinary Disorders"

# Bladder Infections
See "Bacterial Infections"

# Bloating and Gas
(See also "Bowel Conditions," "Constipation," and "Diarrhea/Loose Stools")

Bloating and gas complaints are common among my clients. They range from mild/occasional bouts to more extreme cases, such as when it exists in conjunction with conditions like Irritable Bowel Syndrome, Crohn's, colitis, and others. (For more information on these conditions, see "Bowel Conditions.")

Bloating and gas occur in your bowel. Because your bowel is one of your first organs to become unhealthy, it is no surprise that problems associated with this organ are some of the most common. (Coupled with the fact that your bowel is also one of your *last* organs to heal.)

While gas and bloating do not add weight to the scale, they do make your clothes tight, and you, uncomfortable. For some of you, they dramatically affect the quality of your life.

## Healing Your Body With This Program Eliminates Bloating and Gas

Bloating and gas can occur when there are too many un-eliminated acids in your bowel. These unformed acids can ferment and turn into gas, and bloating. Healing your body with this program eliminates the acids that contribute to gas and bloating.

## Healing Your Bowel With This Program Eliminates Bloating and Gas

Your bowel bacteria help with the digestion of insoluble fiber in your diet (especially prevalent in foods like corn, beans, lettuce and other raw vegetables, whole grains, and seeds.) When your bowel is unhealthy, these fibrous foods are not completely digested, resulting in the production of gas, and bloating.

Your bowel bacteria are also responsible for fighting bad bacterium, whose presence are a third possible trigger of bloating and gas.

In addition to its many other important functions, a healthy bacterial environment in your bowel is a necessity for the complete elimination of acids (toxins, heavy metals, pesticides, etc.) from your body. When these are not eliminated, they can trigger fermentation and the production of gas, and bloating.

# Why My Crutches Work for Bloating and Gas

*Body Bentonite* binds to acids (toxins, heavy metals, chemicals, etc.) in your bowel, preventing them from triggering fermentation, and bloating and gas.

*Unique Healing Calcium Citrate* is an alkalinizing mineral that helps neutralize the acids that your bowel does not eliminate. When these acids are neutralized, they do not ferment and cause gas and bloating.

*Unique Healing Colloidal Silver* has natural anti-bacterial, anti-fungal, anti-parasitic properties, and it eliminates the gas and bloating caused by these infections.

## How much do I take?/Questions about using these

See Chapter 5 for information on using these crutches, including recommendations on the amount to use, as well as a discussion of the misunderstandings about the particular crutch that may, if not understood correctly, cause you to fail to look and feel better while you heal your bowel and body with this program.

## How long will I need to use crutches for my bloating and gas?

Bloating and gas occur at Level 4 of your pipe. It is the last area of your body to heal (assuming that other areas are unhealthy too). Refer to the diagram "Sequence of Healing" in Appendix A at the end of this book to better understand this concept, as well as to Chapter 1 under this subject heading.

The bacterial environment in your bowel also affects bloating and gas. To better understand how long you may need crutches for this, refer to Chapter 1 under this subject heading.

# Misunderstandings About Bloating and Gas and Other Information for Your Success

## Keep your stools well-formed

Because bloating and gas are caused in part by un-eliminated acids, and because well-formed stools reduce the presence of these acids, you will suffer from the least amount of bloating and gas if you keep your stools well-formed while you are healing your bowel and body.

If you do not have a very good handle on how to define well-formed stools, review Chapter 6 of *Unique Healing* now. (And remember, when your stools are hard and slow you are eliminating more acids, and will therefore feel better, than when your stools are one or more times a day but not all extremely well-formed.)

If your stools are not well-formed, the following changes can help: increase your *Body Bentonite* intake; reduce your carbohydrate intake (pasta, breads, grains, cereals, yogurt, etc.); reduce your sugar intake (including natural healthy sugars such as agave, honey, raw sugar, cane juice, etc.); reduce your alcohol, salt, coffee, and/or soda intake; do not have a massage, chiropractic adjustment, or any other body work; drink a lot of water; rest; and keep your exercise aerobic (see Chapter 4 for more information on how to attain this, and why it is important.)

If these changes do not noticeably help the form of your stools in two days, take them further (i.e. take more *Body Bentonite*, reduce your carbohydrate intake more, etc.)

Out of all of these recommendations, increasing your *Body Bentonite* intake is one of the most productive and helpful. It heals your body, unlike many of the other recommendations. It will do the most to lead you to a place where looking and feeling good is effortless, and some of the other suggestions, such as reducing sugar intake, are simply "too hard to do when your blood is too acidic."

(Note: the exception to this information is when your poorly formed stools are caused by an infection, in which case *Unique Healing Colloidal Silver* is needed to reduce your symptoms. Refer to Chapter 5 for information on when and how to use this crutch.)

## *Body Bentonite* does not cause bloating and gas

On the contrary, this product can reduce or eliminate these symptoms. Never blame it for causing them. On the other hand, it does nothing to eliminate the bloating and gas caused by undigested fiber or an infection, so if you have these problems, make sure you are using the right crutch to eliminate them.

## Consider using *Bowel Strength* over probiotics to heal your bowel

One of my intentions in designing *Bowel Strength* was to include some crutches to help you look and feel better while you are healing your bowel. *Bowel Strength* contains an anti-gas herb that is *not* found in probiotics.

In other words, *Bowel Strength* can immediately reduce your symptoms of bloating and gas; probiotic usage cannot.

## Reduce your dietary fiber intake for now

Until your bowel bacterial environment is healthier, you may experience less bloating and gas if you reduce your fiber intake.

High fiber foods include salads, most vegetables (especially when eaten raw) and most fruit. The vegetables that are highest in fiber are: beans, broccoli, brussel sprouts, cabbage, carrot, eggplant, greens (collards, kale, turnip greens), tomato (the skin), mushrooms, potato (skin), pumpkin, peas, peppers, rhubarb, spinach, and sweet potatoes. The fruits that are highest in fiber are: apples (the skin), avocado, bananas, berries (blueberries, blackberries, raspberries, etc.), dried fruits (figs, raisins, apricots, dates, etc.), guava, kiwi, orange, pears (the skin), and prunes. Also high in fiber are nuts and seeds, beans, popcorn, and high fiber cereals, including oatmeal, and high fiber breads.

Salads and other high fiber foods are great for you, but if you have these problems, stop them, and other high fiber foods, for a few days to see how you feel. If you have less bloating and gas, then it is up to you to decide how to proceed (cut out the fiber until your bowel is healthier, or add it back now and deal with some bloating and gas, but at least with the comfort of knowing that *one day*, because of this program, you will be able to eat these foods without any problems.) Most of all, it is important to stop eating high fiber foods for a few days if you are tempted to blame any of the recommendations or products I have made, so that you can see that they are *not* the cause of your symptoms.

For now, substitute healthy, lower fiber foods for the higher fiber ones you currently eat, like nut butters instead of nuts, cooked fruits and veggies in place of raw, white rice in place of brown, and sourdough (made with a starter, not yeast) in place of whole grain breads. (See Chapter 9 of *Unique Healing*, for more information and advice on these foods.)

Look at the label of the foods you eat. If it contains more than 2 grams of fiber/serving, it may cause you bloating and gas.

## Heal your bowel and body, because high fiber diets are healthy

When your bowel bacterial environment is unhealthy, you may tend to avoid healthy, high fiber foods because of the discomfort caused by eating them. Or your doctor or alternative health practitioner might have told you that you must avoid these foods forever. This is unacceptable.

Because many very healthy foods are high in fiber, it is a problem if you are advised to avoid these foods, and nothing is done to create a healthy bowel. While I also advise the minimal intake of high fiber foods, at least with this program, you are healing your bowel as well, so that one day you will be able to eat a healthy high fiber diet without discomfort (a situation that will *not* occur if you simply avoid fiber and don't concurrently heal your bowel, as is the case with the most common approach to these symptoms that is recommended by other practitioners.)

## Raw food diets often trigger *more* bloating and gas

Raw food diets are very high in fiber and therefore they can be especially gas and bloating-producing. I have worked with many clients who could not stick to this diet because of the discomfort caused by it. I have had many clients experience immediate relied from gas, bloating and discomfort as soon as they stopped eating this very high fiber diet.

An argument in favor of these diets is that ill health is caused by a lack of enzymes, and that cooking food eliminates these enzymes. Raw food consumption can help with enzyme levels, and it is a healthy diet, but it cannot heal your bowel and body, like this program does, and an unhealthy bowel and body cause your digestive problems in the first place. An unhealthy bowel and body, not a lack of enzymes, cause ill health.

## Undigested food in your stools is a sign of an unhealthy bowel

Many of my clients see undigested food in their stools, and most of them (and you) have no idea that this is unhealthy. Undigested food in your stools is primarily undigested fiber (tomato skins, seeds, lettuce leaves, corn, etc.) Notice that you never see a non-fibrous food, like chicken or cheese, in your stools.

As you heal your bowel bacterial environment with this program, the presence of undigested food in your stools will stop occurring. This is a sign that your bowel is healthier. While you might not care about undigested food in your stools, your unhealthy bowel that is causing it, and the resultant symptoms, weight problems, illness, and addictions that occur as a result, *will* bother you.

I am an immense fan of "Jersey corn," and every year when we vacation at the south Jersey shore, I eat it in large amounts (as I only have one week to enjoy it!). On many days, it is common for me to eat three ears a day. I am also terrible at chewing my food well, so *a lot* of corn kernels enter into my digestive system partially chewed; yet I never see them in my stools.

100

## Bloating and gas are normal, but not healthy

Dr. Oz states that is it normal and healthy to pass gas 14-16 times a day. This may be normal, as it is normal to have an unhealthy bowel and body, but when your bowel and body are healthy, the release of gas will not occur at all. *It is healthy to pass gas zero times a day.* If you pass gas more often, this is a sign that your bowel and body are not as healthy as they could, and should, be.

## You can be bloated and have no gas

Bloating and gas do not always co-exist. You can be bloated and be *retaining* a lot of gas, but never pass it (and not realize that you are gassy after all.) When a baby has colic, it finds relief once the gas triggering this discomfort is passed. While you will feel better if you pass gas and do not retain it, gas never should be created in the first place.

## Other crutches that have some value

For bloating and gas that is caused by un-eliminated acids, herbs like peppermint, chamomile, fennel, and ginger, as well as digestive enzymes, as found in the health food store, can offer mild help for these problems. Gas-X, a product found in grocery and drug stores, may also be helpful, although this is a less preferable crutch as it contains a small amount of toxic food colorings. "Beano," as found in health food stores, contains enzymes that help with the digestion of fiber (not just that found in beans, but as found in vegetables, nuts, etc.) Taken as directed, it can help reduce the bloating and gas caused by undigested fiber. Colonics and enemas may also reduce gas and bloating, but they are uncomfortable and are a much more expensive bloating and gas crutch than the crutches listed above.

## The limited value of digestive enzymes

When your bowel bacteria are healthy, you have a healthy supply of enzymes. Healing your bowel bacterial levels, which naturally improves your enzyme levels, is far superior to addressing this problem by ingesting numerous digestive enzymes. (A bandwagon that existed many years ago when I was sick, which many of you are being led to jump on right now.)

Digestive enzymes are crutches that treat symptoms and do not heal the underlying cause of the problem, and over twenty-five years of professional, and early personal, experience with enzymes has shown me that these have limited value in treating these symptoms, anyway.

## A connection to eating disorders and underweight problems

Bloating and gas can result in under eating, leading to problems with healthy weight gain.

Also, eating disorders are prevalent when food consumption causes discomfort and bloating. These symptoms can be relieved, in part, by not eating; if food triggers these symptoms, it can be appealing to eliminate food and thus eliminate these discomforts.

All of the clients I have seen who have anorexia or bulimia have extremely unhealthy bacterial environments in their bowel. For more information on why this program eliminates eating disorders, see "Eating Disorders" later in this chapter.

## Success With Bloating and Gas

"When I came to Donna I had severe stomach pains, gas, and bloating. I dealt with this almost every day. It stopped me from doing my job and it made travelling very difficult. Now I hardly ever have this problem. It is like night and day. I have my life back."

"Once I started taking *Body Bentonite*, my bloating immediately went away."

"I was eating a lot of salads, knowing they were good for me and trying to improve my health. I was bloated all day, and when I reduced these, and took the *Body Bentonite*, the bloating went away. Now, after healing my bowel and body for a while, I can eat salads and the bloating stays away."

### Watch my Video, "Why This Program Eliminates Bloating and Gas."

This video, and all of my videos, can be found at ***www.UniqueHealing.com*** or at ***www.YouTube.com/UniqueHealing***.

## Blood Pressure (Hypertension/Hypotension)

Whether your blood pressure is too high or too low, it can cause you to be uncomfortable (although, readings that are on the low side are often wrongly disregarded as "no big deal."). Likewise, whether yours is too high or too low, the underlying cause is the same, and healing your bowel and body with this program will stabilize it. If you start this program with blood pressure that is too high, you will eventually see it reduce to normal; if you start this program with blood pressure that is too low, you will eventually see this increase to normal.

## Healing Your Body With This Program Eliminates Blood Pressure Problems

Blood pressure issues generally stem from three physiological conditions: water retention, dehydration, and unhealthy kidneys.

You kidneys may react to un-eliminated acids by retaining water, which dilutes these dangerous acids, but which can also increase your blood pressure. (Hence the common recommendation to reduce salt intake, as it has been shown to increase water retention and blood pressure.)

In cases of blood pressure that is too low, un-eliminated acids also trigger this, but in this case, it is too little water, or dehydration, that usually triggers this condition. (See the section later on "Dehydration" to better understand how this program eliminates it.)

Your kidneys produce an enzyme called rennin, which plays a role in the release of aldosterone, a hormone that helps control your body's sodium and water balance. When sodium and water levels are out of balance, this can create water retention and greater pressure in your blood. The fewer acids there are, the better this hormone is regulated.

Healing your body with this program eliminates the acids that trigger water retention and dehydration. Healing your body with this program heals your kidneys so that even if there are acids, your body is strong enough to handle them without a reaction (it fixes the holes on your roof so that even if it does rain, your house does not get wet).

## Healing Your Bowel With This Program Eliminates Blood Pressure Problems

In addition to its many other important functions, a healthy bacterial environment in your bowel is a necessity for the complete elimination of acids (toxins, heavy metals, pesticides, etc.) from your body. A healthy bowel eliminates the acids that cause water retention and increased blood pressure. It also eliminates the acids that cause dehydration, and a blood pressure reading that is too low as a result. **You need healthy kidneys to** have normal blood pressure, and a healthy bowel helps create healthy kidneys by eliminating the acids that cause them to become unhealthy in the first place.

## Why My Crutches Work for Blood Pressure Problems

*Body Bentonite* binds to and eliminates acids (toxins, heavy metals, chemicals, etc.) from your body. It helps prevent them from becoming re-absorbed into your bloodstream, where they trigger a response by your body to protect you from them. It eliminates the acids that trigger the retention of water or dehydration, and subsequent rise or reduction in your blood pressure.

*Unique Healing Calcium Citrate* Calcium is an alkalinizing mineral that helps neutralize the acids that your unhealthy bowel is not eliminating. When these acids are neutralized, your body will not retain water, or become depleted of water; your blood pressure will be stable.

### How much do I take?/Questions about using these

See Chapter 5 for information on using these crutches, including recommendations on the amount to use, as well as a discussion of the misunderstandings about the particular crutch that may, if not understood correctly, cause you to fail to look and feel better while you heal your bowel and body with this program.

### How long will I need to use crutches for my blood pressure problems?

Blood pressure problems occur at Level 4 of your pipe. It is the last area of your body to heal (assuming that other areas are unhealthy too). Refer to the diagram "Sequence of Healing" in Appendix A at the end of this book to better understand this concept, as well as to Chapter 1 under this subject heading.

## Misunderstandings About Blood Pressure Problems and Other Information for Your Success

### Keep your stools well-formed

Because un-eliminated acids cause too high or too low blood pressure, and because well-formed stools prevent the re-absorption of acids into your blood, you will have the most stable blood pressure if you keep your stools well-formed while you are healing your bowel and body.

If you do not have a very good handle on how to define well-formed stools, review Chapter 6 of *Unique Healing* now. (And remember, when your stools are hard and slow you are eliminating more acids, and will therefore feel better, than when your stools are one or more times a day but not all extremely well-formed.)

If your stools are not well-formed, the following changes can help: increase your *Body Bentonite* intake; reduce your carbohydrate intake (pasta, breads, grains, cereals, yogurt, etc.); reduce your sugar intake (including natural healthy sugars such as agave, honey, raw sugar, cane juice, etc.); reduce your alcohol, salt, coffee, and/or soda intake; do not have a massage, chiropractic adjustment, or any other body work; drink a lot of water; rest; and keep your exercise aerobic (see Chapter 4 for more information on how to attain this, and why it is important.)

If these changes do not noticeably help the form of your stools in two days, take them further (i.e. take more *Body Bentonite*, reduce your carbohydrate intake more, etc.)

Out of all of these recommendations, increasing your *Body Bentonite* intake is one of the most productive and helpful. It heals your body, unlike many of the other recommendations. It will do the most to lead you to a place where looking and feeling good is effortless, and some of the other suggestions, such as reducing sugar intake, are simply "too hard to do when your blood is too acidic."

(Note: the exception to this information is when your poorly formed stools are caused by an infection, in which case *Unique Healing Colloidal Silver* is needed to reduce your symptoms. Refer to Chapter 5 for information on when and how to use this crutch.)

## You can be at risk of heart disease if you have normal blood pressure readings

Blood pressure readings are similar to blood test readings in that they do not accurately reflect the health of your body. Normal blood pressure does not always correlate to a lower chance of heart attack, as is so widely implied. Likewise, high blood pressure does not always correlate to a greater risk, either.

## A risk when coupled with an unhealthy heart

In other words, high blood pressure by itself is not normally a problem; it is dangerous when it accompanies an unhealthy heart and clogged arteries. Un-eliminated acids in your blood cause blood pressure problems, but it is the presence of un-eliminated acids in your *arteries* that is most problematic.

You can have high blood pressure and a healthy heart; you can also have normal blood pressure but an unhealthy heart and an increased risk of heart disease and death by heart attack.

Here is another good reason to have a heart scan, as described in the section on "Cholesterol." If your arteries are clogged, high blood pressure is a riskier condition than if they are not.

## Your blood pressure may go up as you heal

Just as your blood cholesterol can change quickly, and can go and up and down depending on the amount of acidity in your blood (and will not *stay* down until your liver is healthy), so too can you experience changes in your blood pressure during this program. These changes can occur while you are healing, *before* your kidneys have healed completely.

In other words, while you are fixing the holes on your roof, the holes over your kitchen will be the last to be fixed. If it rains while you are still fixing these holes, your kitchen may get wet. While you are healing your body with this program, your kidneys, which regulate your blood pressure, are among the last to heal. So while you are in this process, if you eat a lot of acidic foods, a cleansing diet, and/or your stools are not very good (especially if they are one or more times a day and not perfectly well-formed), your blood pressure may go too high or too low. This can be quickly improved by reducing the acids in your diet, and life, eliminating cleansing foods, and increasing your *Body Bentonite* dosage until your stools are firmer and better formed.

To date, I have never had a client experience high blood pressure during this program where it became dangerous/caused a problem.

## Too low blood pressure is not healthy either

While high blood pressure gets the most attention and causes the greatest alarm, blood pressure that is too low is unhealthy and a sign of poor health, and this should also be respected.

The medical profession considers normal blood pressure to be around 120/80. Really, a reading close to this range is healthy. A reading above

125/85 is too high, and a reading below 105/65 is too low. During my most ill days, my blood pressure was usually 90/60, or too low.

Just as diarrhea and constipation, and low blood sugar and high blood sugar, seem to be entirely different from each other, they are actually extremely similar, and stem from the same cause. Likewise, both high and low blood pressure can occur when your blood is too acidic, and eliminating acids from your body improves both blood pressure states.

Finally, just as diarrhea is worse than constipation and high blood sugar is worse than too low blood sugar, high blood pressure is worse than low blood pressure and can signal a greater level of ill health. On the other hand, blood pressure that is *very* low and can be a sign of severe dehydration and danger.

Whether your blood pressure is too high or too low, healing your bowel and body with this program will correct it.

## Reducing salt can help high blood pressure, but it requires much more than this

Common table salt is highly acidic, and because acids negatively affect your blood pressure, the consumption of table salt does too.

The common advice to reduce salt to lower blood pressure therefore has some merit, but by itself, it is not effective, or adequate.

*It is not the sodium in salt that increases your blood pressure, but the acidity of salt that causes this problem.* And, you could eliminate all salt from your diet, yet still consume a highly acidic diet, or a highly cleansing diet (one that dumps acids into your blood), and as a result, your blood pressure could increase. You could eat healthy cherries all day, with no salt, and have high blood pressure, for example, because of the release of acids from your organs into your blood that occurs with cherry consumption.

Of course, the simple advice to stop eating salt also does nothing to heal your bowel, which should be eliminating the acids that cause high blood pressure in the first place.

## Salt cravings

In my experience, people with excess acidity in their blood, which can trigger high blood pressure, crave salt. Your body wants natural salt but *you* have to make that choice; your body will simply ask for salt, you have to give it the right kind (i.e. sea salt).

It is much easier, therefore, for someone with high blood pressure to replace their refined salt with sea salt (see below) than to ask them to stop eating salt altogether. It is much more helpful, too.

## Natural sea salt/sodium *improves* blood pressure

The advice to eliminate salt does not differentiate between unhealthy, acidic table salt and healthy, alkalinizing sea salt.

While you are healing, increasing your consumption of natural sodium from sea salt will help stabilize blood pressure levels that are too high or too low. This is because sea salt is alkalizing; it buffers the acids that cause blood pressure problems.

## Even doctors are questioning their salt reduction recommendations

Some doctors and researchers have recently stated that salt consumption is not what causes high blood pressure. They theorize that high blood pressure is due to an overactive hormone system, or an imbalance in the production of that hormone aldosterone, that helps regulate water balance/blood pressure.

When your kidneys are not healthy, your ability to regulate this hormone will be negatively affected. And while salt contributes to unhealthy kidneys, so do *all* acidic foods and beverages, as described earlier.

Just as eating cholesterol-containing foods does not cause high cholesterol levels; eating salt does not cause high blood pressure, either. Both of these can be triggers, but they are not the cause.

## The "DASH" diet (Dietary Approach to Stop Hypertension)

This has been studied extensively in the medical community and has been shown to be helpful for lowering blood pressure. It is high in potassium, magnesium, and calcium, which are alkalinizing minerals that buffer the acids that cause your blood pressure to rise. While it is low in sodium, this is because, as described above, the wrong conclusion has been made that since refined salt increases blood pressure, all sodium is bad.

## Your I.V. in the hospital probably contains sodium!

Surely someone in the medical field has to question the "sodium is bad" concept when sodium is routinely used in the I.V.'s in hospitals to help save your life and recuperate from surgery, illness, etc.

Sodium is great for you health, as the medical profession has clearly observed for a very long time. It is acidic, refined salt that is not healthy.

## Don't eat more salt if you have low blood pressure

The advice I have heard from some doctors to treat low pressure by eating more salt is very wrong and I strongly discourage you from taking it if you are in this place. When your blood pressure is too low, you are unhealthy, and consuming *more* unhealthy foods, like salt, will only make things worse in the long run.

This program eliminates the acids that cause low blood pressure.

## Elimination of acids through breathing and sweating lowers blood pressure

A recent ad in the *New York Times* advertised a medical device called Resperate, which has been proven to lower blood pressure with no side effects. It regulates your breathing, so you take deep breaths. Their explanation for why this works is that it relaxes the smooth muscles of your arteries. More accurately, deep breathing helps your body eliminate acids, as described and encouraged in Chapter 8 of *Unique Healing*. A reduction in acids reduces inflammation all over your body, including your arterial muscles.

Along this same line of thinking, a report in 2002 described a study in which Japanese researchers enlisted 35 men, two-thirds of whom had at least one coronary risk factor, such as smoking. They all spent fifteen minutes a day in a sauna for two weeks. Afterward, researchers found that all of the men, even those with a risk-factor, had better functioning blood vessels and some showed signs of lowered blood pressure.

Your skin is an organ of elimination, and the use of a sauna encourages elimination of blood-pressure raising acids from your body through your pores, just as deep breathing eliminates them through your lungs.

## Stress is a trigger too, but not the cause, either

Stress is the "rain that hits your roof and makes your house wet," but this only occurs if you have holes in your roof. Stress makes your blood more acidic, and if you cannot eliminate these acids, and your kidneys are not healthy, you can experience blood pressure problems. Stress cannot be completely avoided; you *can* create a healthy bowel and body that eliminates blood-pressure affecting acids, as this program does. As always, stress is a trigger to many problems, like blood pressure, but it is not a cause.

On the other hand, if you suffer from a noticeable increase in emotional or mental stress during this process, and it is negatively affecting your blood pressure, consider using a natural, non-toxic relaxant, like "GABA" (you can find this a the health food stores). Buy GABA that contains 750 mg/capsule and take three two hours before bed and two in the morning. If your blood pressure is triggered by emotional stress, this recommendation will help lower it.

## High protein diets to control blood pressure are dangerous

Like your blood tests, symptoms, and weight, your blood pressure can be manipulated with diets, most notably high protein ones, giving you the dangerous sense that you are much healthier, and safer, than you really are.

If you limit carbohydrates, you may have low levels of acids in your blood and normal blood pressure, but this can cause high levels of acids in your arteries, and a higher risk for heart attack (just as you can have normal blood cholesterol levels but concurrently, very clogged arteries and be at a high risk of heart attack.)

If you ever become convinced this approach is the "answer," ask for *mortality statistics* before you embark on it. You should only feel safe following this approach when you can be shown that this approach reduces blood pressure *and reduces death by heart attack.* (This concept applies to all of the conditions that these program treat, at the expense of your longevity). Of the thousands of studies I have read, I have yet to find one that these diets increase the length of your life (on the contrary.). Don't be fooled.

## Buy a blood pressure monitor

A blood pressure monitor is an inexpensive device that can be purchased at any drug or large discount store. Because your blood pressure reflects un-eliminated acids in your blood (just like a blood test), if you have high or too low blood pressure, this can be used as a way to measure your effects of the crutches I recommend. You can't have a blood test done everyday, but you can easily do a blood pressure test daily.

For example, take your blood pressure daily for a week, then start this program, and once your stools have improved (as described in Chapter 6 of *Unique Healing*), take your blood pressure. It should improve, if it is too low or too high to begin with.

If this gives you a better understanding of how your body, and this program, works, and it empowers you and gives you comfort, then it will have been worth the investment.

# Success With Blood Pressure Problems

"My blood pressure increased while I was healing my bowel and body with this program, and it was concerning at first. I had numerous medical tests done to check the health of my heart and they all came back showing that I was extremely healthy. As I continued to heal my body with this program, it eventually became normal, and I have never felt better!"

"As my blood pressure went down with this program, so did my weight."

"I was able to stop my blood pressure medications that I was told I would need my entire life (in fact, the amounts I was needing were increasing prior to this program.) Even if I am stressed or eating sugar, which used to make my blood pressure go up, it now stays stable and healthy."

## My story

Throughout much of my illness, my blood pressure remained at around 90/60. It went lower than this at times as well. At its lowest, I felt my worst. Many doctors took my blood pressure and commented on how low it was, but no one ever suggested that this was a concern, and they certainly never had a solution for correcting this. I knew better, however. So for many years I monitored my blood pressure and for many years I tried every alternative program in the book, yet my blood pressure remained too low. After healing my bowel and body with this program, my blood pressure rose to around 120/80. Not coincidentally, my symptoms disappeared as well. Additionally, as I healed my body and bowel and my kidneys became healthier, my taste for salt diminished greatly. I "taste" the excess salt in food immediately, and can watch others eat the same salty foods with pleasure (I even "wipe" salt off of foods like pretzels, as I just don't like the taste).

## Watch My Video, "Why THIS Program Eliminates Blood Pressure Problems."

This video, and all of my videos, can be found at *www.UniqueHealing.com* or at *www.YouTube.com/UniqueHealing.*

# Bone Health
See "Osteoporosis"

# Bowel Conditions
## Celiac, Colitis, Crohn's, I.B.S., Hemorrhoids, Polyps, and Others
(See also, "Bloating and Gas," "Constipation," and "Diarrhea")

Because I have always promoted my program as one that heals your bowel, I have inevitably been swamped with clients looking to improve their bowel problems (and have had a relatively smaller number of clients who have been made aware of the fact that a healthy bowel heals every condition under the sun, not just bowel problems). Bowel conditions are therefore the ones I have the most experience with, and an enormous amount of success with, as well.

Below I describe the most common bowel conditions, but this is not to imply that this program is limited to only helping these. Also, while the above conditions have different names, they are really quite similar in that they have many symptoms in common, and can include abdominal pain, gas, bloating, inflammation, diarrhea, and/or constipation (unhealthy elimination).

Like most of the other conditions covered in this book, bowel conditions have increased over the years as well. A record number of people are suffering from these, and they are extremely common. For example, 1 in 133 people in the U.S suffer from celiac disease. This is a very large percentage of you.

# Healing Your Body With This Program Eliminates Bowel Conditions

Un-eliminated acids can causes fermentation in your bowel, which can trigger gas, bloating, and cramping. These acids may also be buffered with inflammatory chemicals, and eliminating these acids with this program eliminates inflammation (especially as occurs in colitis and irritable bowel syndrome, or I.B.S.). Constipation is caused by excess un-eliminated acids as well, as are many cases of loose stools.

A healthy body has healthy tissues, including healthy tissues in your bowel, which prevents hemorrhoids.

A great accumulation of built-up of acidity increases your risk for polyps. Healing your body with this program eliminates these acids, and your polyps.

Healing your body with this program eliminates the acids that trigger gas, bloating, cramping, loose stools, constipation, inflammation, hemorrhoids, and polyps, for example. Healing your body with this program heals your bowel that even if there are acids, your body is strong enough to handle them without a reaction (it fixes the holes on your roof so that even if it does rain, your house does not get wet).

## Healing Your Bowel With This Program Eliminates Bowel Conditions

Celiac is a condition where one is intolerant to gluten-containing foods. A healthy bowel is responsible for the digestion of gluten, and hence the elimination of this condition.

Colitis and some other bowel conditions are triggered by bacterial, fungal, or parasitic infections. A healthy bowel fights these infections and keeps them from causing problems, especially diarrhea.

A healthy bowel digests the fiber in your diet, eliminating the gas and bloating associated with undigested fiber.

In addition to its many other important functions, a healthy bacterial environment in your bowel is a necessity for the complete elimination of acids (toxins, heavy metals, pesticides, etc.) from your body. A healthy bowel prevents the re-absorption of acids into your blood that cause gas, bloating, cramping, loose stools, constipation, inflammation, hemorrhoids, and polyps.

## Why My Crutches Work for Bowel Conditions

***Body Bentonite*** binds to and eliminates acids (toxins, heavy metals, chemicals, etc.) from your body. *Body Bentonite* forms these acids into a stool that is very easy for your body to eliminate, resulting in less constipation and firm stools that are not loose. It eliminates the acids that trigger gas, bloating, cramping, and inflammation.

***Unique Healing Calcium Citrate*** is an alkalinizing mineral that helps neutralize the acids that your bowel does not eliminate. When these acids are neutralized, your body does not produce gas and bloating, nor does it need to create inflammatory chemicals to buffer them. When these acids are neutralized, they are less irritating to your bowel, resulting in less constipation and less loose stools.

***Unique Healing Colloidal Silver*** has natural anti-bacterial, anti-fungal, anti-parasitic properties. It eliminates the infections that trigger conditions like colitis, diarrhea, and gas and bloating.

## How much do I take?/Questions about using these

See Chapter 5 for information on using these crutches, including recommendations on the amount to use, as well as a discussion of the misunderstandings about the particular crutch that may, if not understood correctly, cause you to fail to look and feel better while you heal your bowel and body with this program.

## How long will I need to use crutches for my bowel condition?

Bowel conditions occur primarily at Level 4 of your pipe. It is the last area of your body to heal (assuming that other areas are unhealthy too). Refer to the diagram "Sequence of Healing" in Appendix A at the end of this book to better understand this concept, as well as to Chapter 1 under this subject heading.

The bacterial environment in your bowel also affects bowel conditions. To better understand how long you may need crutches for this, refer to Chapter 1 under this subject heading.

There are no crutches for degenerative conditions and accumulations of acidity in your organs, like polyps and hemorrhoids. Crutches can offset the effects of acids in your blood, or the effects of poor function of your bowel bacterial environment (as these can be quickly altered), but degeneration is caused by depletion and damage to your organs, and organs take time to heal.

# Misunderstandings About Bowel Conditions and Other Information for Your Success

## Keep your stools well-formed

Because bowel problems are caused in part by un-eliminated acids, and because well-formed stools prevent the re-absorption of acids into your blood, you will suffer from the least amount of these problems if you keep your stools well-formed while you are healing your bowel and body.

If you do not have a very good handle on how to define well-formed stools, review Chapter 6 of *Unique Healing* now. (And remember, when your stools are hard and slow you are eliminating more acids, and will therefore feel better, than when your stools are one or more times a day but not all extremely well-formed.)

If your stools are not well-formed, the following changes can help: increase your *Body Bentonite* intake; reduce your carbohydrate intake (pasta, breads, grains, cereals, yogurt, etc.); reduce your sugar intake (including natural healthy sugars such as agave, honey, raw sugar, cane juice, etc.); reduce your alcohol, salt, coffee, and/or soda intake; do not have a massage, chiropractic adjustment, or any other body work; drink a lot of water; rest; and keep your exercise aerobic (see Chapter 4 for more information on how to attain this, and why it is important.)

If these changes do not noticeably help the form of your stools in two days, take them further (i.e. take more *Body Bentonite*, reduce your carbohydrate intake more, etc.)

Out of all of these recommendations, increasing your *Body Bentonite* intake is one of the most productive and helpful. It heals your body, unlike many of the other recommendations. It will do the most to lead you to a place where looking and feeling good is effortless, and some of the other suggestions, such as reducing sugar intake, are simply "too hard to do when your blood is too acidic."

(Note: the exception to this information is when your poorly formed stools are caused by an infection, in which case *Unique Healing Colloidal Silver* is needed to reduce your symptoms. Refer to Chapter 5 for information on when and how to use this crutch.)

## Hemorrhoids are not caused by constipation

Hemorrhoids are caused by acid irritation to the fragile lining of your intestinal wall, which causes it to become inflamed. Clients with hemorrhoids typically have daily, but poorly formed stools, which allows for acid irritation to the colon, and the possibility of hemorrhoids. Clients who heal their bowel and body with this program consistently find that when their stools become firmer with this program, *eventually* their hemorrhoids get better.

However, if you start this program with a fragile colon/hemorrhoids, you may experience an aggravation of these while you are healing, due to the valuable "firming-up" of your stools that occurs with this program. It is a bit of a catch-22 in that you need to firm your stools to heal your colon from hemorrhoids, but for a while, this forming-up of your stools may cause discomfort.

Two remedies can prevent uncomfortable hemorrhoids from occurring while you are healing your bowel.

For one, straining to eliminate can aggravate hemorrhoids, because when you put pressure on your weak and fragile colon, it can become irritated (hence the popular prescription of stool softeners and laxatives for people with this condition.) The problem is that these do nothing to eliminate the acids that are causing your hemorrhoids in the first place. Also, straining to eliminate is often the product of fear. I've met many clients who were threatened as a young child when they did not have a bowel movement. (Please do not ever put your own child into his situation. You cannot force someone to go to the bathroom. Their lack of going has nothing to do with their intentions or behaviors; it is a product of an unhealthy bowel and body. Fix these and you will never have to "threaten" your child again).

If you do not have a bowel movement every day while you are doing this program that is okay. You will still be healing your bowel and body if you do not. There is zero value in forcing yourself to go, only the potential for discomfort. If there is formed stool in your colon, eventually it will come out on its own. The acids in formed stools are not re-absorbed; the acids in un-formed ones are. Do not strain to eliminate.

And two, if you experience any discomfort with hemorrhoids while doing this program, consider using magnesium citrate (1,000 mg/day, or more if needed) to soften your stools and make you more comfortable while you are healing your bowel and body. One day, as a result of this program, magnesium will not be needed. One day, even if your stools become too large or hard, you will not experience hemorrhoids as you eliminate these stools.

## Polyps may not be cancerous, but their presence should alert you of danger ahead

A polyp develops after many years of accumulated acidity in your bowel. If one or more are found at your colonoscopy, respect the red flag and warnings of it, and heal your bowel and body with this program. Non-cancerous "things" often turn into cancerous ones later on. Cancerous polyps occur when there is an *even grea*ter accumulation of acidity in your body and are signs of even greater danger. Likewise, if you have a history of cancerous polyps when you start this program, they will likely become non-cancerous before they go away completely.

## Removing polyps does not extend your longevity from all diseases

Again, polyps are warnings that your body is becoming very acidic and unhealthy. Removing the polyps simply removes a side effect of this acidity, but it does nothing to heal your bowel and prevent acids from continuing to accumulate to deadly levels, nor does it do anything to help you remove the vast accumulation of acids in the rest of your body that also leads to danger down the road. Removing polyps allows you to ignore the major cause of premature death—your unhealthy bowel and body.

You should never feel safe just because your polyps were removed.

## And colonoscopies do not accurately reflect the health of your bowel, anyway

A lack of polyps or cancer detected during a colonoscopy does not mean your colon, or bowel, is healthy. If you suffer from Irritable Bowel Syndrome (IBS), a colonoscopy will not show any bleeding or disease, either.

A colonoscopy cannot measure the intestinal bacterial health of your bowel. It cannot detect large levels of acidity (until it has become extremely large and dangerous).

The best test of your bowel health is defined in Chapter 7 of *Unique Healing*, and it is the one you should use.

## Gluten does not cause celiac; it is merely a trigger

If you are diagnosed with celiac, I advise you to avoid gluten-containing foods (like wheat, oats, rye, barley, etc.), until your bowel has healed. But too many practitioners are blaming gluten for these problems, when the true blame lies in your unhealthy bowel.

When you simply avoid gluten, you avoid the fact that your bowel is unhealthy. This means that your unhealthy bowel continues to allow acids to be re-absorbed, leading to more symptoms, weight problems, addictions, and disease down the road. It allows your unhealthy bowel to continue to malfunction, and as a result, your vulnerability to other problems associated with an unhealthy bowel, like hormonal cancers, infections, osteoporosis, etc., is not reduced (as it is with this program). Simply avoiding gluten also is extremely hard to do in the long run. It is much easier to heal your bowel and body with this program than it is to avoid gluten forever.

Avoiding gluten may minimize your symptoms, but it does nothing to heal your bowel and body.

## Celiac, Crohn's, and I.B.S., etc. are signs of an extremely unhealthy bowel, but this can be changed

I have seen numerous clients who were led to believe that these conditions were "forever." I have seen clients who were told that their condition would never go away. As is true of all of the conditions covered in this book, this is not true. Again, this is the area I have the greatest experience in, and these are problems that I have seen eliminated countless times.

## Mal-absorption is another term for an unhealthy bowel

If someone diagnoses you with mal-absorption, they have diagnosed you with an unhealthy bowel. Your bowel bacteria are responsible for the absorption of numerous nutrients in your body. When it is unhealthy, this is hampered, and mal-absorption occurs. This program heals your bowel, and therefore, it eliminates mal-absorption.

Programs that simply give you handfuls of digestive enzymes and nutrients are crutches that do nothing to heal your bowel (the cause of your mal-absorption), or your body. They may help you feel better, but they do not help you permanently eliminate your condition, nor do they prevent you from early disease or the development of newer, and worse, symptoms, and weight problems, as this program does.

## Appendicitis is a warning that your "bowel trashcan is getting full"

Your appendix is one of the "small trashcans in your body." It stores un-eliminated acids. If it gets too full, it can burst, and these poisonous acids can dump into your blood and cause severe discomfort, and possibly be very dangerous. You can live without your appendix, but it is preferable to have this organ. The more "trashcans" you have, the more trash, or acids, you can accumulate before it causes degenerative problems, like cancer and heart attacks.

I had my appendix removed when I was 11 years old. No one told me (likely, because no one, i.e. the doctors, knew, as they don't seem to know now, either), that my bursting appendix was a sign that my body was highly acidic/toxic and that if I did not do something about this, something "worse" would likely develop in my body (and it did, as twelve years later I was disabled with a devastating autoimmune disease. Today a new client shared that her appendix was removed at age 12 and she now has an autoimmune disease, too. I believe "this" is a common story.)

## Success With Bowel Conditions

"I had a diagnosis of celiac when I first came to Donna. I had to avoid wheat, and still, I had diarrhea frequently. Now I eat wheat products in large quantities, and my bowels are better than ever."

"Just had my colonoscopy this morning and had no polyp, just like you said. I am so excited!!!!"

"I am 45 years old, and my last colonoscopy revealed polyps. I just had one done again and they are gone!"

"I suffered from hemorrhoids after my children were born. It was extremely painful, and the doctors had suggested surgery, but I did this program instead, and here I am, years later, with no surgery and no hemorrhoids."

"I was diagnosed with I.B.S. twenty years ago. I tried *every* alternative program out there to get better, and occasionally I was ok, but most of the time, I was not. I lived in constant fear of an attack. This program worked. I can now even eat whatever I want and still be ok. It is amazing!"

"My daughter was diagnosed with colitis at age 16. It was hard for me to get her to follow this program, but Donna kept assuring me that even if we went slowly, eventually she would get better. It took some time, but now she is a different girl, with a future ahead of her that before, was uncertain and scary (for her dad and I)."

"My last colonoscopy showed pre-cancerous polyps, which were removed. I have done this program for a short time and my latest colonoscopy showed non-cancerous polyps. What a great improvement."

## Watch My Video, "Why THIS Program Eliminates Bowel Conditions"

This video, and all of my videos, can be found at *www.UniqueHealing. com* or at *www.YouTube.com/UniqueHealing.*

## Breast and Other Female Cancers
### Endometrial, Uterine, Ovarian, and Others
(See also "Cancer")

More than 1 million women worldwide are diagnosed with breast cancer each year, and more than 500,000 die from it. It is occurring more often, and at younger ages, than ever before. It is a huge epidemic that generates a great amount of fear.

*My professional experience is that breast and other hormonal cancers are very easy to prevent.*

## Healing Your Body With This Program Eliminates Breast and Other Female Cancers

Breast and other hormonal cancers are the result of hormonal imbalances, and these are caused by an unhealthy bowel (see below). A healthy body does not prevent these cancers, but a healthy body does help prevent *death* from *all* cancers, hormonal cancers included.

A healthy body eliminates the acids that cause dehydration. A study conducted at the Centre for Human Nutrition at the University of Sheffield in England found that women who stayed sufficiently hydrated reduced their risk of breast cancer by 79 percent. (For more information on how this program eliminates dehydration, see Chapter 3.) And, cancerous breast tissues have over four times higher levels of pesticides than do non-cancerous breasts. A healthy body eliminates pesticides and other chemicals from your body.

Of course, it is much more complex than this. For more information on how this program eliminates *death* from *all* cancers, hormonal ones included, see the following section titled "Cancer."

# Healing Your Bowel With This Program Eliminates Breast and Other Female Cancers

As a woman, you make estrogen in your ovaries, a few other organs, and body fat. Estrogen flows through your body one time, stimulating your breasts, uterus, ovaries, and skin. After one passage through your bloodstream it goes to your liver, where it is attached to another substance and conjugated, or "bound." Conjugated estrogen, which is not absorbable, is excreted into your bowel to be eliminated through your stools.

Unfriendly bacteria deconjugate estrogen, or free it up, and allow it to pass through your body again, contributing to disease. Excess re-absorption of estrogen is implicated in the majority of *ovarian, uterine, and breast cancers.*

A healthy bowel bacterial environment eliminates excess estrogen from your body and prevents it from being re-absorbed, preventing these conditions and diseases. In other words, when your bowel is unhealthy, it allows this dangerous excess estrogen to become reabsorbed.

While studies on the connection between an unhealthy bowel bacterial environment and hormonal cancers are nowhere to be found, one study did find that the use of antibiotics, which contribute to an unhealthy bowel by reducing good bacteria, was associated with increased risk of incident and fatal breast cancer. (JAMA, 2003; 291(7): 827-35.)

# Why My Crutches Work for Breast and Other Female Cancers

**Natural progesterone cream** provides progesterone, which can offset the cancer-causing effects of excess estrogen. Until your bowel is healthy and regulating estrogen healthfully on its own, your use of natural progesterone is extraordinarily helpful (and highly recommended) for preventing breast and other hormonal cancers.

***Body Bentonite*** While this helps heal your body, and a healthy body does not necessarily prevent hormonal cancers (as a healthy bowel does), *Body Bentonite* does help prevent death from *all* cancers, including breast and other hormonal cancers.

## How much do I take?/Questions about using these

See Chapter 5 for information on using these crutches, including recommendations on the amount to use, as well as a discussion of the misunderstandings about the particular crutch that may, if not understood correctly, cause you to fail to look and feel better while you heal your bowel and body with this program.

## How long will I need to use crutches for my breast and other female cancers?

The bacterial environment in your bowel affects breast and other female cancers. To better understand how long you may need crutches for this, refer to Chapter 1 under this subject heading.

If you currently have breast or another hormonal cancer, and you are *not* taking a medication to reduce estrogen re-absorption, it is critical that you use natural progesterone cream. I recommend the use of natural progesterone cream on a daily basis for two years after your diagnosis. If you do not have a current or recent diagnosis of one of these cancers, using natural progesterone cream daily for one year while you are healing your bowel with this program is strongly recommended.

# Misunderstandings About Breast and Other Female Cancers and Other Information for Your Success

## Drugs like Tamoxifen reduce estrogen

In the medical community, estrogen has long been known to be a huge risk factor for breast and other female cancers. The popular drug Tamoxifen takes advantage of this knowledge, as it blocks the action of estrogen, which has been shown to inhibit uncontrolled cell (cancer) growth. Other drugs are being developed for preventing breast cancer that also work by blocking estrogen absorption. (The safest and most effective way to do this is by healing your bowel with this program and relying on it to regulate your estrogen levels for you.)

## Reduce your consumption of products that contain synthetic hormones

In 2004, Daniel Cramer of Harvard and his colleagues reviewed data from the 80,326 participants in the long-running Nurses' Health Study and found that the risk of serious invasive ovarian cancer increased by 20% for every glass of skim or low-fat milk the women drank each day. A well-designed study of 61,084 women in Sweden also concluded that two or more glasses of milk a day doubled the risk of this common subtype of ovarian cancer. It is a popular assumption that the reason for this increase is due to the estrogenic hormones commonly added to, and ingested in, dairy products.

Many dairy and meat products contain synthetic hormones, and your consumption of these should be minimized as much as possible. Buy ones that are hormone-free, whenever possible.

## Natural progesterone *reduces* the harmful effects of excess estrogen

Excess progesterone is often found at the breast cancer site, which has led researchers to wrongly conclude that progesterone is dangerous. Progesterone is often at the site, as it is "called upon" to help offset the harm caused by excess estrogen. Progesterone is the good guy, not the bad guy. Just because there are firemen at the fire does not mean that they started it. On the contrary, they arrived on the scene to put the fire out, and you'd better not kick them out! Progesterone can put your hormonal cancer "fires" out, and you better not "kick it out" either!

*Just because two variables co-exist does not mean that one caused the other, as is constantly implied in the health field.*

Likewise, a study in the *International Journal of Cancer* suggests that women who took black cohosh, an herb that reduces estrogen, just like natural progesterone does, were 47% less likely to have breast cancer at the time of the study.

My hope and dream is that someday, someone with the resources to do so will conduct a study on the effects of natural progesterone on breast and other female cancer rates. (Or even better, a long-term study on the effects of healing your bowel and body with this program and the effects on not just hormonal cancer rates, but overall mortality from cancer deaths as well.)

## Studies showing the connection between hormone use and female cancers

The landmark Women's Health Initiative study found that women who took hormone therapy were diagnosed with more advanced stages of breast cancer than women who did not (42% of hormone users had invasive breast cancer diagnosed versus 34% of the non-hormone users. 24% of hormone users had their cancer spread to their lymph nodes versus only 16% of the non-hormone users, for example). (*Wall Street Journal*, 10/20/10: "Research Finds Hormone Therapy Speeds Up Breast-Tumor Growth").

Most importantly, women who took hormone therapy for an average of 5.5 years had a higher *mortality* rate than those who did not. Twenty-five women in the hormone group died of breast cancer versus 12 in the non-hormone-taking group.

Hormone drug sales from Pfizer were $213 million in 2009.

Note: Synthetic hormones, which are associated with a greater risk of female cancers, and natural hormones, like natural progesterone cream, which are associated with a reduction in female cancers, are completely different. Synthetic substances are toxic and harmful; natural ones are not.

## You *can* die of breast cancer even if you do not have any breasts!

A relative (who declined my offer of help) was diagnosed with advanced metastatic breast cancer, even though she had breast cancer two times previously, a double mastectomy, and was an excellent medical patient.

When her two breasts were removed, she was led to believe that she had addressed the cause of her cancer. She truly thought she couldn't die from breast cancer. However, at the young age of 53, after a horrible battle with breast cancer again, she did just that. This is not an isolated story.

With this program, you have the opportunity to *truly* feel safe and secure if you are a previous cancer patient.

## Lower protein diets equal less breast cancer-causing estrogen

According to the American Cancer Society, vegan women (who eat no animal protein foods), have *four times as much estrogen in their stool* as women who eat the typical Western diet. This means that they eliminate a lot more of cancer-causing estrogen than meat-eating women.

When your bowel and body are unhealthy, higher animal protein diets help you look and feel better, and therefore they become very appealing, but this increases your risk of breast and other hormonal cancers. When my women clients heal their bowels and bodies with this program, they automatically desire less animal protein.

## High fiber diets reduce harmful estrogen re-absorption

Low protein diets are usually high in fiber. A recent study out of France, titled "Dietary lignan (fiber) intake and postmenopausal breast cancer and progesterone receptor status," found an 18-23% lower risk of breast cancer in the women who consumed the highest amount of plant lignan, or fiber.

In a study of 16 pre-menopausal women, the daily consumption of 10 g of flaxseed daily showed increased elimination of estrogen from their body. Some women were also given an additional 28 g of wheat bran daily, which was not shown to have any effect. "The Effect of Flaxseed and Wheat Bran Consumption on Urinary Estrogen Metabolites in Premenopausal Women," Haggans CJ, Travelli EJ, Thomas W, et al, ***Cancer Epidemiol Biomarkers Prev***, July 2000; 9:719-725.

A healthy bowel digests fiber so that you do not become gassy, bloated, or uncomfortable after eating it. A healthy bowel "helps you" be able to eat this cancer-protecting high-fiber type of diet.

## The melatonin connection

Dr. Christine Horner advises sleeping between 10 pm and 6 am, because sleeping during these hours optimizes the body's production of melatonin, a hormone thought to lower breast cancer risk by reducing estrogen production.

A healthy bacterial environment keeps your melatonin levels high.

## Vitamins and breast cancer

A recent study out of France found that women who consumed the most dairy products, and therefore calcium, had the lowest rates of breast cancer. ("Dairy products, calcium and the risk of breast cancer: results of the French SU.VI.MAX prospective study." Kesse Guyot E, Bertrais S, et al, Annals of Nutrition and Metabolism, 2007; 51(2): 139-145.) A similar study conducted at the Harvard Medical School found that pre-menopausal women who consumed the highest amounts of calcium had 39% lower risk of breast cancer. This study needs to be viewed with caution, however (as they all do!), because other studies find that a higher consumption of dairy products increases breast cancer (likely due to the hormones added to the dairy products, so my guess is that the dairy products consumed in France, and in this study, were hormone-free).

Another study out of Sweden titled, "Serum calcium and breast cancer risk: results from a prospective cohort study on women," also observed that breast cancer rates were lower among women with the highest serum calcium levels.

If you have or have had breast cancer, you will find numerous recommendations for the ingestion of a mass quantity of vitamins/supplements, calcium included, to "protect you." Vitamins and supplements are crutches that can help you look and feel better, but they *do not* eliminate estrogen from your body, and they *do not* eliminate the acids from your body that cause death from all cancers, hormonal cancers like breast cancer included.

Reducing breast cancer rates does not necessarily mean that you have reduced the rate of death from breast cancer. *This* is the result you must demand when you embark on a program that claims to help reduce your risk of cancer (see discussion below as well).

## Does chemotherapy increase your longevity?

If caught early, as is often the case nowadays, many cancers would take years to kill you, whether you did chemotherapy or not. It is extremely dangerous to think that chemotherapy will, and can always, save you. Many people die every year while under expert medical care and chemotherapy treatment.

Regardless of the form of cancer you had, if it is cured by chemotherapy but you do not heal your body and bowel, which keep excess estrogen, and acidic toxins, from becoming re-absorbed in your body and causing cancer, it will likely come back. It often comes back in a more deadly form, because while chemotherapy kills cancer, it also kills some of the beneficial bacteria in your bowel, and some of your cells, and together, these allow for a faster, more aggressive re-absorption of hormones and acids, which means a more rapid movement towards medically incurable cellular damage and death.

## The cure isn't as great as you think

To expand upon the above concept, and to generalize, cancer can occur under two different conditions: one, when there is degeneration of your body, which eventually leads to cellular weakness and susceptibility to mutations and cancer; two, when hormonal imbalances, like excess estrogen, trigger abnormal, cancerous cellular growth.

If your breast cancer is the result only of the hormonal imbalances in your body, your chances of surviving this are much greater than if the hormonal imbalances are accompanied by deeper, cellular depletion. In other words, with Stage I cancer, there is less accumulated acidity than in Stage III cancer. But because nothing is ever done to eliminate this acidity—only the cancer is treated—many people who previously have had a Stage I cancer eventually die from a Stage IV one.

In other words, if your bowel is very unhealthy but you have managed to eat well and have done other things to keep the acids from accumulating to the "top of your pipe," you will have a greater chance of surviving your cancer longer than if not. The conventional treatments in these cases are heralded as miraculous, although I wouldn't call them that.

If your breast cancer is "incurable" or if you do not survive it, you may have been confused into thinking that the conventional treatments "might work," as they have for so many others. You are led to believe that you never know, because "chemotherapy has saved lots of lives." The fact that these treatments work for some and not for others is not just a matter of luck; it is likely a reflection of the overall degree of degeneration in one's body. Therefore, if you have "medically incurable" breast cancer, you would be wise to get on this program fast! Many people have died from cancer because drugs cannot, and will never be able to, reverse the internal physiological depletion of your body. And it is this depletion, not the cancer itself, which ultimately causes death.

In other words, these cancers are warnings that your bowel is unhealthy, which allows for the more rapid accumulation of death causing acids than a healthy bowel does. *This* is the danger of these cancers, and a danger when your bowel is not healed when you get diagnosed with one of them.

On the other hand, if you have been diagnosed with a hormonal cancer, you have a massive opportunity to listen to this warning and heal your bowel and body now, before it is too late.

## Where is the proof that mammograms reduce death?

In an article from the *Wall Street Journal* (9/23/10), the following significant comment about a study that looked at the benefits of mammograms in women over age 50 was made: "It's not the great lifesaver that people think it is. It's not a magic bullet," says Dr. Jeanne Mandelblatt, Georgetown University researcher.

Also, it was found that mammograms reduced mortality by only 2/4 deaths per 100,000 women. In an accompanying editorial, Dr. H. Gilbert Walch of Dartmouth Medical School noted that some 2,500 women would have to be regularly screened over 10 years to save one life from breast cancer! At this low level, one must also ask, is this paltry death reduction due to the mammogram, or better care? Or do these women change their lifestyles, or diet, in response to an earlier diagnosis?

Again, the question that you must ask is not "Do mammograms detect breast cancer earlier?" but rather, "Do mammograms reduce death from disease?" Just because cancer is caught earlier does not mean that your lifespan has increased as a result (as these studies imply).

Ask your doctor, "Where is the proof that this test/treatment/or whatever he/she advises, will extend my life?" (Dying of brain cancer, instead of breast cancer, at age 54 is death too soon, regardless of the type of cancer you had. You need to demand that *all* cancers are reduced with any treatment you follow, as is true with this program.)

Hormonal cancers are a warning that your bowel is unhealthy, and a warning that needs to be respected. Your unhealthy bowel allows for the more rapid accumulation of death-causing acids than a healthy bowel does, and *this* needs to be your concern, and priority.

### You are not safe just because it does not "run in your family"

Sometimes I hear the comment from a woman that she is not worried about breast cancer because it does not run in her family. Do you think that women with breast cancer come from a line of women where the mother, and grandmother, and great-grandmother, and great-great-grandmother, and so on, all had it?—Of course not. It started somewhere, and it could start with you.

Likewise, a genetic inheritance toward this disease is not a life sentence for you, either. You certainly inherited an unhealthy bowel from your mother if she had one herself, for example, and I agree you are more vulnerable to it as a result, *but only if you do not take active steps to heal your bowel.*

## Success With Breast and Other Female Cancers

In the 19 years of this work, I have only had two female clients, out of thousands, diagnosed with breast cancer while I was working with them. In one case, this was questionable, and in the other, the woman was told that the cancer was there for a while and simply missed on the previous mammogram (and therefore, existed prior to our working together.) In neither of these cases was the client using the natural progesterone cream crutch, highly recommended in *Unique Healing*, and in this book, as well.

Considering the many hundreds of women that I have worked with (many of whom are in the "prime breast cancer age"), statistically speaking, my record with preventing this condition is profoundly remarkable.

## Watch My Video, "Why THIS Program Eliminates Breast and Other Female Cancers"

This video, and all of my videos, can be found at *www.UniqueHealing.com* or at *www.YouTube.com/UniqueHealing*.

# Bronchitis
See "Bacterial Infections"

# Bulimia
See "Eating Disorders"

# Bumps on Skin
See "Skin Conditions"

# Bursitis
See "Aches and Pain"

# Cadmium Toxicity
See "Heavy Metal Toxicity"

# Caffeine Addictions
See "Addictions"

# Cancer
(See also "Breast Cancer," and "Prostate Disorders")

(For specific information on breast, ovarian, endometrial, uterine and other female hormonal cancers, see "Breast Cancer." For information on prostrate cancer see "Prostrate Cancer.")

Over thirty percent of Americans say that their biggest fear is getting cancer. No surprise, as many have died from this often-horrible disease (which often includes months, if not years, of chemotherapy and other grueling treatments, and the ordeal of facing one's mortality and dealing with a great deal of fear and stress during this treatment, as well).

It is no surprise that cancer is feared, because it seems so prevalent nowadays. (Thirty years ago I could count on one hand the number of people I knew of, older adults included, who had it; now that number is in the many handfuls.) And it is not just older people who are getting cancer, and who are fearful of it. 72,000 Americans aged 15 to 39 are diagnosed with cancer every year and more than 10,000 of them die from it.

When I was young, I was fearful of it. When I first became very ill at the age of twenty-two, I was scared to death that I had cancer. I lived with this fear daily. Intellectually, I knew that I had taken things too far with all of the damage I had done to my body, and it stood to reason that I was likely paying the price for those actions. (As little as I did know about health back then, I did get that cancer did not occur in a healthy body, and I knew my body was extremely unhealthy at this time.)

Eventually I was diagnosed with an autoimmune disease, not cancer, and was told that I would have to live with my unbearable symptoms forever. I was thrown into a scary and uncompassionate world. At times, I wished I *did* have cancer. At least then there would be a probable "cure," and at least then others would be understanding and sympathetic towards my condition (neither of which was the case in my current situation). Also, the cancer patients that I knew were not completely disabled "the rest of their life." Many survived their cancer diagnosis and were back to their old lives and able to work and function, unlike myself, with my "non-cancer" diagnosis. I had no life. I was completely unable to function at all.

Later on, as I became aware of the ineffectiveness and politics of the medical system, and as I discovered the power of healing myself, I was very grateful for what I had. By this time I was fully committed to, and had complete faith in, using alternative methods to heal my body. I knew that I was going to journey down a different road; one that was lonely and would take a massive amount of strength and conviction and commitment, and a diagnosis of cancer may have prevented me from accomplishing this. It might have evoked a fear in me that would challenge me and cause me to easily lose my faith in the alternative road I had chosen.

Even though I was never diagnosed with cancer, I feared that my immune system was much worse off than the very limiting medical testing acknowledged (as the medical tests that were done were mostly blood tests; I never had an MRI or scan, which *may have* shown something worse than an autoimmune disease), so I spent a lot of time studying not only about the immune system, but cancer too. This included my attending "Cancer Control Society" meetings in southern California, which consisted of speeches by representatives from the Mexico cancer clinics and other very unaccepted, "radical" cancer therapies. At one point, I went to a nutritionist who had spent years working in these clinics. I followed many "cancer cures" but I never got better.

My immune system never got better with all of the alternative treatments I aggressively followed with immense discipline, and my fears remained. Eventually, I developed this program, which not only healed my bowel and body and immune system, but which gave me a peace of mind that never existed before.

Today my immune system is stronger than ever, and my fear of getting cancer is completely non-existent. This is priceless.

(If you do not have or have never had cancer, read the following section anyway. I hope to show you how this program can prevent you from ever having this diagnosis.)

## Healing Your Body With This Program Eliminates Cancer

Cancerous cells are unhealthy cells. Cells become unhealthy only after many acids—from diet, stress, drugs, and the environment—have not been eliminated from your body.

As described in Chapter 3 of *Unique Healing*, it is only after your organs of elimination)"bottom of your pipe", and then your liver, adrenal glands, pancreas, stomach, and small intestine ("middle of your pipe") can no longer keep your blood pH balanced that your body turns to its alkaline reserves—calcium, magnesium, sodium, and potassium ("top of your pipe")—to help do this job. This is your body's "last line of defense" against excess acidity. A reduction in these alkaline minerals results in damage and destruction to your cells, and cells that are prone to cancer and death.

Note that the most common types of cancer are lung, colon, skin, kidney, breast and prostate—cancers of your organs of elimination, and hormonal cancers, caused by an unhealthy bowel, i.e., the "bottom of your pipe," which is the first area of your body to become unhealthy when acids are not eliminated. This reflects the miracle of the human body, as your organs of elimination are the "least necessary." You can live without a part of your colon, or prostate, or with just one lung or kidney. When you are diagnosed with a cancer closer to the "middle or top of your pipe," like liver, pancreatic, or bone, this is much more deadly. Also, you cannot live without any of these organs.

Healing your body eliminates the acids that cause alkaline minerals to become depleted, and your cells to become diseased and cancerous. Crutches—diets, vitamins, drugs, chiropractic, acupuncture, massage, exercise, etc. do not do this.

Cancer is anaerobic, which means that it cannot live in an oxygenated environment. Think about it. Have you ever heard of heart cancer? Your heart needs, and receives, a lot of oxygen, and if your total oxygen levels are low, all of your *other* organs are shut off from this supply first. Many alternative treatments and clinics in Mexico take advantage of this knowledge and give oxygen treatments to their cancer patients for this reason. Providing the cancerous body with external oxygen is valuable; creating a healthy body, as this program does, that can eliminate the acids that *cause* low oxygen levels in the first place, is much more effective, and permanent. Also, it results in higher amounts of oxygen in your body *24 hours a day*, not just the limited hours and days the oxygen treatment is administered. (See Chapter 3 for more information on how this program increases oxygenation.)

A healthy body eliminates the acids that cause dehydration. A study at the Fred Hutchinson Cancer Research Center in Seattle found that, after controlling lifestyle factors such as diet and activity levels, women who drank more than five glasses of water a day had a 45 percent reduced risk of colon cancer compared with women who drank two or fewer glasses a day. Those numbers are impressive. Keep in mind that hydration is a complex matter that is affected not only by water consumption, but also by bowel function (the better formed your stools are, the less dehydrated you are, contrary to many misunderstandings about this). (See Chapter 3 for more information on how this program eliminates dehydration.)

# Healing Your Bowel With This
# Program Eliminates Cancer

In addition to its many other important functions, a healthy bacterial environment in your bowel is a necessity for the complete elimination of acids (toxins, heavy metals, pesticides, etc.) from your body. It eliminates the acids/toxins that, if not eliminated, eventually cause the alkaline minerals in your cells to be utilized for acid neutralization, and your cells to become cancerous as a result. A healthy bowel eliminates the acids that cause low oxygen levels. Again, cancer cannot live in an oxygenated environment. It eliminates the acids that cause dehydration. It eliminates the acids that weaken your immune system. It eliminates the extra estrogen and testosterone that is implicated in breast, ovarian, prostate, and other hormonal cancers, as described in the last section.

## A sampling of studies regarding bowel health and cancer

Studies that focus on the connection between a healthy bowel and cancer are lacking. Most studies are looking for a drug or supplement to treat a symptom and are not focused on healing your bowel. It is virtually impossible to conduct a study that focuses on healing your bowel, as this is an individualized, complex, lengthy process. Healing takes time, and the longer a study lasts, the more expensive it is. You cannot patent *Bowel Strength* or probiotics, and therefore, the likelihood that studies on their effectiveness at preventing and treating cancer will be done is slim.

I found a few studies that suggest a connection between a healthy bowel and the reduction of cancer, and are a reflection that others believe that one might exist.

- Wormwood, or artemisia (as found in *Bowel Strength*), has been found to kill cancer cells. It has been found to even be able to kill cancer cells that were resistant to chemotherapy. (Sadavaa D, Phillips T, Kane SE, et al., Transferrin overcomes drug resistance to artemisinin in human small cell lung carcinoma cells, Cancer Letters, 2179: 151-156, 2002.); (Singh NP, Lai H, Selective toxicity of dihydroartemisinin and holotransferrin toward human breast cancer cells, Life Sci 70: 49-56, 2001.); (Woerdenbag HJ, Moskal TA, Konings AW, et al., Cytotoxicity of artemisinin-related endoperoxides to Ehrlich ascites tumor cells, J Nat Prod 56:

849-856, 1993.); (Efferth T, Dunstan H, Chitambar CR, et al., The anti-malarial artesunate is also effective against cancer, Intern J Oncol 18, 133-139, 2001.); (Singh NP, Verma KB, Case report of a laryngeal squamous cell carcinoma treated with artesunate, Arch Oncol 10;4:279-280. 2002.)

- A study published in the 2007 American Journal of Clinical Nutrition titled, "Dietary synbiotics reduce cancer risk factors in polypectomized and colon cancer patients," found that supplementation with "synbiotics" (a combination of probiotics and prebiotics), may help to reduce risk factors for colorectal cancer. (My knowledge and experience is that probiotics and prebiotics are equally helpful in healing your bowel; one is not necessarily better than the other and it is not necessary to use both to heal your bowel.)

- Dr. Claudio DeSimone, an immunologist at the University of Rome, has found that eating yogurt boosts blood levels of gamma interferon, a component of the immune system that rallies killer cells to fight infection and possibly cancer. Yogurt contains live cultures that enhance the population of good bacteria in your bowel.

- The summer 2004 issue of *AICR Science Now*, a publication of the American Institute for Cancer Research, starts off with the headline: "Could a diet high in animal protein and fat increase colon cancer risk by suppressing 'good' bacteria and promoting the growth of 'bad' microbes that damage the colon?" Stephen J. O'Keefe, MD, is trying to find out. "When Dr. O'Keefe worked as a gastroenterologist in South Africa, he was 'astounded' by how rarely he saw native African patients with colon cancer or colon polyps. Out of 100 native Africans over age 50, two or three might have colon polyps. By contrast, in the U.S. population as a whole, colon polyps may be found in three or four out of every 10 otherwise healthy patients over age 50 (or, 30-40 people out of 100 compared to just 2-3 people out of 100 in Africa)." When Dr. O'Keefe searched for the dietary link that might explain this vast difference, the number one explanation that surfaced was animal protein consumption. Africans consume very little animal products, whereas Americans consume very large amounts, relatively. As you increase your intake of animal protein, the amount of beneficial bacteria in your bowel decreases. Many other studies have shown the correlation between increased animal protein intake and increased rates of colon and other cancers; this study differs because it looks at the role that your intestinal bacteria play in causing cancer. (Most likely, the drug companies are looking for a drug that can affect these bacterial levels.)

- In the book "The Cure for all Cancers" by Hilda Clark, Clark claims numerous successes in treating cancer by using herbs, like wormwood, cloves, and black walnut, which kill harmful bacteria in your bowel. Unfortunately, to prevent cancer *deaths*, you can't just kill bad bacteria, you have to also support and strengthen the good bacteria, which this does not do. My program does both. She also advises strict, military-like avoidance of all toxic chemicals, a feat very few people will be able to accomplish. When your body and bowel are healthy this is not necessary, and success is much more attainable. Finally, avoiding new toxins/acids is advisable, but it does nothing to eliminate the *existing* ones that constitute your "total toxic load," and which makes you vulnerable to cancer.

## Why My Crutches Eliminate Cancer

Cancer occurs when there is an accumulation of great amounts of acidity, and **Body Bentonite** eliminates these acids. But this takes time, so while it eliminates acids, it cannot quickly or immediately eliminate cancer. (Your focus should be on eliminating acids, not on quickly eliminating cancer, as all other approaches do. These approaches have not necessarily been proven to be life saving.)

*In other words, cancer is the product, or symptom, of an overly acidic body, and it is your acidic body, not the cancer itself, that most threatens your life.*

(I realize this concept may take some time to grasp, so re-read this statement, and section on cancer, repeatedly until it makes sense.)

*Using Body Bentonite to extend your life and reduce cancer mortality sounds simple, and for this reason, I understand you may be suspicious of its effectiveness and power. But I stand by it. It really is this simple.*

Because it eliminates acids, *Body Bentonite* can also improve your blood tests and reduce your symptoms while you have cancer, and as such, it is valuable as both a crutch and as a healing agent.

While *Body Bentonite* is *by far* the most effective crutch for improving your blood tests and symptoms when you have cancer, it is also helpful to consider the following.

## Dietary crutches for cancer

For the most part, diet is a crutch that does not eliminate the acids that cause death from cancer, but it can improve your blood tests, make you feel better, and reduce the future accumulation of acidity in your body. As such, dietary crutches, like alkaline diets, serve a valuable purpose. (Review Chapter 9 of *Unique Healing* for more information on alkaline diets. You will also find an enormous amount of information online about the value of eating an alkaline diet when you have cancer, but be careful that you use this only as a crutch and not as a "cure," as it is often touted as being.)

An alkaline diet contains a lot of fruit and vegetables, no sugar, no refined salt, no hydrogenated fats, no carbonated beverages, no alcohol, no coffee, and little to no animal protein. It can contain nuts, seeds, olive oil, soy, some grains, and some dairy.

Fruits and vegetables have been repeatedly linked to reductions in cancer deaths. Consistently, high alkaline foods have been shown to reduce cancer deaths, while high acid diets, like high protein diets, have been shown to increase cancer deaths.

Green tea is also alkalinizing, and its consumption has been linked to a reduction in colorectal cancer in women, for example. (Why not men, you may ask? Likely, the answer is the same for any other study in which only one gender is tested, which is that men simply have not been tested. If a similar study was done on men my guess is that you would see similar results. Tests are very expensive and often require the funding of a company or organizations that can profit from the results. This results in a great limitation of variables that are tested. The lack of a test does not mean that a correlation does not exist.). In other words, often when you read a study about diet and its ability to reduce cancer, the food that is tested, which yields this result, is an alkalinizing food.

On a cautionary note, however, while alkaline diets are healthy diets, they are also very cleansing diets. Remember, a cleansing diet moves acids from your organs into your bloodstream, which will make you feel and look bad when they are not eliminated when they reach your bowel. So while this diet can reduce the *future* accumulation of cancer-causing acids, when it makes you look and feel bad, and your blood tests to become worse, you will likely become wrongly, but understandably, concerned and stop it.

Also, this diet does not do much to help eliminate the *existing* cancer-causing acids.

Healing your body with *Body Bentonite* eliminates both *future and existing* cancer—and death-causing acids.

Watch my video, "Diets Don't Heal" available at ***www.YouTube.com/UniqueHealing.*** If you insist on making your diet a priority in this situation, I applaud you, but proceed carefully. And if you really want a diet that will help you while you heal your bowel and body with this program, consider fasting on a regular basis (i.e. no food, just water for 3-4 days, 2-3x/month), as this will not "over-cleanse" you, and a fast is the most helpful diet for aiding in the elimination of acids from your body.

On the other hand, trust that your diet will improve while you do this program, and that your results are largely dependent on your consuming large amounts of *Body Bentonite,* which, when consumed at the levels I recommend, are powerful enough to remove old accumulations of acids, as well as any new acidity that enters your body through a "less than perfect" diet (and stress, chemicals, etc.).

## Vitamin/supplement crutches for cancer

If you have or have had cancer, you will find numerous recommendations for the ingestion of a mass quantity of vitamins/supplements, as well. The list is endless, and includes numerous ones that are said to "strengthen your immune system," "fight cancer," etc.

Vitamins and supplements are crutches that can help you look and feel better, but they *do not* eliminate cancer-causing acids from your body; they *do not* eliminate the acids from your body that cause death from all cancers.

In 1985 at Memorial Sloan-Kettering Cancer Center in NYC, scientists chose 10 subjects who had colon cancer in their family and gave then 1,250 mg. of calcium a day and took samples of their colon linings before and after treatment. After two to three months on calcium, cell proliferation had slowed by more than 40 percent. This is impressive, but again, the important question to ask is, and "Did this reduce *death rates* from this cancer?"

Vitamin and supplement crutches can wrongly make you, and others, think that you are "healing" yourself and extending your life, so be careful.

Ask the right question. "Do these vitamins reduce death from cancer" (yes I am repeating this, because it needs to be repeated!)

If you want to take a bunch of supplements/if you feel "safer" doing so, go for it. Take *Unique Healing Calcium Citrate* in large, safe doses of 4,000 mg/day or more. It buffers the acids that cause cellular damage. But never let the time or money you spend on this and other crutches, if taken, interfere with the time and money you spend on taking *Body Bentonite* (that must be your priority), and never think that you are "at risk" if you do not take other vitamin crutches, or think less of this program because I do not recommend other vitamin crutches, like so many others do. I have a massive amount of knowledge and experience about supplement usage. My failure to recommend them is not because I am uneducated or unaware of them; I do not recommend them because they do not work. This program works.

## How long will I need to use crutches for my cancer?

There are no crutches for degenerative conditions like cancer. Crutches can offset the effects of acids in your blood, or the effects of poor function of your bowel bacterial environment (as these can be quickly altered), but degeneration is caused by depletion and damage to your organs, and organs take time to heal. In other words, the above recommendations can quickly make you feel better, and your blood tests to come back better, but none of them can quickly eliminate cancer from your body.

# Misunderstandings About Cancer and Other Information for Your Success

### Fear is your greatest enemy to longevity

I do not get the opportunity to work with many cancer patients, which is extremely sad and frustrating for me. I am very qualified to do so, and in fact, I strongly believe that the only way to live a long, cancer-free life is to heal your bowel and body with this program.

But with cancer, the fear tends to be greater than in most diseases. The greater the fear, the more likely one is to look for a savior, and modern medicine is often seen as this.

When you are immobilized by fear, you are less likely to succeed with this program, which is very "unconventional." You are more likely to "need" a quick, "everyone is doing it" fix, and conventional medicine, as well as alternative medicine that relies on crutches too, may seem desirable to you, even though these are failing to prevent death from cancer. Crutches—chemotherapy, vitamins, acupuncture, low carbohydrate diets, etc.—may temporarily reduce the presence of cancer, but they have not been shown to be very effective at eliminating *death* by cancer.

If you are overwhelmed with fear, you may think that the more you do, the better. You may think that you need to do every alternative "treatment" out there. You want lots of workmen under the sink trying to fix the leaky pipe, but this easily backfires. Treating symptoms can take priority over healing your body, and because of all of these reactions, the fear often does indeed manifest itself, as you find your cancer eventually returning, or progressing.

When overwhelmed with fear, many of you will give all of your power to doctors, or God. Millions of you who have prayed to God to save you have died prematurely of cancer. Please find strength in your God, and ask to be given the faith and patience to heal your bowel and body with this program. *Listen to your God, who sent the life-saving information in this book to me, and is sending this life-saving information to you, too.*

I love the story of the man on an island, with floods causing the water to rise, and his desperate cries to God to be saved. As the water grows higher, a boat passes by, and he continues to cry to God to be saved. Just as the water begins to engulf him, he screams to God, Why didn't you save me?' to which God replies, "I tried to save you. That's why I sent you a boat." This program was my boat, and it can be yours, too.

A strong religious faith, and positive support groups, can minimize fear. If you have cancer and you have not tapped into these already, make this a priority. Read about people who beat all odds; surround yourself with positive, supportive friends and family. When I was very ill, I attended support groups that consisted of nothing but negative, "woe is me" attendees. They were one big pity party. I heard a lot about people's problems and nothing about their successes. I quickly stopped going to these meetings and read as many books as I could find about people who had succeeded in healing themselves. This was a far cry from the groups I had found and a necessary part of my success in healing. People stuck in pity are usually stuck in a state of non-action; to heal and live, you must take action.

Fear is more readily existent where there is a lack of knowledge about how your body works. Of the many intentions of this book, one of them is to educate and empower you so that you, like me, are completely fearless about getting cancer. So that if someone you love gets this diagnosis, you can help get them "driving down the right road."

To heal your bowel and body and not be one of the millions who have died prematurely of cancer, you must let go of fear. Fear is your greatest enemy if you have cancer.

## The focus needs to be on longevity, not cancer

The information in this section pertains to the *elimination of death by cancer*. Way too much focus is dangerously placed on eliminating cancer, but this does not necessarily mean that *death* by cancer has been eliminated.

Millions of people who have "fought the cancer" have died from it, even when it was "cured." How many people do you know, or have you heard of, whose cancer was sent into remission, only to reoccur, and send them to their death, just weeks later? Killing cancer does not get rid of the acids that kill you.

*We need to measure death rates, not cure rates, for cancer.*

## Studies on longevity from drug treatments are lacking

An article in the *Wall Street Journal* (2/9/11) discussed the number of cancer drugs on the "fast track" for approval, but reported that *many of the companies making cancer drugs fail to provide follow up studies on their effectiveness or safety*. Since the 1990's, the FDA has granted accelerated approval to several dozen cancer drugs *based on preliminary evidence only*. "We are willing to accept drugs with the most minimal evidence," said Silvana Martino, who runs the breast cancer program at the Angeles Clinic and Research Institute in Santa Monica, California. (Several companies said they had difficulties finishing some studies because they couldn't find enough patients to generate reliable results.)

## Medical and alternative cancer treatments

Conventional cancer treatments, like chemotherapy, radiation, and surgery, are crutches that treat cancer, but they do nothing to eliminate the acids that *cause* cancer, and cause death. Chemotherapy and radiation are very toxic, and they *increase* the accumulation of acidity/make your body less healthy, meaning that your future risk of cancer can be increased after the treatment is complete. When the acids that caused your cancer are not eliminated, cancer can eventually come back. It often does.

When someone who goes through chemotherapy and radiation is found to have extended their life, is it due to the treatment, or to another variable? Many people with cancer drastically change their lifestyle and diet, reducing the acidity/toxicity they are exposed to (they stop eating junk, stop drinking alcohol and soda, etc.), so how can one say for certain that it was not the lifestyle change that caused the improvement in one's longevity, and not the treatment itself? (Likewise, when studies find that vitamins extend one's life with cancer, they cannot control for the fact that vitamin-takers often change their diet and lifestyle as well, and in fact these studies often comment on the dietary changes that accompany the vitamin usage.)

In the short-term, treating cancer is different from treating other symptoms, because of the fear and at times, urgency, of the condition. I understand the popularity and security of choosing conventional treatments. While I would never chose this path, I do respect you if you have, as long as your underlying bowel and body health are soon after, or concurrently, addressed and healed.

On the other hand, if you are very ill with cancer or have been given less than one year to live, I believe that your chance of living is very low if you use chemotherapy or radiation, as at some point, the ability of these to make you more acidic is greater than the ability of this program to eliminate the death-causing acids from your body. They can cause you to retain more acids than you can eliminate with this process, and the continued accumulation of acids may lead to death.

The benefit of alternative cancer treatments is that they are non-toxic and do not weaken your health in the attempt to kill the cancer. The downside, however, is that these approaches are also largely based on treating the symptoms of excess acidity (cancer), and not the cause, as drugs do. They usually rely on strict diets and/or massive supplementation, and require that this be followed indefinitely. A very small percentage of you will succeed with this. Also, because your bowel is not healed, even if the program is followed, the cancer can return. If the holes are not fixed in your roof and you simply try to keep your house dry by avoiding the rain, you have a high likelihood of encountering rain, even given your best efforts, and having your house become flooded (with cancer) again. And again, the focus needs to be on eliminating death by cancer, not just eliminating cancer, as most of these programs do.

## It takes more than vitamins (or acupuncture, chiropractic, massage, etc.) to survive cancer

As mentioned earlier, common recommendations for people with cancer include the ingestion of large quantities of antioxidants and other nutrients that "support the immune system."

Vitamins like calcium, enzymes, antioxidants, selenium, zinc and medicinal mushrooms can help neutralize the acids that create an environment in which cancer flourishes, but they do not eliminate these acids from your body, as this program does. Neither do physical modalities like acupuncture, chiropractic, or massage. And it is my experience that it is the continued accumulation of acidity that causes death.

In fact, in a study involving 77,719 subjects between the ages of 50 years and 76 years, *no significant associations were found between multivitamin or vitamin E supplementation and cancer mortality*, yet most of you are led to believe otherwise.

("Use of supplements of multivitamins, vitamin C, and vitamin E in relation to mortality," Pocobelli G, Peters U, et al, Am J Epidemiol, 2009; 170(4): 472-83)

## Are incurable cancers really incurable?

There are certainly some cases of cancer that occur when one's body is extremely unhealthy and depleted and it is just too late to help, such as when someone is given only six weeks to live. On the other hand, an "incurable" cancer, or one that does not bring immanent danger of death but that also can't be "cured" with medical treatments, is a situation where this program is most needed (and requires an aggressive, individualized program with personal consultations with me on a regular basis). Personally, I was told by many doctors that my autoimmune disease and alcoholism were "incurable," and I proved that to be incredibly wrong. I would never take someone's medically "incurable" diagnosis as a life sentence. In these cases, a more appropriate statement would be "incurable *with medical procedures*." Just because "they" don't have the answer does not mean that one does not exist.

## This program enhances conventional cancer treatments; it cannot interfere with them

Sometimes a client with cancer is told to stop this program as their doctor is not familiar with it and somehow believes it may negatively affect the client's outcome. This is entirely untrue. On the contrary, this program can only *increase* your chance of responding well to chemotherapy, radiation, etc. And it can only help extend your life. *Body Bentonite* does not and cannot "soak up" the chemotherapy drug's effectiveness; it can "soak up" the toxic by-products of this drug. It cannot stop the drugs from killing your cancer; it can only reduce the illness and weakness that these drugs can cause.

## Early detection does not necessarily mean "death prevention"

Some of the "success" of cancer treatments comes from the fact that drugs and treatments have been developed that more specifically target cancer cells and are less damaging to the rest of your cells, and health, of your body. But most of it comes from the fact that early diagnoses are more prevalent now than they used to be. Because most untreated cancers take many years to kill you if left untreated, the earlier a cancer is diagnosed, the longer you will "live with it." The earlier it is diagnosed, the better the treatment for it looks!

For example, as reported in the *Wall Street Journal* (11/5/10); "Early detection screening for lung cancer in healthy people isn't commonly done because X-rays haven't shown to be effective and . . . studies involving CT scans haven't shown that screening saves lives, rather than simply finding cancer earlier."

Cancer takes a very long time to develop in your body. It can also, in some cases, take a very long time to cause death as well. Given this, the current definition of a cancer cure, "cancer-free five years after treatment," needs to be revised to "cancer-free ten or more years after treatment." If this were revised, our statistics on current treatments would look much grimmer than they do now.

Discovering cancer early on means that, even without treatment, a person will live longer after it is diagnosed than if it is caught later on. Let's say that someone gets cancer at age 40 and they die at age 50. If it is diagnosed at age 43, and they die seven years later, they will be called cured. If this same person is diagnosed at age 49, and dies at age 50, they are not called cured.

## A new definition of success

If you get treated for cancer, either conventionally and/or with alternative medicine, and the cancer comes back, it means that the program you followed did not heal your body. The approach you took failed you.

You treated the symptoms of cancer with crutches, but you did not eliminate the underlying accumulation of acidity that allowed it to happen in the first place.

A good cancer program not only has the ability to reverse cancer but to keep you free from it for life. If you are told you are vulnerable to it forever it is because only your symptoms have been treated. A tarp has been placed on your roof but the holes have not been fixed.

The pharmaceutical companies and medical profession can't lose because we expect to die from cancer, so no one gets mad when their approach doesn't work. We do not really believe there is a cure when we are told there isn't one. They have the ultimate win-win situation. If you live, they are the heroes. If you die, well, "there was nothing else that could have been done."

The same thing happens when alternative treatments fail to keep someone alive, but this should be unacceptable.

## It's not about being a "fighter"

I am very disturbed every time I read about someone with a deadly cancer, and the conviction from their friends and family that this person is going to survive because they are a "fighter." While a positive, strong attitude is wonderful, it alone will not save you.

I understand that in many cases these statements result from fear and a need to believe one's friend or family member will survive, but it is harmful. It is harmful because it allows one to believe that attitude alone will save them—it won't—and that they don't have to do anything else to live—they do! It bothers me because I have seen dying people who felt the pressure to maintain a positive attitude for friends and family while they were dying, and I think it is horribly unfair and wrong to put someone in this place. Maybe we wouldn't be so afraid of death in this country if we approached it differently, and one difference could be that we sympathized with the dying and allowed them to express their sorrows and fears, rather than pressuring them to stay positive (because, who does that really benefit anyway?).

It bothers me because it implies that people who have died were somehow inferior, and not "fighters." This is simply not true. Have any of you lost a loved one to cancer who was a "fighter," and if so, how does it make you feel when you read that *this* person, usually a celebrity, who is newly diagnosed with cancer, will not die like others before them, because they are a "fighter?"

This same mentality holds true for people who say that they will live because they are praying to God. Many people with cancer who have prayed to God have died from it. What makes someone think they will have a different outcome? It implies that they feel "more worthy" than someone who prayed and died. This is really disturbing to me. I know many wonderful, morally sound people who have died of cancer while praying to be healed.

## Low carbohydrate diets increase cancer deaths

Lately, a lot of dietary focus has been geared towards manipulating your looks and symptoms, and not towards eating for health. I think you buy into the high protein "is good for preventing cancer" agenda because when you have an unhealthy body and bowel, you look and feel better eating this way. You have been led to believe that looking and feeling better means you are healthier. (If you snorted cocaine all day long you would lose weight and have a lot of energy, but this does not mean you are healthy.) You want to buy into it. But be careful. It is very dangerous to buy into the idea that a low carbohydrate diet will keep you alive for a long time, when in reality, it is just the opposite.

I routinely receive pamphlets from the American Institute for Cancer Research (AICR). This is a government-sponsored organization that employs doctors and medical researchers for the purpose of supporting cancer research and providing education in the area of diet, nutrition and cancer. (If you would like to receive their pamphlet you can order one by calling 800.843.8114, or visiting their website, *www.aicr.org*.) For many years I have been receiving their information. They have always promoted a low-protein (no more than 10% of calories), grain-based diet, even in this hey-day of high protein diets. They have even gone as far as to promote a plant-based diet, which is simply a nice term for a largely vegetarian diet. These recommendations are made by scientists whose entire purpose is to analyze studies and determine how best to prevent death from cancer.

These researchers cannot deny the overwhelming evidence that a low-animal protein diet significantly reduces one's risk of cancer.

T. Colin Campbell, Ph.D., author of *The China Study*, says, "Cancer begins when a harmful agent, like a toxic chemical, alters a normal cell. But a cancer won't persist and grow without certain nutrient conditions."

His number one recommendation, based on his findings, is the switch from a meat-based to a plant-based diet—from a high protein to a low protein diet. (I love this book, but the problem is, if it motivates you to switch to a plant-based diet, this motivation may be short-lived once you experience the weight-gain and symptom increase that usually occurs when you switch to a healthy, but very cleansing, plant-based diet when your bowel and body are not healthy and able to eliminate the acids/ toxins that this switch "stirs up." When you heal your bowel and body with this program, then you will be able to eat this "cancer-preventing" diet and not look or feel worse doing so. The chicken needs to come before the egg; this program needs to come before the diet change, and in fact, it will automatically come as you heal your bowel and body with this program, anyway.)

From the Harvard School of Public Health: Researchers tracked 88,000 women who enrolled in the Nurses Health Study in 1980. After 14 years, they found that women who reported eating red meat (beef, pork, or lamb) as a main dish at least once a day had a risk of non-Hodgkin's lymphoma roughly twice that of women who ate red meat less than once a week. Many people have veered away from red meat over the last five to ten years, but I thought I'd throw this in anyway, just in case the high-protein diet craze has led some of you to forget that red meat is a definite "disease-enhancer."

There are hundreds of studies that show a positive correlation between animal protein intake and cancer rates.

Whatever you do, get rid of the mentality that if you look and feel good you are healthy and if you don't you are not. I know of people with cancer who have fallen for the high protein diet because in the short-term they look and feel better this way, and this is wrongly interpreted as "being healthier." Eventually, cancer usually returns with these programs. Earlier this week I heard about a man who had contacted me seven years ago with hepatitis and rather than working with me, he went to someone who authored a high protein diet book. He recently died. This is a story you won't hear from people who have diligently followed my program.

## Go low protein now if your cancer is deadly

This is not the time to "worry about eating enough protein." If you are dying from cancer, you have probably already eaten way too much. You have a significantly higher chance of dying from cancer than you do of a protein deficiency.

If you have a deadly form of cancer, ignore the "don't reduce your protein " recommendation given in *Unique Healing*, and contact me for an appointment immediately.

## There is not one "toxic trigger"

We get lost and confused about cancer when we do studies that look for the "one cause" of it. There is not one cause and we will never find one. Here again is a situation where studies are dangerous. The nature of a study is that it has to isolate only one variable at a time. Studies that find that pesticides do not cause cancer are correct, in that it takes numerous toxic, acidic substances, along with an unhealthy bowel and body, to cause cancer. But to then conclude that pesticides, or any other toxic agent, is "safer than we think" is dangerous and wrong. It takes a lot of straws to break the camel's back, and while no one straw breaks it individually, collectively, they all do, and therefore each individual straw contributes to it.

## Focus needs to be on health, not the "cause"

Most of the current focus on preventing cancer is directed towards identifying the rain hitting the roof, or the "toxin" or "cause" of the cancer. It is not focused on fixing the roof. The trigger is irrelevant. All of the time and money spent looking for this would be much better spent on helping to fix the holes in the roof. You will never be able to avoid all of the "cancer-causing" toxins in life, and you won't have to if you create a very strong roof. This bowel and body-healing program creates a strong roof!

As long as we keep focusing on cancer and not on the elimination of acids, millions of people are going to die needlessly from this disease.

## Cancer is more than an unhealthy immune system

We often describe cancer as a weakness in the immune system, but this is very misleading. A weak immune system, in the absence of unhealthy cells, does not result in cancer; someone with a weak immune system and lupus, for example, does not necessarily have cancer. And people with cancer do not necessarily have symptoms of "classic" immune weaknesses, like a cold, sore throat, allergies, etc.

Cancer occurs when the immune system is weak *and* your cells are degenerative.

## Be careful, cancer can "sneak up on you!"

Have you ever heard someone say, "I feel like I have cancer growing in my body?" No. There is not a feeling to this. In fact, many people who are diagnosed with cancer are completely shocked, as they didn't have "symptoms," whatever that means, prior to their diagnosis. (It usually means that they looked and felt okay and rarely had colds, for example.)

Likewise, when you heal your body and bowel with this program, the first order of priority in your body is to replace any damaged cells with healthier ones. Just as there is no symptom associated with the breakdown of cells, there is none associated with the healing of them, either.

In the beginning of this process some of you will wonder if anything is getting better, as the cellular healing will not be obvious to you. But cellular healing is your body's priority, and I believe it is for this reason that my clients, even those who do not complete this program, are not getting diagnosed with deadly cancers while I am working with them.

## Drive as far as you can

If California represents the state of cancer, then you would be safer if you drove all the way to Nantucket than if you just drove across the border to Utah.

In other words, if cancer represents a very unhealthy and acidic cellular system, you can heal your body with this program for a few months and drive away from cancer, but still have it within your reach. If you heal your body with this program for a few years, you will be much further from this state. The longer and more completely that you heal your body and bowel with this program, the better.

## It is easier to heal than you think

The "top of your pipe," where cellular degeneration like cancer develops, is a dangerous situation, but also your body's first priority when healing.

When you begin to heal your body and bowel with this program, the first area of your body that heals is the "top of your pipe," or your cells. This is good news for anyone who is battling cancer and/or is concerned about getting cancer. Your cells are constantly changing. Cancerous ones can become non-cancerous ones.

## But then of course, it's much more complicated than this

Cancer requires an extremely aggressive approach to healing as well as an extremely aggressive "crutch program." If you currently have cancer, do not attempt this program without consulting with me personally.

If you currently have cancer, especially one that keeps coming back with conventional treatments or is considered incurable by the medical profession, and you are not willing to give up, and you understand (hopefully!) why this program can save your life, you need to consult with me on an aggressive, individualized basis.

# Success with Cancer

As I already said, I have not worked with a large number of clients with cancer, but I have worked with a large number of clients, and they are not getting and dying from cancer while they are under my care. That is not to say they never do, because I cannot control how quickly they heal their body, how much they heal it, or what they do after they leave my office. Do they leave with impatience and embark on a high-protein diet that sends them zooming towards cancer? *But in the 19 years that I have done this worked, I have never had a client get cancer and die from it while under my care.* (And I have many older clients, and clients that I have worked with for several years.)

I am not surprised by this outcome, but I think it should get your attention. Statistically speaking, these results are remarkable.

It is a necessity that you contact me and work with me directly, and consistently, if you have a dangerous diagnosis of cancer.

## Watch my Video, "Why THIS Program Works for Cancer"

This video, and all of my videos, can be found at *www.UniqueHealing.com* or at *www.YouTube.com/UniqueHealing*.

# Candida
See "Fungal Infections"

# Cataracts
See "Eye Problems"

# Celiac Disease
See "Allergies (food)" and "Bowel Disorders"

# Chemical Allergies
See "Allergies (Environmental)"

# Cholesterol (high)/Heart Disease/Stroke (Atherosclerosis, Arteriosclerosis)

About twenty years ago, heart disease became a common concern, and a widely discussed condition.

We witnessed an increase in heart disease diagnoses, and not just among the elderly. In 1993, it was reported that autopsies on 1532 people ages 15 to 34 that had died largely of homicides, accidents and suicides found that *all* of them had arterial fat deposits. And in 1992 a California study found that 17 percent of elementary school children had cholesterol readings in the high-risk range of 200 or above. These shocking statistics got our attention, and more blood test variables, in addition to the already measured blood cholesterol level, were designed to assess heart disease risk.

We also began to hear a lot more about the importance of diet as related to heart disease and cholesterol, and we were told that cutting out butter, eggs, and cholesterol-containing foods, and fats, would reduce our risk.

Given all of this "progress" in knowledge, awareness, and the adoption of a "heart-healthy" diet, we haven't made much progress in reversing cholesterol levels, or more importantly, death from heart disease. More than half of men and 40% of women will go on to develop it during their lifetime (according to the Centers for Disease Control). And more alarmingly, greater numbers of younger adults are dying from heart attacks than never before.

Consuming fat or high cholesterol foods, genetics, stress, a lack of exercise, etc. does not cause high cholesterol and heart disease. The wrong "things" have been blamed, as the results confirm. Success in eliminating death from heart disease will only occur once the *right* thing is blamed.

Un-eliminated acids cause high cholesterol and heart disease.

This program heals your bowel and body and eliminates these acids, and as a result, your cholesterol levels will go down. More importantly, the build up of cholesterol in your arteries, the kind that leads to heart attacks and death, will also go down. This is *not* the case with the majority of advice given for lowering cholesterol and heart disease. In fact much of it results in lower blood cholesterol levels but an *increase* in the cholesterol in your arteries, *increasing* your risk of death by heart attack!

## Interpreting your blood cholesterol results

When you have your blood cholesterol levels checked, some of the information that you will be given is: total cholesterol, HDL, LDL, risk ratio, and triglycerides.

**Total Cholesterol.** Many years ago the only heart disease risk variable measured was the amount of cholesterol circulating in your blood, or your total cholesterol number. And while other heart disease risk variables have been added to the blood heart profile, this continues to be the number that most of you are most familiar, and concerned, with.

**HDLs, LDLs, and risk ratio.** Back when blood tests only measured cholesterol levels, medical doctors found many "confusing" cases of heart disease; some people with high blood cholesterol levels were not having heart attacks, and others with low blood cholesterol levels were.

Soon we heard about HDLs and LDLs. LDLs are lipoproteins that affect the transport of cholesterol into your arteries. HDLs are lipoproteins that transport the cholesterol away from your arteries, and away from danger. If you have high blood cholesterol levels but also high levels of HDLs, in other words, you may have a low risk of dying from a heart attack, even though your cholesterol reading is high. HDLs carry cholesterol from your arteries to your liver to be combined with bile so that it can be carried away in the stools.

The *risk-ratio* number on your blood work is your total cholesterol number divided by your HDLs (CHO/HDL). This is thought to represent the amount of cholesterol that is being deposited in your arteries. It the cholesterol that is being deposited in your arteries, and not the cholesterol circulating in your blood, that can kill you.

**Triglycerides.** Triglycerides are the chemical form in which most fat exists in food, as well as in your body. High triglyceride levels have been associated with higher rates of heart disease.

Ideal ranges for all of these measurements are listed on your blood test results, and these differ, depending on the lab and the latest scientific findings, so check your blood tests for the ideal ranges being used. Always ask for a copy of your test results so you have record of them. Often, you will only be notified if these results are considered risky, however the more information that you have about your health, the more empowered you will be to improve it.

**C-reactive protein.** A few years ago, a doctor on television was discussing new research in measuring heart-disease risk, as the current approach seemed to be missing this risk in a number of individuals. He said that a test called CRP (C-reactive protein), that signals possible arterial inflammation, was thought to more likely predict heart disease than cholesterol count.

I have not seen this test performed on many of my clients, and I have not heard much more about it since this initial discussion. I think the test was developed as an attempt to sell an anti-inflammatory drug to people concerned about their heart disease risk. Whatever the story that is behind it, the "search" for more and newer blood tests to predict heart attacks is frustrating and dangerous, given that a heart scan (see more on this later) is available, and provides more accurate information regarding your heart attack risk than any blood test likely ever will.

## Strokes

A stroke occurs when your brain does not receive adequate oxygen, and as a result, there is damage to the tissues of your brain. Strokes are included in this section because clogged arteries, which block the flow of oxygen to your brain, cause 90% of these (just as clogged arteries can block the flow of oxygen to your heart, causing heart attacks).

Stroke takes its highest toll on older people. For those over 65, there were nearly 300 stroke cases among 10,000 hospitalizations in the more recent period studied. Yet strokes are rising dramatically among young adults, and middle-aged women. Numbers recently reported at an

American Stroke Association conference reported government researchers compared hospitalizations in 1994 and 1995 with ones in 2006 and 2007, and find the sharpest increase (51 percent) was among men 15 through 34. Strokes rose among women in this age group, too, but not as fast (17 percent). For males 15 to 34, there were about 15 stroke cases per 10,000, and for girls and women in that age group there were about 4 per 10,000.

"It's definitely alarming," said Dr. Ralph Sacco, American Heart Association president and a neurologist at the University of Miami. "I'd say at least half of our population (of stroke patients) is in their 40s or early 50s, and devastating strokes, too," says Allison Hooker, a nurse who coordinates stroke care at Forsyth Medical Center in Winston-Salem, N.C.,

## Healing Your Body With This Program Eliminates High Cholesterol/Heart Disease/Stroke

Arteries become blocked with deposits of plaque, cholesterol, and fat, and these deposits cause them to narrow, making it difficult for oxygen to get to your heart or brain, leading to an eventual heart attack or stroke.

As even Dr. Oz explains it, plaque is deposited at certain places in your arteries to "fix a hole" in them, like a Band-Aid. To quote Dr. Oz, "Rusting of the arteries is caused by *toxic elements* in the blood." He says that holes in your arteries are caused by damage from acids! Un-eliminated acids, that is. Healing your body with this program eliminates the acids that damage your arteries, and cause these "holes." It eliminates the acids that cause the production of plaque, fat, and cholesterol, which are simply "protection" against these acids. Without these acids, these artery-clogging products do not accumulate.

For example, your liver regulates cholesterol metabolism. It manufactures about 80% of the cholesterol that is in your body at any given time. Your liver responds to un-eliminated acids with the production of cholesterol, which buffers these acids in your blood. Cholesterol is made to "protect you" from un-eliminated acids, but in time, this deposits in your arteries, and eventually increases your risk of heart attack and stroke.

When you heal your body with this program, acids are eliminated, and as a result, your oxygen levels increase. That is because oxygen becomes depleted when acids are not eliminated, as oxygen gets "used" to buffer and protect you against them. Higher levels of oxygen flowing through your blood means there is more available for your heart and brain, both of which need oxygen to live. Also, some heart attacks occur when a blood clot forms, blocking oxygen flow to your heart. Blood clots form when your blood is highly acidic, which robs it of oxygen, and causes your red blood cells to clump or stick together. Eliminating acids from your body eliminates blood clumping and clots.

When your body is healthy, you can eat a low protein, high fiber diet without feeling uncomfortable or gaining weight. These diets have been shown time and time again to help dramatically reduce heart disease and, more importantly, death from heart attacks.

## Healing Your Bowel With This Program Eliminates High Cholesterol/Heart Disease/Stroke

A healthy bowel produces sufficient levels of vitamin B-12. Vitamin B-12 is involved in the conversion of homocysteine into methionine. Homocysteine, an amino acid produced by ineffective protein metabolism, can, in high levels, damage blood vessels. Every month I review several dozen new research studies on health and nutrition. In the last ten years, many of these have shown a correlation between high homocysteine levels and increased risk of heart disease and stroke. Vitamin B-12 is one of the nutrients commonly cited for its ability to reduce homocysteine levels. Healing your bowel with this program creates a healthy bacterial environment, and this is needed for the production of vitamin B-12.

A study in the Journal of Dairy Science, March 2000, showed a 17% improvement in the ratio of HDL to LDL in mice that were fed a probiotic.

Healthy bacteria help your body break down bile, and bile has been shown to help remove bile excess cholesterol. High bilirubin levels in blood work and/or yellow in the whites of your eyes are symptoms of improper bile break down, and therefore, of an unhealthy bowel.

The bacteria/heart disease relationship has also been explained as the bacteria taking up residence in your coronary arteries where they create damage to them, thereby causing your body to accumulate cholesterol in an attempt to patch up this damage. Regardless of the explanation, it has been observed that an abundance of bad bacteria exists in the systems of individuals with heart disease.

When your bowel bacterial environment is healthy, you ability to digest your food is improved. Incompletely digested fats, carbohydrates and sugars have been implicated as elements that can raise cholesterol and triglyceride levels. Choosing easy to digest foods, as you are instructed to in this program, and strengthening your digestion, a side effect of a healthier bowel, eliminates this variable as a causative agent. In other words, less of these foods become converted into toxic substances, like excess cholesterol, in the first place.

One hundred percent of the clients I have seen who had a heart scan which showed narrowing of their arteries had very unhealthy levels of beneficial bacteria in their bowel.

In addition to its many other important functions, a healthy bacterial environment in your bowel is a necessity for the complete elimination of acids (toxins, heavy metals, pesticides, etc.) from your body. A healthy bowel prevents the re-absorption of acids from irritating foods into your blood that cause an unhealthy body, and trigger plaque, cholesterol, and fat production, as well as low oxygen levels. When your bowel is healthy, it eliminates the acids from your body that otherwise eventually "attack" your heart, or arteries (the "top of your pipe," as I refer to it.)

## Why My Crutches Eliminate High Cholesterol/Heart Disease/Stroke

*Body Bentonite* binds to and eliminates acids (toxins, heavy metals, chemicals, etc.) from your body. It helps prevent them from becoming re-absorbed into your bloodstream, where they trigger a response by your body to protect you from them. It eliminates the acids that trigger the production of artery-clogging cholesterol and fat by your body to protect you from them. It eliminates the acids that reduce oxygen levels, and therefore it reduces your risk of blood clots.

*Unique Healing Calcium Citrate* is an alkalinizing mineral that helps neutralize the acids that your bowel does not eliminate. When these acids are neutralized, your body does not need to produce cholesterol, or "use up" oxygen, to buffer them.

155

*Unique Healing Methyl Vitamin B-12* provides your body with easy to assimilate levels of this nutrient, which has been shown in numerous studies to reduce homocysteine levels and your risk of cardiovascular disease.

Note: Clogged arteries that cause heart attacks and stroke are degenerative conditions, and there are no crutches for degenerative conditions. Crutches can offset the effects of acids in your blood, or the effects of poor function of your bowel bacterial environment (as these can be quickly altered), but degeneration is caused by depletion and damage to your organs, and organs take time to heal. It will take some time for your arteries to "un-clog" with this program.

## How much do I take?/Questions about using these

See Chapter 5 for information on using these crutches, including recommendations on the amount to use, as well as a discussion of the misunderstandings about the particular crutch that may, if not understood correctly, cause you to fail to look and feel better while you heal your bowel and body with this program.

## How long will I need to use crutches for my high cholesterol/ heart disease/stroke?

High cholesterol occurs at Level 2 of your pipe. It is the second area of your body to heal (assuming that other areas are unhealthy too). Refer to the diagram "Sequence of Healing" in Appendix A at the end of this book to better understand this concept, as well as to Chapter 1 under this subject heading.

Again, there are no crutches for degenerative conditions and accumulations of acidity in your organs like clogged arteries/heart attack/ stroke; however, degenerative conditions are the first to become eliminated as you heal your bowel and body with this program.

# Misunderstandings about High Cholesterol/Heart Disease/Stroke and Other Information for Your Success

## Keep your stools well-formed

Because high cholesterol and blood clots are caused by un-eliminated acids, and because well-formed stools prevent the re-absorption of acids into your blood that trigger this condition, you will have lower cholesterol readings on your blood tests, and fewer clots, if you keep your stools well-formed while you are healing your bowel and body.

If you do not have a very good handle on how to define well-formed stools, review Chapter 6 of *Unique Healing* now. (And remember, when your stools are hard and slow you are eliminating more acids, and will therefore feel better, than when your stools are one or more times a day but not all extremely well-formed.)

If your stools are not well-formed, the following changes can help: increase your *Body Bentonite* intake; reduce your carbohydrate intake (pasta, breads, grains, cereals, yogurt, etc.); reduce your sugar intake (including natural healthy sugars such as agave, honey, raw sugar, cane juice, etc.); reduce your alcohol, salt, coffee, and/or soda intake; do not have a massage, chiropractic adjustment, or any other body work; drink a lot of water; rest; and keep your exercise aerobic (see Chapter 4 for more information on how to attain this, and why it is important.)

If these changes do not noticeably help the form of your stools in two days, take them further (i.e. take more *Body Bentonite*, reduce your carbohydrate intake more, etc.)

Out of all of these recommendations, increasing your *Body Bentonite* intake is one of the most productive and helpful. It heals your body, unlike many of the other recommendations. It will do the most to lead you to a place where looking and feeling good is effortless, and some of the other suggestions, such as reducing sugar intake, are simply "too hard to do when your blood is too acidic."

(Note: the exception to this information is when your poorly formed stools are caused by an infection, in which case *Unique Healing Colloidal Silver* is needed to reduce your symptoms. Refer to Chapter 5 for information on when and how to use this crutch.)

## Blood tests are harmful predictors of heart attacks or strokes

Forty percent of people with coronary artery disease have "normal" cholesterol levels, and forty percent of first time heart attacks end in death, with "no warning." In a large percentage of cases, a heart attack is the first sign that anything is wrong.

Why then are most of you led to believe that you are safe and healthy if your cholesterol number is normal, and why are many of you obsessed with, and fearful of, numbers that are high?

The cholesterol number on your blood test reflects the amount of cholesterol circulating in your blood. But this blood cholesterol does not kill you; the cholesterol stuck on the walls of your arteries can, and a blood test does not measure this.

The reason that a high blood cholesterol level is cause for concern, therefore, is because it may be assumed that the high levels in your blood will eventually settle onto your arterial walls, narrowing them and creating a high risk for heart disease or stroke. Unfortunately, this is a poor assumption when it is made for those of you who are following this program (see "blood tests may get worse as you heal" later in this section for an explanation for this).

Worse, and more commonly, the opposite scenario occurs, whereby you are led to believe you are safe from a heart attack and death if your blood cholesterol levels are normal. Again, a large number of people have died of a heart attack who had normal blood cholesterol readings. If you are following a low carbohydrate diet (and many of you are), this can reduce blood cholesterol levels but *increase* harmful artery-clogging cholesterol, and the assumption that you are safe from heart attack and death is incredibly dangerous and not at all true. (More on this later.)

Also, the medical community keeps changing its opinion on "acceptable" heart disease risk variables. For example, medical guidelines for acceptable triglyceride levels used to consider amounts below 200 as normal, yet researchers found that people with levels as low as 100 were more than twice as likely to suffer from future heart disease than those with lower levels. By accepting a level of 200 as safe, the medical community led many of you to falsely believe that you were safe too. So how can you comfortably believe that any current acceptable blood test levels are really safe?

# The value of a heart scan

A heart scan shows the amount of stenosis, or plaque build up and narrowing, of your arteries, and your subsequent risk of death due to a lack of sufficient oxygen to your heart and brain because of this. Blood cholesterol tests cannot measure this risk, and they cannot accurately predict if you have narrowing of your arteries and if you are at risk of death.

Laboratory results are also not perfect. Some medical statistics show that about 30% of the test results have errors in them. While a heart scan is not a "perfect test" either (there is some margin of error in them), they are still extraordinarily more valuable than a blood cholesterol test. Even with room for error, they are not going to be too "far off." A low *blood* cholesterol level can exist when there is a large amount of cholesterol clogging your arteries putting you at risk of heart attack. On the other hand, a heart scan may show minimal amounts of deposits in your arteries, and even if this is read that 10% of your arteries are clogged, but it is really 15%, this discrepancy, or error, is irrelevant, and this test can safely be interpreted as your having a low risk of heart attack.

If your total cholesterol number is high, your doctor may pressure you to take cholesterol-lowering drugs. Before you embark on this risky and sometimes unnecessary path, get a heart scan done. If you have any concerns about your heart and risk for heart attack, get a scan done. Do not use your blood cholesterol readings as a measurement of your health and safety from heart disease.

Cholesterol-lowering drugs are acidic and harmful to your health, and it is best to avoid them as much as possible. If you ever feel pressured to take these drugs, get some more information about your heart first. Scans can cost anywhere from $200-$500, and for now, insurance generally doesn't cover this. A few hundred dollars will buy you information that could save your life! Also, it would be a lot cheaper than the cost to your health of taking unnecessary cholesterol-lowering drugs. I have never had a client get a heart scan and regret it. In every case, the comfort of having a relatively accurate measure of whether they were at risk of a heart attack was more than worth the money spent on this test.

Even if your cholesterol levels are normal, consider this test. Many people with normal blood cholesterol levels have been found to have life-threatening amounts of build-up in their arteries.

## A healthy heart does not mean a healthy body

If you have a heart scan done and it shows no or very little build-up in your arteries, that is great news. *It could take many years at that point for them to become clogged to a dangerous degree*, which means you have many years to heal your bowel and body, and keep them clear.

At the same time, while a heart scan is an excellent predictor of your short-term risk of death from heart disease, it does not reflect the health of your other organs in your body. The top of your pipe may be clear, but the middle and bottom may be very acidic/unhealthy. In other words, a good heart scan is excellent news, but it does not mean that you are as healthy as you can be. It does not mean that you can't look and feel better. It does not mean that you don't need this program.

## EKGs/stress tests

These do not measure the dangerous build-up of plaque in your arteries, either. You may pass this test even if you are at risk of a heart attack or stroke, which make this a dangerous way to assess your risk.

Several years ago, it was released that newsman Tim Russert, who died of a heart attack at the young age of 58, had recently passed a stress test. Just last week, a client's dad died of a heart attack just two days after passing this test! These are in no way isolated stories.

## Lower cholesterol readings are not always better

Your doctor will be happy if your blood cholesterol reading is less than 200 mg/dl, although many health practitioners consider a reading closer to 160-180 mg/dl better/safer, myself included. Your doctor may also be happy if your number is extremely low, but you should not be. Numbers lower than 160 mg/dl are not necessarily safer, and could be a sign of health problems and/or danger.

Cholesterol is necessary for the production of various steroids and hormones in your body, and too little could mean a reduction in these. Also, cholesterol levels that are too low have been associated with a higher risk of some cancers.

I have never seen a concrete explanation for why lower levels can be risky, but my guess is that these can occur when too much cholesterol is clogging your arteries and not enough is in your circulation waiting to be eliminated. There can be very little cholesterol in your blood, because it is all stuck in your cells and arteries.

A low blood cholesterol test may occur when your cells and arteries are acidic, which is associated with greater cellular damage and subsequently higher levels of heart attacks, stroke, and disease, like cancer.

When I was extremely ill and unhealthy, my reading was around 130 mg/dl, when I was placed on a high protein diet, a diet that caused an increase in the seriousness of my condition.

*If you too have a total cholesterol level below 150 mg/dl and are eating a high protein diet, a heart scan may be a lifesaver for you.*

Likewise, if you are on cholesterol-lowering drugs and your levels have gone below 150mg/dl, my experience is that this is not healthy. You may be suffering from some negative side effects of this "too low cholesterol," like increased inflammation. It is your doctor's responsibility to make the recommendation to lower the amount of the cholesterol drug you are taking in this situation. But then again, it is your responsibility, and yours alone, to make decisions about what is best for your health.

Lower is simply not always better, or safer.

## High cholesterol is not caused by eating too many cholesterol-containing foods

The "eat less cholesterol-containing foods" approach to lowering cholesterol levels has failed because high cholesterol is not caused by the consumption of foods that contain cholesterol; un-eliminated acids cause it. Blood cholesterol levels increase when there are excess acids in your blood.

Some foods, like eggs, contain cholesterol but do not increase blood acidity, and therefore cannot raise blood cholesterol levels; and some foods, like fruit, contain no cholesterol, but increase blood acidity due to the cleansing affect of it, and therefore consuming them can increase blood cholesterol levels. (If you still do not understand this cleansing concept and why healthy foods can make you look and feel worse, and cause higher blood cholesterol levels while you are healing your bowel and body, watch my videos and read my books repeatedly until you do.)

Likewise, some foods, like animal proteins (chicken, turkey, beef, etc.), can reduce blood acids levels but *increase* the acids in your arteries, increasing heart attack risk.

## Clogged arteries are not caused by taking calcium supplements

Calcium deposits are found in arterial deposits, calcium does not cause these deposits, nor is it harmful to your heart. In fact, of the thousands of studies I have read, I have never seen one that found that calcium supplementation increased heart disease; on the contrary, some have found that it reduces the incidence of it. (Just yesterday an older, not very healthy client, who has been taking large amounts of calcium per my advice, had a heart scan and his doctor was very surprised that he had zero calcium deposits.)

Yet, you may be warned against calcium use by your doctor, who has been trained to believe that when two variables co-exist, one is probably the cause of the other (this is a redundant theme and mistake, and a dangerous one that is often made.)

Excess acids cause deposits on your arteries. Your body uses calcium, an alkaline mineral, to protect you from these acids. It is the good guy. Taking more calcium, via supplements, offers you *greater* protection from these harmful, artery-clogging acids.

## Are high fiber diets really helpful?

Many studies have found a positive relationship between high fiber diets and a reduction in cholesterol levels. For example, in one study, rice or oat bran at 84g/day reduced LDL-cholesterol by 13.7% in the rice bran group and 17.1% in the oat bran group. ("Full-Fat Rice Bran and Oat Bran Similarly Reduce Hypercholesterolemia in Humans," Gerhardt,Ann L.). In the second, a study of 573 adults between the ages of 40 and 60 showed a significant inverse association between intima-media thickness progression of the common carotid arteries and the intake of viscous fiber, formally called water-soluble fiber. (Wu H, Dwyer KM et al, Am J Clin Nutr, 2003, 78:1085-1091; *jimdwyer@usc.edu.*)

The technical explanation for why this occurs is that fiber is fermented by *bacteria* in your colon into short chain fatty acids, which then turn down the action of your body's enzyme HMG COA reductase, thereby suppressing cholesterol synthesis in your body.

My explanation goes as follows: a high fiber diet acts like a broom that sweeps acids in your blood, that cause high cholesterol levels, out of your blood into your bowel (hence the possibility that when your blood is tested, these acids, and therefore excess cholesterol, won't show up.) But it doesn't always work that way. Fiber does not eliminate "cholesterol-causing" acids from your body. When fiber "sweeps" the acids that cause cholesterol into your bowel, they are usually not eliminated by your bowel once they get there, and ultimately, they return to your blood, causing your cholesterol levels to eventually rise again. This program eliminates these cholesterol-causing acids, and therefore your results with not only lowering your blood cholesterol levels, but your risk of heart attack as well, is far superior than using a fiber diet, or product, to do this for you.

Foods high in fiber, like grains and vegetables, are also low in acids, and a low-acid diet, not necessarily a high fiber one, has been shown to reduce *death* from heart disease. For example, a study at Harvard Medical School that tracked 68,000 nurses for a variety of lifestyle and disease risk factors over a ten-year period found that the nurses who consumed just two servings of whole grains a day (i.e. one cup of cooked oatmeal) were 30% less likely to develop heart disease, but is that result due to the oatmeal, or is due to the oatmeal "replacing" a highly acidic food that was previously in their diet, like sausage and bacon? I suggest that it is likely the latter.

## High protein diets: lowering your cholesterol does not always mean you have lowered your heart disease risk

In 2004, Bill Clinton had quadruple bypass surgery. An article about this in *People* (September 20, 2004) showed him when he was heavy and had a high cholesterol reading of 226. He was eating a lot of unhealthy food and not exercising. Years later, he began an exercise program and the South Beach diet (aka, High-Protein diet). He had been following this for several years, trimmed down, and "looked great." However, the surgeons commented that well over 90% of his arteries were blocked. Dr. Allan Schwartz, chief of the hospital's cardiology division, said "There was a substantial likelihood that he would have had a substantial heart attack in the near future."

Now think for a minute. If his arteries were well over 90% blocked, and if this situation would result in almost imminent heart failure, it *had* to mean that his arteries had been becoming *more* clogged over the past several years in which he was exercising and following a high-protein diet.

Hundreds of studies show that when people follow a high-protein diet there is a noticeable increase in deaths from heart attacks.

Another "heart and nutrition medical expert" commented that well gee, in truth, diet and exercise alone may not be able to completely stop arterial plaque formation. This doctor also commented that Clinton's South Beach diet was a "step in the right direction." This sends the message to millions of you that the South Beach diet is healthy and protective to your heart, and that you'd better be scared to death because there really isn't anything you can do to prevent a heart attack.

Even the American Heart Association, a government organization that examines the scientific data on diet and heart disease, among other things, has concluded that a low protein diet is extremely important for reducing heart disease risk and *death* from heart attacks. Even throughout the entire recent high protein craze, they have stuck by the recommendation that you consume no more than 10% of your calories from protein. (Versus the 40-60% recommended by most "health" authors and practitioners.)

On a high protein diet, blood cholesterol levels typically go down, dangerously leading millions to believe they are safer as a result.

Blood cholesterol levels go down on lower carbohydrate diets because this diet reduces the amount of cholesterol floating around in your blood, where blood cholesterol is measured, but it *increases* the amount that is stored in your arteries, which blood cholesterol does *not* measure. This is life threatening. High protein diets "shove the acids" from your blood into your cells; cholesterol in your cells can kill you, not cholesterol in your blood.

If you do not understand this "cleansing concept," go back and re-read *Unique Healing*, and watch all of my videos at ***www.YouTube. com/UniqueHealing*** until you do. Your understanding of this concept is by far the most important one for your success in preventing symptoms, disease, addictions, and weight problems.

If you have a history of high cholesterol and have not had a heart scan done yet, schedule one now. This is especially crucial if you are eating a high-protein or low carbohydrate diet to reduce your blood cholesterol levels. Encourage friends and family to do the same; it could save their life. (See Chapter 5 of *Unique Healing* for a definition of a high protein or low carbohydrate diet.)

## Increasing your HDL levels is not the magic solution to preventing heart attacks, either

I've seen many clients return from a physical with their doctor's recommendations for increasing their HDL levels, with great emphasis on this variable, as though elevated HDL levels are *the* answer to preventing heart attacks. In my experience, there is not a strong correlation between these levels and heart attack risk.

In fact, in a recent study of an experimental HDL-boosting drug called Niaspan, it was found that participants experienced about a 20% increase in their HDL levels, but a 0% reduction in heart attack risk.

Drugs do not eliminate the acids that cause heart attacks; this program does.

## Confusion, frustration, and more drugs and surgery

Historically, a high blood level of cholesterol has been a true concern, and a somewhat accurate indicator of future risk from a heart attack. If you are *not* eating a high protein diet, but your bowel is unhealthy, your blood cholesterol levels will rise before excess cholesterol becomes deposited in your arteries. Typically, high blood cholesterol precedes a heart attack.

But history is changing, largely due to the mass consumption of high protein diets. When you eat a high protein diet, this pattern does not hold true anymore. On the contrary, many people with low or normal blood cholesterol levels have died from heart attacks, and I predict that even more will in the future.

I predict that this will baffle the medical profession, many of who still believe that low blood cholesterol levels means you are safe from a heart attack. I think you will then be told, "Dietary changes are of no help in preventing heart disease." Rather than understanding that the fault lies in the diet itself (the high protein diet), I think you will instead hear the message that diet simply doesn't prevent heart disease. The answer that likely will be given to you is that drugs and surgery, therefore, are your only choice.

## Reversing heart disease

Dr. Dean Ornish is a well-known doctor and author who developed a natural approach to reversing heart disease. He recommends a low protein, vegetarian, high fiber diet. Low protein diets are less acidic than high protein diets, and therefore, they can reduce the *future* build-up of plaque on your arterial walls, but they do not necessarily eliminate the *existing* build-up of plaque on your arterial walls.

Also, many of you will abandon this program because this is a cleansing diet, and when your bowel and body are not healthy, this can cause a lot of discomfort, weight gain, as well as a rise in your blood cholesterol levels (as he has recorded), sending you into a wrongful state of fear that you are harming yourself with this diet.

Finally, the greatest disadvantage of this diet is the fact that a cleansing diet does not *eliminate* the acids from your arteries and body in the way that healing your bowel and body with this program does.

Ideally, if you have heart scan done and it shows that your arteries are becoming dangerously blocked, switch to a lower protein, higher fiber diet. A low protein diet helps clear the deposits on your arteries into your bloodstream. If your arteries are badly clogged but not bad enough to have them unclogged medically, reduce the amount of fish, turkey, pork, chicken, and beef that you are eating now. Eat a lot of fruit, vegetables, beans, nuts, and whole grains. Do this, even if it means you might get more bloated, and your blood cholesterol levels may increase, as well as your weight. Bloating, blood cholesterol, and extra weight won't kill you; the blockage in your arteries can. (And your bloating, elevated blood cholesterol, and extra weight will eventually go away as you heal your bowel and body with this program, anyway.)

(Note: You are likely to be led to be alarmed if you follow this heart-healthy diet and your cholesterol numbers increase, so I strongly advise you to consult with me if you are in this state and choose to reduce your protein intake prior to healing your bowel and body with this program.)

In the perfect world, you would not have these blockages and not "need" to choose between a better heart and a worsening of other symptoms, like bloating and increased cholesterol numbers and weight, but it is not a perfect world. If your scan shows no blockages, you can afford the luxury of healing your bowel and body before eating less protein and more fiber; if you have the time (i.e. you are not in immediate danger of dying from blocked arteries) to wait until your bowel and body are healed, these dietary changes won't make you uncomfortable or cause weight gain.

Low protein=less cholesterol blocking your arteries, more cholesterol in your blood.

High protein=more cholesterol blocking your arteries, less cholesterol in your blood.

Blood cholesterol does not kill you; cholesterol clogging your arteries can kill you.

You will have *both* less blockages in your arteries *and* low blood cholesterol levels when you heal your bowel and body with this program.

## Your arteries are your body's first priority when you heal

When you heal your bowel and body with this program, your heart, bones, and cells heal first. When you unplug the bottom of your pipe, the top of it clears out first. Your body heals your heart and cleans out your arteries, if needed, before healing your other organs.

Your body is amazing and heals the most important things first. (Believe it or not, it is not always a client's top priority. If given lower cholesterol, or less bloating and water retention, many clients will choose the later. Yet, it is no good to be thin, and yet die of a heart attack!)

If you are concerned about your heart, know that your body is too, and that on this program, your heart is getting top attention.

## Your blood tests may get worse as you heal your heart

Remember, cholesterol in your arteries and cholesterol in your blood are not related, and they have two separate causes. The cholesterol in your arteries reflects the "top of your pipe" and the cholesterol in your blood reflects the "middle of your pipe," and the top of your pipe heals first. If you heal your heart/arteries, which reduces your chance of death by a heart attack or stroke, but eat a cleansing diet that dumps excess acids into your blood, you may see your cholesterol levels rise or remain high, as it takes more time to heal the middle of your pipe, which needs to be healed before your body stops producing excess cholesterol in response to acids. When you fix your roof with this program, the holes over your bedroom get fixed first, but if it rains before the holes over your living room are fixed, it may get wet (even though the bedroom, which is the most important room, stays dry.)

If your blood cholesterol levels increase on this program, it is extremely likely that you ate a cleansing or highly acidic diet before you were healthy enough to do so without having this reaction. Get a scan done before you assume the worst. If your scan is great, do not over-react to these blood tests.

## Don't yank out your crutches too soon

Crutches do not heal; they merely treat a symptom. If you stop a crutch, the symptoms will return. If, when you start this program, you have been eating a high protein diet, taking red yeast rice, or exercising daily, for example, to reduce your cholesterol levels, and you stop or reduce these crutches before your bowel and body are strong enough to function without them, your cholesterol will likely go up.

If this happens, do not blame this program. It is not the cause. It would have gone up had you stopped those crutches and not done this program. If your levels go back up, get back on your crutches and wait another year before stopping them. Because you are healing your bowel and body, *eventually* you will be able to stop them and not have this occur.

## The failure of most approaches to heart disease

The primary reason that people continue to suffer from very high rates of heart disease is because you keep being led to focus on your blood cholesterol levels. You wrongly and dangerously believe that if your blood cholesterol levels are low, you are healthy and safe, and you keep searching for the quick fix to these problems. And maybe you fail because you are confused and frustrated with all of the contradictory advice that you have had to sort through over the years. First margarine is good for your heart, then it is bad, for example. How many of you have simply stopped listening to all of this advice, because every time you do, it changes?

When advice is geared to treat a symptom and not the cause of the problem, it will keep changing. When advice is given that helps to make your body healthier, it won't. My advice to clients about their heart health has never changed in the over nineteen years that I have been advising clients. I am certain it will not change in the next nineteen either, but then again, I have always focused on helping clients create a healthier body, not just eliminating their symptoms.

## Cholesterol drugs/statins

You've heard the statement, "When diet and exercise are not enough" to reduce your cholesterol levels, you need a drug. I imagine many people like to hear this; they like to believe that changing their lifestyle can't help them so they don't have to hassle with it. If you are reading this book, this is not who you are. You know that you have control over your heart health, like all other aspects of your health, and you won't bow out so quickly. Lucky for you, because while taking a drug for your cholesterol seems easy and effective, it is not. In the short-term you may feel safer because your cholesterol levels went down, but you *shouldn't* feel so safe.

There are significant problems with cholesterol-lowering drugs. All drugs have potential side effects. Some can aggravate or cause liver disease. This is very undesirable and ironic, as you have learned that a healthy liver is needed to keep your cholesterol levels low naturally. (Just because your doctor checks your blood work for liver enzyme levels and they are normal does *not* mean your liver is healthy and that the drug is not hurting it.)

Worst of all, to my knowledge, while these drugs have been shown to lower cholesterol, they have not been proven to prevent heart disease and death. A review of cholesterol drug studies published in the October 3, 2006 issue of the Annals of Internal Medicine found no health or *mortality* benefit (i.e. they did not help people live longer) to artificially lowering cholesterol levels using statin drugs. The next time you see a commercial on television for you, read the fine print a the bottom that states this drug has not been proven to reduce your risk of a heart attack, that is, if you can see it and read it fast enough. You are taken advantage of; your belief that lower cholesterol always means less death from heart disease is exploited.

When someone is diagnosed with high cholesterol, this often prompts lifestyle changes, so who is to say that any observable improvement in cholesterol readings and/or reduction in heart attacks is from the drug or from these changes, anyway?

## Beta blockers

Beta-blockers are drugs that decrease your heart's need for blood and oxygen. That is certainly one approach to reduce heart attacks and stroke, and potentially valuable if you are unhealthy and your oxygen levels are inadequate for healthy heart function. A healthier and better approach is to improve the amount of blood and oxygen available to your heart and brain in the first place by healing your bowel and body with this program.

## Surgery/angioplasty

If your arteries are clogged you can have surgery to open them/unclog them. During this, plaque is physically removed from your arterial walls. This is a very risky, expensive, and stressful operation. What's more, it does absolutely nothing to prevent your arteries from clogging again in the future, and in many cases, that is exactly what happens. How many surgeries do you think you can endure? Having said that, if my arteries were dangerously clogged, I would get the surgery done, and then work on healing my bowel and body with this program.

In 1998 Dr. Dean Ornish published a study in the Journal of the American Medical Association, which showed that people who had regular cardiology care actually *increased* the frequency of their angina 165% and also increased the dangerous narrowing of their arteries. And a 2002 article in the New England Journal of Medicine showed that patients who had arthroscopic surgery did no better than patients who had "sham" surgery (Lancet).

## Antibiotics for heart disease?

Research by Dr. Peter Salgo, associate director of the Open Heart ICU at New York Presbyterian Hospital and clinical professor of medicine and anesthesiology at Columbia University, shows that Chlamydia pneumonia (not the sexually transmitted Chlamydia), a germ that infects 50% of Americans, infects heart blood vessels and causes inflammation linked to heart disease. He proposes giving everyone over 40 years of age antibiotics to kill this germ. (So far, no one has followed his recommendations.) Taking antibiotics to treat this bug is wrong anyway. In the short-term, the bug may be killed and your heart may do better, but in the long-term, antibiotics cause *further* susceptibility to future infections because by killing off beneficial bacteria, as they do, they leave your system *more* vulnerable to future attack by bad bacteria, or Chlamydia. Nevertheless, this theory is relevant in that it supports the role of a healthy bowel bacterial environment, as created in this program, and the development of heart disease.

## Exercise crutches for high cholesterol/heart disease/stroke

Exercise can reduce stress and improve the oxygenation of your blood, and the amount of oxygen going to your heart and brain. But oxygen buffers the acids that clog arteries; it does not *eliminate* them, as this program does. Which means exercise has some heart value, but its value is limited. Also, what happens the 23 hours of the day you are not exercising? When you heal your bowel and body with this program, your heart will be oxygenated 24 hours a day, not just 23.

The problem with relying on exercise, as many of you do, to reduce your heart disease risk is that it is a crutch. In order to keep benefiting from the protective effects of exercise, you need to keep doing it all the time. This can create stress in and of itself. Also, what happens when you break your leg and can't exercise? You could be in danger if you can't use this crutch. This is especially true if you have not improved the internal health of your body.

If you exercise to the point where you have a hard time breathing, then instead of improving the oxygenation of your heart, you may reduce it, putting yourself at *greater* risk of a heart attack. (Just the other day a new client contacted me who had recently had a heart attack that occurred during a new, intense exercise program, which he now wisely avoids!) There is a reason why you are urged to check with your doctor before beginning an exercise program. If it were completely safe and helpful, this warning would not be issued.

Unfortunately, many of you exercise to this point of stress. Many of you have been led to believe, "More is always better." If you are going to exercise for its health benefits, low intense exercise is best. Exercise so that you can still talk and breathe deeply while doing it. Consider purchasing a heart rate monitor and using that to ensure that your exercise does not become too anaerobic ("robbing of oxygen").

When done correctly, exercise is a non-toxic way to help oxygenate your heart. It is still a crutch however; when your bowel and body are healthy, you won't need exercise to oxygenate your blood, heart, and brain.

## Diet crutches for high cholesterol/heart disease/stroke

As described earlier, foods high in cholesterol, or even fat, are not necessarily unhealthy and harmful to your heart; they are only unhealthy and harmful if they are acidic. Some foods that are low in cholesterol and fat, like sugar, are acidic and negatively affect your heart health, even though they have no fat or cholesterol. Other foods, like butter, are very low in acidity, so while it contains cholesterol and fat, it does not hurt your heart or health. Hydrogenated fats/trans fats, alcohol, sugar and excessive amounts of refined carbohydrates—all highly acidic substances, are also readily converted into triglycerides.

A low acid diet protects your heart, as described earlier. For example, it was found that even common distilled vinegar (which is acidic, but contains no fat or cholesterol) as found in salad dressings, condiments, and other foods, becomes *converted* into cholesterol in your body.

Therefore, the recommendations I made in Chapter 9 of *Unique Healing* apply here as well. Butter, cheese, cream, olive oil, nuts, avocadoes, vegetables, sea salt, balsamic vinegar, eggs, and fish are some of the best foods for lowering your cholesterol levels and heart disease risk as you heal your bowel and body with this program.

To completely reduce your heart disease risk, you must *eventually* eat a low protein diet. When you heal your bowel and body with this program, you will be able to eat this heart attack and stroke-preventing low protein diet without looking and feeling bad doing so. (If you *still* do not understand why this "cleansing" type of diet is close to impossible to follow when you are unhealthy, re-read my books repeatedly until you do.)

An unhealthy body is at risk of heart attack, so your dietary focus needs to be on foods that help create health, not on foods that manipulate your blood cholesterol tests in the short run.

## Eat more nuts (as long as you are not allergic to them)

In an extensive Adventist Health Study, men and women who consumed nuts four or more times per week were compared to those who rarely ate nuts. The nut-eaters lowered their risk of heart disease by 50%, and *increased their life expectancies by several years.*

The Archives of Internal Medicine (June 24, 2002) showed that men who ate nuts at least twice a week lowered their risk of heart attack by 47% and reduced the risk of general coronary heart disease by 30%.

And another study found that a diet rich in peanuts and peanut butter significantly lowered total cholesterol and LDL, the "bad" cholesterol. (American Journal of Clinical Nutrition, December 1999).

Nuts are low in acidity and easy to digest, which are qualities of a food that extend your lifespan, and reduce disease.

## The benefits of black tea for your heart

Fifteen participants aged 35 and older had mildly elevated cholesterol levels. They were either given caffeinated black tea or a caffeine-free placebo beverage five times a day for three weeks. Black tea reduced total cholesterol by 3.8% and LDL cholesterol by 7.5 % compared to the decaffeinated placebo.

Black tea is alkalinizing and coffee is acidic, *whether it is caffeinated or not*. High-acid foods contribute to heart disease, while alkalinizing foods reduce heart disease. ("Black Tea Consumption reduces total and LDL cholesterol in mildly hypercholesterolemic adults," *Journal of Nutrition*, 2003.)

## Supplement crutches

Research shows that folic acid, vitamin B-6 and vitamin B-12 helps keep homocysteine from building up in your blood. Participants who eat fruits and vegetables have higher levels of folic acid, and homocysteine, than those eating the typical diet, which is lacking in fruits and vegetables. Lower homocysteine levels have been correlated with lower rates of heart disease.

Alkalinizing minerals, like calcium, magnesium, and potassium, also lower cholesterol levels, as they bind to the acids that, if not eliminated, can trigger the production of cholesterol. A study published in the *American Journal of Clinical Nutrition* found that dieters who took 600 mg of calcium and 200 I.U. of vitamin D reduced LDL levels by 14%. Overall cholesterol was lowered by 9%. Researchers say that calcium may help prevent some fat from being absorbed, however I find it works by buffering the acids in your blood that contribute to the excess production of cholesterol by your liver in the first place.

A study published in 2006 titled the "Coronary Artery Risk Development in Young Adults Study" (CARDIA) found that magnesium might cut the risk of conditions linked to heart disease and diabetes. At the end of a 15-year study of 4,.637 participants it was found that those in the top fourth in magnesium intake had a 31% lower risk of developing three or more of these conditions than those in the lowest fourth.

In 2003 scientists tracked 5,600 adults for 4-8 years and found that those who didn't eat enough potassium were 1.5 to 2.5 times more likely to suffer from a stroke, even if they were on medications to help prevent one.

Other popular supplements that have been recommended over the years to reduce blood cholesterol levels are red yeast rice, lecithin, and niacin.

It is extraordinarily more helpful and life saving, however, to eliminate the acids that trigger cholesterol, heart disease, and stroke, than to simply buffer them with supplements. It is much better to get the trash out of your house, as this program does, than to simply spray it with perfume, as these supplements do. However, if you insist on taking additional supplements, I strongly recommend *Unique healing Calcium Citrate* (see Chapter 5 for more information on its use.)

## If possible, use these non-toxic crutches

Exercise, diet, and supplement crutches for high cholesterol levels, *except* for high protein diet crutches, are preferable to using drugs and surgery for heart health, as the former are not toxic and harmful to your body.

If a nontoxic crutch reduces your cholesterol levels and prevents you from taking a toxic drug or having invasive surgery, even though it is only a crutch, it has served a valuable purpose.

Nevertheless, they are still crutches that treat the symptoms and not the cause of your problem. They are crutches that have the same problems that all other crutches do.

## It's not about genetics

If you have tried diet and exercise to reduce your cholesterol and they have failed, this *does not* mean that your high cholesterol is due to genetics and unavoidable (a conclusion that is often made when these crutches do not work.)

Diet and exercise are crutches, and crutches don't always help, that is true. Healing your body and bowel does.

If you have "tried everything" to reduce your cholesterol without success, I am positive that you have not followed the approach in this book.

# Success with High Cholesterol/Heart Disease/Stroke

"I was told that I had 'genetically high cholesterol,' but this program lowered my cholesterol levels!"

"My cholesterol went down 30 points in three months."

"My cholesterol went form 218 to 172 from last year to last month."

"My cholesterol was at 214 and my bowels were not well formed. Donna told me that once they got slower and firmer my cholesterol would go down. I didn't believe this and I didn't understand this, but sure enough, when I had my test re-done I was constipated and my cholesterol was at 187."

"A heart scan showed that my arteries were 60% clogged. I am now told that they are completely clear."

"I got off my cholesterol-lowering drugs and haven't needed them since."

"I took red yeast rice, exercised, ate no butter or eggs, and my cholesterol was still really high. Donna had me take a lot of bentonite and had me eat a lot of eggs and butter, which was scary, but it worked. My cholesterol went down to the lowest it has been in 5 years."

In the last 18 years, I have never had a client die from a heart attack or stroke while I was working with them.

## Watch my Video, "Why THIS Program Eliminates High Cholesterol/Heart Disease/Stroke"

This video, and all of my videos, can be found at *www.UniqueHealing. com* or at *www.YouTube.com/UniqueHealing*.

## Chronic Fatigue Syndrome
See "Autoimmune Diseases"

## Circulatory Problems
See also "Blood Pressure"

## Cirrhosis
See "Liver Disease"

## Coffee Addictions
See "Addictions"

## Cold hands/feet
See "Circulatory Problems"

## Colds
See "Viral Infections"

# Colitis
See "Bowel Conditions"

# Colon Polyps
See "Bowel Conditions"

# Constipation
(See also "Bowel Conditions")

Constipation is a condition that causes great anguish among many of my clients. While this can cause physical discomfort, it causes even greater mental and emotional discomfort, or stress.

Ironically, while constipation is not ideal elimination, this state is much healthier, and you eliminate more symptom, addiction, weight, and disease-causing acids, than when your bowels are daily but your stools are not very well-formed, which is the state that most clients (and most of you) present themselves in. Yet this does not create nearly the same degree of anxiety as constipation does. Wrongly, you have been told to fear constipation. You have been told that it is harmful, but you have not been told that your daily, not perfectly-formed stools are even *more* harmful.

I consistently find that when a client is overweight, has headaches, skin problems, etc., these are very much improved when they enter the "constipated stage" (If you have frequent but poorly formed stools when you start this program, you will likely experience constipation "on the road to improvement." Review Chapters 6 and 7 of *Unique Healing* to better understand this). For clients who present themselves with a fear of constipation, sometimes I can't say this enough to ease their fears. So I urge you to read this section and watch my videos on constipation over and over again until you "get it."

On the other hand, constipation is not ideal elimination, and in this state, there is a re-absorption of acids, leading to symptoms, addictions, disease, and weight gain. So while it should not evoke the fear that it does, it should evoke action on your part to correct it. This program eliminates constipation in a way that laxatives, colon cleansing products, etc. cannot, and it eliminates acids in a way that these cannot, either.

Constipation was covered extensively in *Unique Healing* in Chapter 6. For more information on it, refer to this section of my book.

# Healing Your Body With This Program Eliminates Constipation

Un-formed acids cause constipation.

When the acids in your bowel are not completely formed into a stool, the result is a stool that is too small, too large, and/or too hard to easily "push out" when your bowel squeezes (an action called peristalsis). Every morning your bowel squeezes gently, but if the stool is small, it won't "find" it when this squeezing action occurs. Or, if the stool is too hard or large, this gentle squeezing action will not be strong enough to eliminate it.

Ideally, all of the acids in your bowel should be formed into a stool, resulting in stools that are "banana-like" and neither too hard, too small, or too hard. This type of stool easily "comes out of you" when your bowel squeezes in the morning.

This program eliminates acids from your body so that your bowel is not "overwhelmed" with them. Stools that are too small, hard, and/or large occur when there are too many acids in your bowel that are not being formed into a stool, and this program eliminates acids so that these "constipating" stools do not occur.

## Healing Your Bowel With This Program Eliminates Constipation

In addition to its many other important functions, a healthy bacterial environment in your bowel is a necessity for the formation of stools in your bowel/absorption of acids. When your stools are well-formed, you will not be constipated.

## Why My Crutches Work for Constipation

***Body Bentonite*** binds to acids (toxins, heavy metals, chemicals, etc.). It forms acids into a stool that is very easy for your body to eliminate, resulting in effortless, daily elimination.

***Unique Healing Calcium Citrate*** is an alkalinizing mineral that helps neutralize the acids that your bowel does not form into a stool, thereby reducing the stress to your bowel, and increasing the ability of it to form acids. (Sometimes calcium is called "constipating" but remember, when something constipates you it is because prior to using it, you had an even worse condition of frequent but poorly formed stools, and this constipation is a step in the right direction of looking and feeling better. Also, remember that if something constipates you, taking *more* of this substance will improve your stools and therefore *reduce* your constipation, not make it worse. If something takes you from "point A" to "point B" then more of it will get you to "point C"—where healthy, un-constipated stools exist.)

### How much do I take?/Questions about using these

See Chapter 5 for information on using these crutches, including recommendations on the amount to use, as well as a discussion of the misunderstandings about the particular crutch that may, if not understood correctly, cause you to fail to look and feel better while you heal your bowel and body with this program.

### How long will I need to use crutches for my constipation?

Constipation occurs at Level 4 of your pipe. It is the last area of your body to heal (assuming that other areas are unhealthy too). Refer to the diagram "Sequence of Healing" in Appendix A at the end of this book to better understand this concept, as well as to Chapter 1 under this subject heading.

## Misunderstandings About Constipation and Other Information for Your Success

### Keep your stools well-formed

Because un-formed acids cause constipation, you will suffer from the least amount of constipation if you keep your stools well-formed while you are healing your bowel and body.

If you do not have a very good handle on how to define well-formed stools, review Chapter 6 of *Unique Healing* now. (And remember, when your stools are hard and slow you are eliminating more acids, and will therefore feel better, than when your stools are one or more times a day but not all extremely well-formed.)

If your stools are not well-formed, the following changes can help: increase your *Body Bentoni*te intake; reduce your carbohydrate intake (pasta, breads, grains, cereals, yogurt, etc.); reduce your sugar intake (including natural healthy sugars such as agave, honey, raw sugar, cane juice, etc.); reduce your alcohol, salt, coffee, and/or soda intake; do not have a massage, chiropractic adjustment, or any other body work; drink a lot of water; rest; and keep your exercise aerobic (see Chapter 4 for more information on how to attain this, and why it is important.)

If these changes do not noticeably help the form of your stools in two days, take them further (i.e. take more *Body Bentonite*, reduce your carbohydrate intake more, etc.)

Out of all of these recommendations, increasing your *Body Bentonite* intake is one of the most productive and helpful. It heals your body, unlike many of the other recommendations. It will do the most to lead you to a place where looking and feeling good is effortless, and some of the other suggestions, such as reducing sugar intake, are simply "too hard to do when your blood is too acidic."

(Note: the exception to this information is when your poorly formed stools are caused by an infection, in which case *Unique Healing Colloidal Silver* is needed to reduce your symptoms. Refer to Chapter 5 for information on when and how to use this crutch.)

## If you are constipated, take *more Body Bentonite,* not less!

Because un-formed acids cause constipation, and because *Body Bentonite* helps form up acids, your constipation will improve if you *increase* the amount of *Body Bentonite* you take, contrary to what may seem instinctual to you in this situation. (It usually takes a doubling of the current amount to experience an improvement.)

Often when a client experiences constipation and reduces their *Body Bentonite* (wrongly, but understandably), they become very confused and frustrated when the desired and expected result—better bowels and fewer symptoms or weight—does not happen. They expect it to happen because they think the *Body Bentonite* is "too strong," and therefore they expect that things will improve with less. This is not the case.

On the other hand, if you increase *Body Bentonite* and your constipation does not improve, consider that you have made other changes at the same time (i.e. changed your diet, had a massage) or that there is another reason you are constipated (i.e. your diet is too high in protein, you are taking muscle relaxants, etc.). In this later case, see the section later on laxative use.

## Your bowels will not become too infrequent as you heal

Healing your bowel will not produce very infrequent bowel movements, or bowels that move only every two days or longer.

If your bowel movements are one or more times a day and not well-formed when you start this program, they will become slower and better formed as you heal, as described earlier, but they will not become very infrequent. You will not miss more than one day in a row of elimination

Frequent bowel movements depend in part on the contraction, or peristalsis, of your bowel. This is an automatic reaction that occurs daily. A few scenarios can cause this peristalsis to be hampered, however, causing very infrequent bowel movements, and include: the use of muscle relaxants and some medications, travelling/time changes, severe illness, and/or surgery.

## Formed acids are not re-absorbed so don't strain to eliminate

Many of you have been taught since a young age that you have to go to the bathroom, or else! Many of you have been conditioned to fear not going, and many of you therefore force yourself to go as much as possible.

There is no value in forcing yourself to go to the bathroom, only discomfort and stress. When you are constipated, some of the acids in your bowel have been formed into a stool. *These will not be re-absorbed*; they will eventually come out of you. You do not need to force this to happen, and in fact, this force can cause hemorrhoids or other discomforts.

## Use a laxative if needed

If you are very concerned about your constipation, uncomfortable, or are suffering from hemorrhoids, a natural laxative may be used. The laxative I recommend is magnesium. Start with 500 mg, increasing to 1,000 mg if this does not help, or reducing or stopping this if your stools become too frequent or loose. Magnesium and most laxatives provide relief usually in 12 hours or so. If you need immediate relief, an enema is your best solution. If you frequently suffer from constipation, you should be able to figure out an amount of magnesium to use on a daily basis to prevent this from occurring until your body and bowel are healthy enough that constipation no longer occurs.

But remember, while laxatives like magnesium (and senna, cascara sagrada, aloe, etc.) may help you "go,' they do nothing to heal your bowel or body. They do nothing to make you healthier. They do nothing to form acids and prevent them from being re-absorbed into your body (leading to symptoms, weight problems, addictions, and disease.) They do not help eliminate acids, and they will not add years to your life.

## High protein diets and constipation

High protein, low carbohydrate diets can be constipating because they reduce your body's cleansing process, which means they slow down the movement of acids, or trash, that enters your bowel. They tend to "keep it in your cells/organs." If no or few acids enter your bowel, no stools can be formed, and therefore there will be none to eliminate when your bowel squeezes in the morning. If there is no trash in your trashcan when the trash man comes, because you did not clean your house, the trash man will skip your house on trash collection day!

Excess dietary protein is likely responsible for the largest number of cases of prolonged constipation in this country, or going more than one day without having a bowel movement.

## Cheese and constipation

Cheese is extremely easy to digest, very low in acidity, and it does not cleanse acids from your organs into your blood and bowel. Some people avoid eating it because they have heard that it is constipating. If you experience harder or less frequent stools when eating cheese, it is because prior to eating it, your stools were frequent and poorly formed. Frequent and poorly formed stools are worse than harder or less frequent ones. *Constipation is a good thing if you previously experienced poorly formed stools.* In other words, the consumption of cheese has *improved,* not worsened, your elimination.

## Your colon will not become impacted

There is sometimes great concern that the use of *Body Bentonite* will cause one's colon to become impacted with stool. People sometimes visualize the clay clogging their colon.

This is not how clay, or bentonite, works. It will not clog your colon. (Please do be sure, however, to drink adequate water when you take it. It is advised that you drink 8 ounces of water with every 10 capsules of *Body Bentonite.*)

At one point when I was ill, I was put on a *high protein diet*, and during this time, I ended up in the emergency room with an impacted colon. *I was not taking bentonite at the time.* Knowing what I do now, had I been taking it aggressively, I never would have landed in this position.

For many years I have recommended amounts of bentonite to clients that are considered extraordinarily large. I have not had a single client experience an impacted colon as a result.

(For more misunderstandings about constipation, see Chapter 6 of *Unique Healing*.)

# Success With Constipation

"I started working with Donna to help my 4 year old son, who suffered from chronic constipation. We went to many doctors and even therapists, who told us it was "all in his head." This was very stressful, and the approaches they advised us on did not work, anyway. Now that he has been doing this program, his constipation is gone and the stress of this is out of our lives."

"I had daily, but very difficult, hard stools. I came to Donna because I had daily headaches and was always bloated, and she told me this would go away when the constipation went away. With this program, I no longer am constipated, and as Donna told me, I also no longer have headaches or bloating."

## My story

"I suffered from constipation my entire life. I was constipated for many years before I became ill, and I was constipated for years after I became ill. I tried every remedy in the book. I took lots of fiber, laxatives, ate handfuls of prunes, and did numerous enemas and colonics. For years, I took massive amount of colon cleansing products. None of these remedies worked. Some of them gave me cramps and loose stools, but this did not feel good, and I knew this was not how things should be. This program eliminated my constipation."

## Watch My Video, "Why THIS Program Eliminates Constipation."

Watch this video, as well as, "Stop Freaking Out About Constipation" at *www.YouTube,com/UniqueHealing*. You can also access this directly from my website at *www.UniqueHealing.com*.

# COPD (chronic obstructive pulmonary disorder)
See "Asthma/Lung Disorders"

# Copper Toxicity
See "Heavy Metal Toxicity"

# Crohn's Disease
See "Bowel Disorders"

# Cystic Fibrosis
See "Bacterial Infections"

# Cystitis
See "Urinary Problems"

# Depression
See "Mental Health"

# Dental Problems
## Cavities, Gum Disease, Infections, and Others

Modern dentistry relies heavily on crutches to treat dental problems, as modern medicine relies on crutches to treat health problems. Both recommend crutches that can cause these problems to worsen over the long-term. Also, when you have a cavity and get it filled, does anyone ever stop to ask what caused that cavity in the first place? (Likewise, when you have appendicitis, for example, does anyone ever stop and ask what caused this in the first place?)

Like many doctors, many dentists make you believe that their procedures are the only available for your teeth, and that problems like cavities and receding gums are the result of stress, old age, bad luck, or other variables that you cannot change or control.

The health of your teeth and gums is 100% in your control.

## A Healthy Body Eliminates Dental Problems

Alkaline minerals, like calcium, are found in large amounts in your teeth. Un-eliminated acids deplete your teeth of these minerals (as your body uses alkaline minerals like calcium to buffer un-eliminated acids), causing your teeth to become weak, unhealthy and decayed. Healing your body with this program eliminates the acids that cause these minerals, and your teeth, to become depleted.

Healing your body with this program also eliminates the acids that reduce circulation and oxygenation. Like all tissues of your body, your gums, and teeth, need adequate blood and oxygen to be healthy.

## A Healthy Bowel Eliminates Dental Problems

A healthy bacterial environment in your bowel prevents the growth of the bad bacteria that cause cavities, infection, and tartar buildup. Tartar is a build-up of bad bacteria. And a healthy bowel bacterial environment makes it easier for your bowel to digest dairy products, allowing you to benefit from the calcium they provide.

In addition to its many other important functions, a healthy bacterial environment in your bowel is a necessity for the complete elimination of acids (toxins, heavy metals, pesticides, etc.) from your body. A healthy bowel prevents the re-absorption of acids into your blood that cause unhealthy teeth and gums.

## Why My Crutches Eliminate Dental Problems

***Body Bentonite*** binds to and eliminates acids (toxins, heavy metals, chemicals, etc.) from your body. It helps prevent them from becoming re-absorbed into your bloodstream, where they trigger a response by your body to protect you from them. It eliminates the acids that deplete your body of the minerals your teeth need to be healthy, that reduce blood flow/circulation and oxygenation, resulting in healthier teeth and gums.

***Unique Healing Calcium Citrate*** is an alkalinizing mineral that helps neutralize the acids that your bowel does not eliminate. When these acids are neutralized, your body does not need to "use up" oxygen to buffer them. Also, your teeth cannot become healthy overnight. You can quickly eliminate problems due to excess acids in your blood, like receding and bleeding gums, and problems due to infections, but the ill health of your teeth is the result of a large quantity of un-eliminated acids, and it will take some time to eliminate these. To make up for the loss of calcium that may have occurred to weaken them, I advise the use of *Unique Healing Calcium Citrate* (2,400 mg/day) for 6-12 months while you are healing your bowel and body with this program.

**Unique Healing Colloidal Silver** has natural anti-bacterial, anti-fungal, anti-parasitic properties. It eliminates the bacterial infections that cause cavities, infection, and tartar build-up.

**Unique Healing Methyl Vitamin B-12** provides your body with easy to assimilate levels of this nutrient, which can reduce sugar, coffee, alcohol, nicotine and other cravings, reducing your consumption of acidic items that damage your teeth and gums.

## How much do I take?/Questions about using these

See Chapter 5 for information on using these crutches, including recommendations on the amount to use, as well as a discussion of the misunderstandings about the particular crutch that may, if not understood correctly, cause you to fail to look and feel better while you heal your bowel and body with this program.

## How long will I need to use crutches for my dental problems?

This condition occurs at Levels 3 and 4 of your pipe. They are the second to last and last area of your body to heal (assuming that other areas are unhealthy too). Refer to the diagram "Sequence of Healing" in Appendix A at the end of this book to better understand this concept, as well as to Chapter 1 under this subject heading.

Some dental problems, like unhealthy teeth, are caused by large accumulations of acidity/degeneration. There are no crutches for degenerative conditions and accumulations of acidity in your organs. Crutches can offset the effects of acids in your blood, or the effects of poor function of your bowel bacterial environment (as these can be quickly altered), but degeneration is caused by depletion and damage to your organs, and organs take time to heal.

# Misunderstandings About Dental Problems and Other Information for Your Success

## Keep your stools well-formed

Because teeth and gum problems are caused in part by un-eliminated acids, and because well-formed stools prevent the re-absorption of acids into your blood, you will suffer from the least amount of problems with your teeth and gums if you keep your stools well-formed while you are healing your bowel and body.

If you do not have a very good handle on how to define well-formed stools, review Chapter 6 of *Unique Healing* now. (And remember, when your stools are hard and slow you are eliminating more acids, and will therefore feel better, than when your stools are one or more times a day but not all extremely well-formed.)

If your stools are not well-formed, the following changes can help: increase your *Body Bentonite* intake; reduce your carbohydrate intake (pasta, breads, grains, cereals, yogurt, etc.); reduce your sugar intake (including natural healthy sugars such as agave, honey, raw sugar, cane juice, etc.); reduce your alcohol, salt, coffee, and/or soda intake; do not have a massage, chiropractic adjustment, or any other body work; drink a lot of water; rest; and keep your exercise aerobic (see Chapter 4 for more information on how to attain this, and why it is important.)

If these changes do not noticeably help the form of your stools in two days, take them further (i.e. take more *Body Bentonite*, reduce your carbohydrate intake more, etc.)

Out of all of these recommendations, increasing your *Body Bentonite* intake is one of the most productive and helpful. It heals your body, unlike many of the other recommendations. It will do the most to lead you to a place where looking and feeling good is effortless, and some of the other suggestions, such as reducing sugar intake, are simply "too hard to do when your blood is too acidic."

(Note: the exception to this information is when your poorly formed stools are caused by an infection, in which case *Unique Healing Colloidal Silver* is needed to reduce your symptoms. Refer to Chapter 5 for information on when and how to use this crutch.)

## It is not just acidic foods like sugar that cause dental problems

Many of you are aware that sugar is bad for your teeth, but there are many other acidic foods, and beverages, that can damage your teeth and gums. (Just as there are many other acidic substances other than alcohol that can damage your liver, etc.)

Excess acids in your blood can cause many dental problems, as discussed above, but acids in your blood come from *new* acids from foods like sugar, vinegar, salt, coffee, and alcohol (as well as from chemicals, metals, pollutants, stresses, etc.), and from *old* acids that are moved into your blood by a cleansing diet. Eating fruit, yogurt, carbohydrates (even gluten-free ones), can increase the acidic load in your blood, as they cause stored acids to move into your blood faster than you can eliminate them, and these foods can therefore also contribute to dental problems.

Healing your bowel and body with this program eliminates the new *and* old acids from your blood that trigger many dental problems.

## Get a second opinion

When my son was eight years old, he had x-rays taken and the dentist proclaimed with absolute conviction that his permanent teeth were coming in perfectly straight and that he would in no way need braces when he was older. Even without the x-rays, this seemed obvious to me. When I looked at his teeth coming in, the spacing and bite looked perfect. One and a half years later we went to a new dentist (because of new dental insurance) and this dentist stated, with absolute conviction, that my son would definitely need braces (and he then handed me the business card of an orthodontist). I was suspicious. I told him that was odd, since the last dentist was 100% convinced he would not. This new dentist simply stared at me and offered no response. We never went back to him. Since writing this, my son has turned sixteen and his teeth have grown in straight, and he has never needed braces.

When my mother moved to Boulder she went to three different dentists who gave her three different reports on her teeth and the work that needed to be done.

If you do go to a dentist and expensive procedures are recommended, especially if this is stated as though you have no choice in the matter, seek a second opinion. You are encouraged to do this with medicine, but many of you do not. Even fewer of you do so with dentistry, but you should do it then, too.

## Get your mercury fillings replaced, if you have to

When I was ill, I took thousands of supplements and tried numerous alternative methods to heal my body and feel better. None of it worked. Early on, a nutritionist said that my failure to respond was due to the mercury from my fillings. I had a lot of fillings and so this made some sense to me. Deep down, I didn't think it was going to cure all of my problems, but I went ahead and had them removed anyway, as I was desperate and hoped it would help. I felt no better after having done this, but I *did* suffer through pain, a root canal, tooth sensitivity for two years, a crown, and the expenditure of a lot of money that I did not have.

To date, I've seen the same poor results in clients who have also traveled this path.

Some dentists state that removing these fillings cure people of disease, but I completely disagree. These dentists also commonly put their patients on large quantities of nutrient/vitamin and diet crutches, so is it the nutrients and diet, or the removal of the mercury that sometimes produces improvements in one's symptoms? I suggest to you that it is the crutches.

Mercury is toxic. I would never put mercury fillings in my teeth again, and I am glad they're out. Mercury is but one of thousands of highly toxic ingredients that an unhealthy body can store; removing just one of these toxins from your mouth isn't enough to heal your body. Additionally, much of the mercury in these fillings has already leached into your organs anyway. You are simply eliminating further leaching when you have your old fillings removed, but this does nothing to eliminate the accumulated mercury that has already settled in your tissues/organs.

Nevertheless, mercury fillings do not last a lifetime. If your fillings are old, I suggest that you wait until they *need* to be replaced before doing so, and then replace them with a non-toxic filling.

Your fillings do not need to be replaced in order to heal your bowel and body; this program will work even in the presence of them.

> Mercury and other highly toxic heavy metals that have become stored in your body are eliminated from your body when you heal your bowel and body with this program.

(For more information on how this program eliminates heavy metal toxicity, see this heading later in this chapter.)

## Fluoridation

Fluoride helps offset acids in your mouth, and reducing these acids reduces tooth and gum decay.

The problem with fluoride treatments is that there is great controversy over the use of fluoride for improving the health of your teeth, and while I have read about the toxicity and harm of it over the years, I am no expert in it.

The safest way to protect your teeth and gums is by creating a healthy bowel and body. There are no risks involved in this.

## Alternative dentistry

An "alternative dentist" usually avoids using mercury fillings, may recommend supplement crutches, and will avoid the use of toxic dental ingredients, like many common toothpaste products.

If possible, find a dentist like this, but keep in mind that they still rely on crutches for dental health, and do not address the cause of your problems. They will not know how to heal your bowel and body.

## Dentistry offers some useful crutches

While modern dentistry relies on crutches, and uses some toxic procedures, like Novocain, x-rays, and fluoride, which can make your dental health worse in the long—term, it also promotes some actions that help prevent tooth decay and gum disease. Flossing, brushing your teeth, and having your teeth cleaned professionally are safe crutches that can help keep your mouth healthy until your healthy bowel and body can do this for you on its own.

On the other hand, while flossing your teeth improves the circulation to your gums, for example, a healthy body that eliminates the acids that reduce circulation does this job much better, and it doesn't require you to floss all the time.

Do you think we were put here on earth with toothpaste and dental floss?

# Success With Dental Problems

"My eight year old son has been doing this program with me for the last two years, and he has never had a cavity."

"At my last visit to my dentist he was shocked by the health of my teeth. The hygienist used to scrap a lot of tartar off of them, and my gums bled a lot during this, too. This time, there was hardly any tartar and my gums barely bled. I anticipate that I will save a lot of money on dental bills in the future!"

"I just wanted to tell you how much I appreciate your wisdom and insight. As you suggested, I took the Colloidal Silver and it really helped me. I have had very little tooth/gum pain since I took it and my endodontist decided to hold off on the oral surgery. Pretty cool, huh?! "

## My story

I'm a bad dental patient. I visit the dentist approximately once every four years or longer for a cleaning (last visit was about six years ago). I brush my teeth only one time a day and I rarely floss, but my gums are healthy, and I have had no new cavities or any other problems with my teeth since healing my bowel and body with this program.

## Watch my Video,
## "Why THIS Program Eliminates Dental Problems"
This video, and all of my videos, can be found at *www.UniqueHealing.com* or at *www.YouTube.com/UniqueHealing*.

# Diabetes and Hypoglycemia
(See also "Adrenal Disorders")

Hypoglycemia, or *low* blood sugar, is implicated in a large number of health conditions, including but not limited to: overweight, fatigue, headaches, allergic reactions, depression, irritability, insomnia, heart palpitations, poor vision, dizziness, anxiety, excessive sweating, decreased sex drive, and others.

Diabetes, or *high* blood sugar, is also implicated in a number of health conditions, including but not limited to: excessive thirst, frequent urination, fatigue, weight loss or weight gain, blurred vision, slow healing, frequent infections, tingling in hands/feet, dry itchy skin, and others.

Adult-onset diabetes is more prevalent than juvenile diabetes (also known as "Type 1") diabetes. (The lifetime risk of developing diabetes for a person born in 2000 is estimated to be about 33% for men and 40% for women.)

Just as diarrhea and constipation are both caused by an unhealthy bowel and body, and are much more similar than they sound, so too is the case with diabetes and hypoglycemia. These conditions are *both* the product of an unhealthy bowel and body, too.

Like many other conditions, the incidence of diabetes keeps increasing. Over the last three decades, the number of cases of diabetes has doubled, and worse yet, the number of children diagnosed with it has increased as well.

### Juvenile versus adult-onset diabetes

Your pancreas produces insulin, which, along with your liver and adrenal glands, helps regulate your blood sugar levels. Juvenile diabetes is an autoimmune disease that is blamed on an inherit weakness in your pancreas, causing it to dysfunction. When your pancreas cannot produce insulin, blood sugar levels cannot be regulated. This condition commonly occurs in young children and teens, and can lead to blindness, kidney failure, heart disease and amputations.

Adult-onset diabetes usually occurs later in life, and it is generally thought to be less dangerous than juvenile diabetes. In this case, a lifetime of unhealthy living (i.e. too many acids) damages your blood-sugar regulating organs. It is generally thought that adult-onset diabetes can be controlled, while juvenile diabetes is out of your control. (I disagree.)

Adult-onset diabetes often occurs only after your body has fought many years of low blood sugar. Just as low blood pressure usually precedes high blood pressure and constipation usually precedes diarrhea, hypoglycemia usually precedes diabetes.

You are generally much healthier if you have hypoglycemia than if you have diabetes.

## Healing Your Body With this Program Eliminates Diabetes and Hypoglycemia

When carbohydrates are eaten, they are converted into glucose, and then turned into ATP, which provides your body with energy. Excess glucose is stored in your liver and muscles in the form of glycogen, which is used to regulate your blood sugar levels if they ever become too low. Your pancreas regulates insulin, which also helps to control your blood sugar levels.

To maintain proper blood sugar levels this system of storage and re-conversion of glycogen to glucose must work properly, and the proper amount of insulin needs to be secreted. Proper function depends on a healthy pancreas, liver, and adrenal glands. Healing your body with this program heals these organs.

The delivery of glucose to your cells and the secretion of insulin are affected by the pH of your blood. The more acidic your blood is, the more disturbed your blood sugar will be.

## Healing Your Bowel With This Program Eliminates Diabetes and Hypoglycemia

Fiber has been shown to increase insulin sensitivity (reduce blood sugar problems). A high fiber diet is well tolerated when your bowel bacterial environment is healthy.

In 2006 researchers from the Joslin Diabetes Center in Boston and Washington University in St. Louis were able to cure diabetes in some mice by giving them a substance called Complete Freund's Adjuvant (CFA), which contains dead tuberculosis *bacteria* and hyper activates certain immune cells. This *implies* a connection between the health of your bowel bacteria and the ability to cure diabetes.

In addition to its many other important functions, a healthy bacterial environment in your bowel is a necessity for the complete elimination of acids (toxins, heavy metals, pesticides, etc.) from your body. A healthy bowel prevents the re-absorption of acids into your blood that cause a disruption in insulin regulation, and damage to your pancreas, liver, and adrenal glands.

## Why My Crutches Eliminate Diabetes and Hypoglycemia

***Body Bentonite*** binds to and eliminates acids (toxins, heavy metals, chemicals, etc.) from your body. It helps prevent them from becoming re-absorbed into your bloodstream, where they disrupt insulin production and regulation, and damage your pancreas, liver, and adrenal glands.

***Unique Healing Calcium Citrate*** is an alkalinizing mineral that helps neutralize the acids that your bowel does not eliminate. When these acids are neutralized, they no longer disrupt insulin levels.

## How much do I take?/Questions about using these

See Chapter 5 for information on using these crutches, including recommendations on the amount to use, as well as a discussion of the misunderstandings about the particular crutch that may, if not understood correctly, cause you to fail to look and feel better while you heal your bowel and body with this program.

## How long will I need to use crutches for my diabetes or hypoglycemia?

Diabetes and hypoglycemia occur at Level 2 of your pipe. It is the second area of your body to heal (assuming that other areas are unhealthy too). Refer to the diagram "Sequence of Healing" in Appendix A at the end of this book to better understand this concept, as well as to Chapter 1 under this subject heading.

# Misunderstandings About Diabetes and Hypoglycemia and other Information for Your Success

### Keep your stools well-formed

Because diabetes and hypoglycemia are caused in part by un-eliminated acids, and because well-formed stools prevent the re-absorption of acids into your blood, you will suffer the least from these conditions if you keep your stools well-formed while you are healing your bowel and body.

If you do not have a very good handle on how to define well-formed stools, review Chapter 6 of *Unique Healing* now. (And remember, when your stools are hard and slow you are eliminating more acids, and will therefore feel better, than when your stools are one or more times a day but not all extremely well-formed.)

If your stools are not well-formed, the following changes can help: increase your *Body Bentonite* intake; reduce your carbohydrate intake (pasta, breads, grains, cereals, yogurt, etc.); reduce your sugar intake (including natural healthy sugars such as agave, honey, raw sugar, cane juice, etc.); reduce your alcohol, salt, coffee, and/or soda intake; do not have a massage, chiropractic adjustment, or any other body work; drink a lot of water; rest; and keep your exercise aerobic (see Chapter 4 for more information on how to attain this, and why it is important.)

If these changes do not noticeably help the form of your stools in two days, take them further (i.e. take more *Body Bentonite*, reduce your carbohydrate intake more, etc.)

Out of all of these recommendations, increasing your *Body Bentonite* intake is one of the most productive and helpful. It heals your body, unlike many of the other recommendations. It will do the most to lead you to a place where looking and feeling good is effortless, and some of the other suggestions, such as reducing sugar intake, are simply "too hard to do when your blood is too acidic."

(Note: the exception to this information is when your poorly formed stools are caused by an infection, in which case *Unique Healing Colloidal Silver* is needed to reduce your symptoms. Refer to Chapter 5 for information on when and how to use this crutch.)

## Another lousy blood test

Blood tests for hypoglycemia are very unreliable, as *all* blood tests are. When your blood becomes too acidic, this impairs your blood sugar levels. Your body will do all it can to try to regulate this low blood sugar imbalance, leading to a normal blood sugar level on a blood test, but the result of regulating this causes symptoms, which are then ignored or deemed irrelevant by a medical doctor checking for low blood sugar.

For example, when your blood sugar levels are low, your adrenal glands may secrete extra adrenaline to stimulate the release of sugar/glycogen into your blood, so your blood sugar level looks normal on a test, but the adrenaline can cause anxiety and nervousness. You may crave sugar when your blood sugar is low, and the consumption of this can increase your blood sugar levels on your test, leading your doctor to pronounce you in good health (and often declaring this state of hypoglycemia as "nonsense").

Like all blood tests, your organs may be very unhealthy, but your blood test can miss this. They do not measure the health of your organs.

## Low blood sugar often precedes high blood sugar, or diabetes

After many years of low blood sugar and damage to your liver, adrenal glands, and pancreas from un-eliminated acids, these organs may become less able to regulate your blood sugar levels. At this point, your blood tests may finally show there is a problem, and by then, it is often labeled as diabetes. When you have hypoglycemia these organs are unhealthy; your body's ability to regulate your blood sugar levels is impaired. When you have diabetes, they are even unhealthier; your body's ability to regulate your blood sugar levels is even *more* impaired.

Blood tests for diabetes are more accurate than those for hypoglycemia, as diabetes represents a state of greater ill health, and it often takes a greater level of ill health before problems/imbalances show up on your blood test.

## Related to alcoholism, sugar cravings, nicotine cravings, and caffeine cravings

Alcohol, sugar, nicotine, and caffeine can all be very desirable when you have low blood sugar, as in one way or another, they all increase blood sugar levels. This can lead to addictions (see the earlier section on "Addictions" for more information.)

## Sugar cravings are not always caused by blood sugar problems

On the other hand, some practitioners wrongly diagnose *all* sugar cravings as being the result of low blood sugar, or hypoglycemia, and then recommend supplement crutches, like adrenal glandulars, to treat these.

Sugar cravings are not always due to low blood sugar problems, however. They can be the result of low energy, and a craving for the energy burst that eating sugar provides to your brain and muscles. In some cases, low levels of vitamin B-12 cause sugar cravings, and *Unique Healing Methyl Vitamin B-12* is needed/valuable to reduce them. (Many of my clients have commented that when they take it, they notice a significant reduction in their desire for stimulating and sugar-producing substances, like sugar, coffee, soda, etc.)

## Desire for sugar is a sign of ill health

With this program, all of your organs and glands are healed, and one-day, your craving, or interest, in sugar will noticeably decline. Clients are often shocked when this happens. And it happens all the time. It is a very empowering experience; it puts *you* in control of what you eat.

When your blood sugar levels are in balance, these sugar-raising items (like sugary foods, sodas, alcohol, nicotine, etc.), take it out of balance, and you feel worse, not better, when you ingest them. Initially, your brain may "remember" the pleasant experiences your brain and body felt when you corrected your low blood sugar problems with the consumption of sugar (or alcohol, coffee, cigarettes/nicotine, etc.), even when your body "no longer wants them." Eventually, your brain will be re-programmed to associate the intake of these substances with negative experiences, and you will find avoiding them is effortless.

I am an ex-alcoholic who craved sugar, and alcohol, which acts like sugar, all the time. I completely eliminated these cravings, and so can you.

## Tolerance of sugar is also a sign of ill health

If you can eat large quantities of sugar and feel fine doing so, you are not healthy (just as you are not healthy if you can drink large quantities of alcohol and feel fine the next day).

When you eat a highly acidic food like sugar, it should take your blood chemistry out of balance, and into an uncomfortable state.

It is the people who can eat vast quantities of sugar and not react that are the unhealthiest.

## You will become more sensitive to sugar intake as you heal

Sugar is acidic, and cleansing. When you eat sugar, your blood becomes more acidic. In a state of ill health, this acidity may disturb the "top of your pipe;" it may clog your arteries, and while this is dangerous, it produces no symptoms of discomfort.

As you become healthier, your organs of elimination become more reactive to acids in your blood. As you unclog your pipe, the trash in it dumps into the bottom of your pipe. When your organs of elimination react to these acids, this produces more discomfort (albeit it is much safer) than when your arteries respond to them. So early in this program, the acids created from eating sugar might be clogging your arteries, but later on, as you become healthier, your skin will begin reacting to them, which can result in symptoms like acne (but no clogging of your arteries).

This reaction may be frustrating, but it is very valuable. It reflects a healthier body than you had before, and the physical annoyance caused at this point creates a situation where your body begins to find unhealthy foods, like sugar, unappealing.

## Low blood sugar is not caused by inadequate protein intake either

High protein diets are a common recommendation made for blood sugar problems, but these are dangerous crutches to use for this, and *any*, condition. Over time they make you less healthy; they make your organs less healthy, which are, ironically and sadly, supposed to keep your blood sugar stable in the first place!

A high protein diet stops the movement of acids from your organs into your blood, and as described earlier, a lack of acidity in your blood results in more stable blood sugar levels. This is done at the expense of the health of your organs, however, and unhealthy organs can precipitate an early death.

Following one of these diets and having normal blood sugar levels does not mean that these diets are healthy for you, or that they will prevent you from suffering an early death. Feeling better when you eat more protein does not mean you have a protein deficiency any more than feeling better when you drink coffee means you have a coffee deficiency. Feeling better when you consume more protein (or coffee, or sugar or alcohol, for example), means your bowel and body are not as healthy as they can be.

Throughout these past years of high protein recommendations, the American Diabetic Association has been unable to ignore the significant body of evidence that *low* protein diets result in the least amount of *death* from diabetes, and they have continued to promote these.

When you heal your bowel and body with this program, you will be able to go the whole day without eating, or without needing to eat protein or sugar, without experiencing weakness, headaches, dizziness, cravings, or any other uncomfortable symptoms (other than hunger!).

If you need to eat protein to keep your blood sugar stable, you are not as healthy as you can be, and you need to heal your bowel and body.

## Diabetes is not just a problem in overweight people

A recent report showed equivalent rises in diabetes in Americans and the people of India, even though the body mass index of the people in India has hardly risen at the same rate as Americans. In other words, diabetes rates are rising in heavy and not-heavy people. I see relatively thin clients with diabetes, and certainly I am not alone in this. So why is this disease largely considered "a fat person's disease?"

Diabetes occurs when your liver, adrenal glands, and pancreas (your blood-sugar-regulating organs) are unhealthy, and when they are unhealthy, you prone to manufacturing large amounts of fat in response to un-eliminated acids, too. So the correlation between overweight problems and diabetes is relevant, but many of you have manipulated your weight with exercise, low calorie diets, and low carbohydrate diets, which have caused weight loss, but not an improvement in the health of your liver, adrenal glands, or pancreas. Hence, you can be relatively thin if you use one of these weight-reducing crutches, yet still have unhealthy organs, and diabetes.

## Pregnancy, high protein diets, and increased rates of diabetes

In a study of 168 men and women, it was found that those men and women whose mother's consumed a diet high in fat *and protein* during late pregnancy had an impairment in the development of their pancreatic beta cells. This can lead to higher rates of impaired glucose metabolism, or diabetes, later in life. ("Diet in Late Pregnancy and Glucose-Insulin Metabolism of the Offspring 40 years Later," Shiell AW, Campbell DM, Hall Mh, Barker DJP, *Br J Obstet Gynaecol*, July 2000; 107:890-895.)

## Juvenile diabetes might not be forever

People with adult-onset diabetes are told that they can control it, but juvenile diabetics are generally considered to need insulin for life. This type of diabetes is much more difficult to help because it reflects severe ill health in your lymphatic system (which prevents autoimmune diseases, of which juvenile diabetes is one), but I think it can be helped. If you are not born with it, then it "developed," which means it should also be able to go away. Developments can be reversed.

In one study, scientists cured mice of juvenile diabetes by injecting them with donor spleen cells. (Your spleen is part of your lymphatic system, a system that heals when you heal your bowel and body with this program.)

In another study, researchers from Massachusetts General Hospital found that a drug used as a vaccine against tuberculosis (BCG), appeared to halt diabetes. In fact, in four of the six patients, who have been living with Type 1 diabetes for an average of 15 years, the treatment enabled the pancreas to temporarily begin producing insulin again. The fact that the pancreas can "start working" again after 15 years was a surprise to the researchers. And it implies that this condition *can* be reversed/healed. Likewise, the fact that a drug used to prevent tuberculosis, which is a harmful bacteria, created this affect implies that a healthy bowel, as created with this program, can create the same "pancreas—healing" properties, as a healthy bowel eliminates bacterium like tuberculosis from your body.

Autoimmune diseases can be cured. I never get the chance to work with kids with juvenile diabetes but would love to have this opportunity. Only after they have healed their bowel and body with this program would I accept that their diabetes was incurable, if indeed it was not eliminated. "Everyone" is treating symptoms with crutches, yet remember, crutches do not "cure" things; healing your bowel and body does.

## Success With Diabetes and Hypoglycemia

"Before I did this program, if I did not eat breakfast, I felt miserable—headachy, tired, and cranky. Now that I have followed this program for several years, I usually don't even want to eat breakfast, and I feel great!"

"I was diagnosed with diabetes right before I came to see Donna. My blood sugar levels were always high. For the last two years now they have been normal, and they stay normal, even if I eat a lot of bread (my favorite) or other foods I was told by the dietician my doctor sent me to I would need to stay away from forever."

"Prior to this program I had to eat protein at least every few hours or else I was tired, achy, had brain fog, and was anxious. It was miserable and I knew it wasn't right. I carried protein snacks with me everyday. The second I missed one of these my symptoms came screaming back. Also if I missed one of these I craved sugar like crazy. I didn't keep it in my house because I didn't want to be tempted, so sometimes I would be driving to the store at 10 pm for a sugary soda. Sometimes I got sick and tired of eating protein all day long. Now I am a different woman. I can't believe I don't want or need to drink soda anymore. I do not have to eat protein at every meal like I used to. I rarely get brain fog or tired or any of the other symptoms I had when I didn't eat. I even went to a wedding the other day and for the first time I can remember I actually didn't want any of the wedding cake. I feel one hundred times better than I did before I started this program."

### My story

I had severe hypoglycemia when I was ill. If I didn't eat something every two or three hours, I became disoriented, irritable, weak, and shaky.

Early in my illness, when I was trying to figure out what was causing my symptoms, I picked up a small book on low blood sugar, and after reading all of the symptoms caused by this, I thought I had found the answer to my problems. I fit the profile of this low blood sugar person perfectly.

I called my doctor and excitedly told him I thought this was the problem. He ordered a blood test to measure my blood sugar, and I anxiously awaited the end to my hell; the answer was soon to be discovered. I was going to be cured!

The test required me to fast and drink a high sugar beverage. I had my blood drawn, and after the test, I felt extremely ill. I was shaky, dizzy, nauseous, and foggy-headed. I had all of the symptoms that I had read were related to this condition.

Soon after the test the results came back I was told my glucose (blood sugar) levels were normal. Normal? I was shocked. That couldn't be. In my heart, I knew that my violent reaction to the sugar drink was significant, but he did not, and not knowing any better, I gave up on this as my diagnosis, and the solution to my nightmare. Afterwards, I spent many years suffering with the symptoms of hypoglycemia.

Now that I have healed my bowel and body with this program, I can go for eight hours during the day without eating (which I admit I do sometimes when I am very busy at work), and the only symptom I experience is hunger.

### Watch my Video,
### "Why THIS Program Eliminates Diabetes and Hypoglycemia."
This video, and all of my videos, can be found at *www.UniqueHealing.com* or at *www.YouTube.com/UniqueHealing*.

## Diarrhea/Loose Stools
### (See also "Bowel Conditions")

Diarrhea and loose stools and are a frequent occurrence with clients, and a good amount of time is spent discussing this situation. Maybe this is because we discuss their bowels at every visit, and they are conditioned to pay close attention to them. I think this is part of the reason I hear about this problem so often, but I think it is also because it is very common.

Diarrhea and loose stools are more than an inconvenience; they usually exist along with other annoying symptoms, like fatigue, aches and pains, mental irritability, bloating, and other discomforts.

They cause even greater problems when clients "blame the wrong thing" for them, and this happens often. Read this section carefully and repeatedly so you do not make this mistake, as it can prevent you from healing your bowel and body with this program.

("Loose stools" refer to stools that are mushy, flakey, or a soft pile while "diarrhea" refers to watery stools.)

## Healing Your Body With This Program Eliminates Diarrhea/Loose Stools

Un-eliminated acids can trigger loose stools. Your bowel may react to these by contracting more often in an attempt to eliminate the irritating effect of them, by secreting water into your bowel to dilute these acids, resulting in greater frequency of elimination, and loose stools. Diarrhea is not usually a product of un-eliminated acids (see below).

## Healing Your Bowel With This Program Eliminates Diarrhea/Loose Stools

For most of you, your loose stools are caused by bacterial, fungal, or parasitic, infections and by pathogens in food. In the majority of cases where there is diarrhea, this is caused by one of these infections. It is the job of your healthy bowel bacteria to fight these "bad" bacteria and keep them from producing symptoms, like diarrhea/loose stools.

Loose stools can also be triggered by the consumption of foods high in fiber, like salads, raw vegetables, beans, and nuts. The healthy bacteria in your bowel are responsible for digesting the fiber in your food, reducing the irritation, and subsequent loose stools, caused by undigested fiber.

In addition to its many other important functions, a healthy bacterial environment in your bowel is a necessity for the complete elimination of acids (toxins, heavy metals, pesticides, etc.) from your body. A healthy bowel eliminates the acids that can irritate your bowel and cause loose stools.

# Why My Crutches Work for Diarrhea/Loose Stools

*Body Bentonite* binds to and eliminates acids (toxins, heavy metals, chemicals, etc.) from your body. It eliminates the acids that trigger the release of water to dilute them, and the loose stools that occur as a result.

*Unique Healing Colloidal Silver* has natural anti-bacterial, anti-fungal, anti-parasitic properties. It eliminates the diarrhea and loose stools caused by bacterial, fungal, and parasitic infections, as well as that caused by contaminated foods, etc.

## How much do I take?/Questions about using these

See Chapter 5 for information on using these crutches, including recommendations on the amount to use, as well as a discussion of the misunderstandings about the particular crutch that may, if not understood correctly, cause you to fail to look and feel better while you heal your bowel and body with this program.

## How long will I need to use crutches for my diarrhea/loose stools?

Diarrhea and loose stools occur at Level 4 of your pipe. It is the last area of your body to heal (assuming that other areas are unhealthy too). Refer to the diagram "Sequence of Healing" in Appendix A at the end of this book to better understand this concept, as well as to Chapter 1 under this subject heading.

The bacterial environment in your bowel also affects diarrhea and loose stools. To better understand how long you may need crutches for this, refer to Chapter 1 under this subject heading.

# Misunderstandings About Diarrhea/Loose Stools and Other Information for Your Success

## Keep your stools well-formed

Because loose stools are caused in part by un-eliminated acids, the information I have provided for you in *Unique Healing*, as well as in this book, on keeping your stools well-formed is especially relevant in this situation.

If you do not have a very good handle on how to define well-formed stools, review Chapter 6 of *Unique Healing* now. (And remember, when your stools are hard and slow you are eliminating more acids, and will therefore feel better, than when your stools are one or more times a day but not all extremely well-formed.)

If your stools are not well-formed, the following changes can help: increase your *Body Bentonite* intake; reduce your carbohydrate intake (pasta, breads, grains, cereals, yogurt, etc.); reduce your sugar intake (including natural healthy sugars such as agave, honey, raw sugar, cane juice, etc.); reduce your alcohol, salt, coffee, and/or soda intake; do not have a massage, chiropractic adjustment, or any other body work; drink a lot of water; rest; and keep your exercise aerobic (see Chapter 4 for more information on how to attain this, and why it is important.)

If these changes do not noticeably help the form of your stools in two days, take them further (i.e. take more *Body Bentonite*, reduce your carbohydrate intake more, etc.)

Out of all of these recommendations, increasing your *Body Bentonite* intake is one of the most productive and helpful. It heals your body, unlike many of the other recommendations. It will do the most to lead you to a place where looking and feeling good is effortless, and some of the other suggestions, such as reducing sugar intake, are simply "too hard to do when your blood is too acidic."

(Note: the exception to this information is when your poorly formed stools are caused by an infection, in which case *Unique Healing Colloidal Silver* is needed to reduce your symptoms. Refer to Chapter 5 for information on when and how to use this crutch.)

## You are NOT eliminating toxins/acids when your stools are loose

When your stools are loose, your body is in "crisis mode." It is dumping a lot of water into your bowel to try to protect you from an irritant/toxin/infection. At the same time, your body reabsorbs this irritant/toxin/infection and attempts to handle it by your other organs, too.

When your stools are loose, you are eliminating water, but very little toxicity/acidity. Only well-formed stools eliminate toxins/acids.

Too many of you have been wrongly told that it is a positive reaction to have loose stools, and that this is valuable for getting toxins/acids out of your body. This is 100% wrong. It is never valuable, and you should "stop doing" whatever it is that causes this, when possible (for example, if a massage or chiropractic adjustment or a "cleanse" causes loose stools, this is causing you more harm than good).

## Loose stools and diarrhea: Is this from these healing products, or something else?

While the bowel-healing products *Bowel Strength* and *Unique Healing Probiotics* can cause loose stools (but not diarrhea, by the way) when they are too strong (not needed), the *majority* of the time that you have loose stools, it will be triggered by another variable.

At the start of this program, and for at least one year after, it is very rare for 12 *Bowel Strength*, 10 *Unique Healing Probiotic Pills*, or 1 teaspoon of *Unique Healing Probiotic Powder* to cause loose stools.

Wrongly blaming these products for causing loose stools is a common reason for failing to heal your bowel.

I have worked with many clients who have taken over 24 capsules / day of *Bowel Strength* or over 20 *Unique Healing Probiotic Pills* a day, for two years, without this becoming too strong. These amounts have proven to be remarkably healing.

(Contact me for an appointment if you have taken these products for less than one year and you think they are too strong/causing problems. Your doing so is vital for your success.)

## Bacterial infections and food-borne pathogens will cause most of your cases of diarrhea/loose stools

Bacterial infections and food borne pathogens are the most common causes of diarrhea/loose stools. While *eventually* your healthier bowel will protect you from these, most of you will be vulnerable to them for at least two years after you start following this program.

One of the most common symptoms of food poisoning is diarrhea occurring more than twice a day. When you have diarrhea, you lose a lot of valuable water and electrolytes, which can lead to dehydration, even death. Diarrhea is a symptom that a strong toxin is in your bowel, and your body is sending water into it in an attempt to dilute it.

In the spring of 2010, it was reported that a scientific test of turkey and chicken products revealed that one-fourth of them were contaminated with staph bacteria. Thirty-six million pounds of turkey were recalled as a result, but not until one month after the first illness from this were reported. For one month, how many of you ate this contaminated turkey and never knew it? (And if you think the government is protecting you, think again. Regarding the contaminated turkey, government officials found the salmonella last year, and during inspections four times this year too, but never acted on it.)

As reported in the *Wall Street Journal* (12/1/10), "There are about 76 million cases of food-borne illnesses every year in the U.S. that result in 325,000 hospitalizations and 5,000 deaths, according to the Centers for Disease Control and Prevention."

From 2009-2010, there were 72 illnesses from cookie dough; 272 from re/black pepper, 1,442 from jalapenos and tomatoes, 3 dead and 199 ill from spinach, 1,600 ill from eggs, and 9 dead and 714 ill from peanut butter and related products.

Contaminated food is a definite problem. Given the large numbers of reported illness caused by food poisoning every year, it is very likely that one of you will be subject to a food-borne pathogen in the near future. If this happens before you have healed your bowel, you will need help.

Bacterial infections can trigger loose stools. These do not always seem obvious, however; these can cause your stools to be loose, but few other symptoms. You can have an infection, for example, even if you don't "feel sick." Surprisingly, symptoms of insomnia, brain fog, and even weight gain can be triggered by these infections, instead.

On the other hand, you might also have other "obvious" symptoms of an infection, aside from loose stools, that give you a clue that this is what is causing these. For example, a bad cough, sinus pain and congestion, bladder discomfort, and/or extreme fatigue and nausea may occur with a bacterial infection, along with looser stools.

At the first sign of loose, watery stools, take *Unique Healing Colloidal Silver* (as directed in Chapter 5.)

If you experience loose, watery stools more than 2x/day for more than two days in a row, and *Unique Healing Colloidal Silver* has not stopped this, a trip to your doctor is recommended. (Healing will not yield persistent, frequent diarrhea, so never assume that this is the problem.)

## Cook your food, but even that can't prevent all food-borne contaminants, and diarrhea

Every year, more than one million people get sick from salmonella poisoning, and it leads to more hospitalizations and deaths than any other kind of germ found in food. "Reducing salmonella infection is hard because it is so widespread," say health officials.

Salmonella can contaminate many foods including meat, eggs, and vegetables. The percentage of infections that come from poultry is highest at 29%, eggs account for 18%, pork 12%, beef 8%, and the other 20% comes from other foods including fish, sprouts, green leafy vegetables, grains, beans, shellfish, oil, and dairy. In other words, if you "eat food," you are at risk!

Cooking food properly can eliminate these infections, but not completely. Also, some foods, like peanut butter, are not cooked, and therefore, salmonella in these foods is never destroyed.

Raw food diets are healthy, although they will not heal your bowel, like this program does, and they do not eliminate massive amounts of acidity from your body, as this program does. But they are also problematic because raw food contains more bacterium than cooked, so if you are prone to diarrhea or loose stools, my advice is that you avoid these diets.

## Other possible sources of infection—your family and pets included

If you are prone to loose stools or diarrhea, be extra vigilant about everything you put into your body. I have had clients get diarrhea from consuming protein powder that was old and expired (check your food labels for expiration dates and throw out everything that has expired). I have had clients get diarrhea from their water bottles. If you use them, or a on the counter water filter, wash these in a dishwasher regularly. Wash your sponges regularly, your cutting boards, your hands, etc.

If your kids or partner is sick, and they have diarrhea/loose stools, you likely got an infection from them. If your dog has diarrhea, you may have gotten it from him too. (Give the infected person, or animal, *Unique Healing Colloidal Silver* at the same time that you take it for best results in eliminating your infection and loose stools/diarrhea that has occurred as a result.)

## Waste carries bacterium

A common cause of bacterial infections and diarrhea or loose stools is contamination from waste products (from feces/stool). Not to sound too gross, but waste from stools can "spread" easily. When someone with an infection uses the bathroom and does not wash their hands, they can spread infections to others with their hands. My dogs sometimes wipe their behinds on my rugs and sofa pillows after a bowel movement—yuck, I know. But this can infect you if you have a similar pet problem!

If you get diarrhea/loose stools often, it is a very good idea for you to buy an anti-bacterial soap and disinfectant and put it in every bathroom, and use it regularly. Maybe you want to carry some in your car or purse to use when you are out (heaven knows what you find in public bathrooms and other places). When your bowel is healthy, you can relax, and you will be able to get away with not being so "paranoid." But for now, respect the value of this common germ-avoiding advice.

## The flu and loose stools

While bacterial infections are one of them most common causes of diarrhea and loose stools, *viral* infections, like the flu, can trigger this too. Often, you can differentiate between bacterial and viral-causing loose stools in that viral infection-causing ones often come with symptoms like a fever, body aches, and vomiting as well, whereas bacterial-causing loose stools often come with other symptoms, but not these.

For loose stools caused by a viral infection, reduce your food intake and increase your *Body Bentonite* intake.

## Foreign travel and diarrhea/loose stools

When you travel out of the United States, you may be subjected to numerous bacteria, parasites, etc. that your body is not used to.

Therefore, if you have travelled out of the country—to Mexico, Peru, China, Chile, India, etc., and your stools have become loose, it is likely that you picked up an infection or parasite while travelling.

I encourage you to automatically take *Unique Healing Colloidal Silver* during your trips out of this country as a preventative measure.

## Fruit and loose stools

Fruit is "good for you so how could it cause loose stools?" is a common question I hear.

Fruit *is* good for you, but fruit is very cleansing. It causes a lot of acidity to be moved out of your organs and "sent into" your bowel. This is good for your organs, because the fewer acids that are stored in your organs, the less damage and disease. The problem is that many of you do not have a healthy bowel, and "throwing" too much acidity into it by eating a lot of fruit can trigger loose stools (and other discomforts).

In the summertime, when fruit is especially plentiful, I run into this scenario often. The fruit that seem most likely to trigger loose stools are cherries, oranges and nectarines, peaches, berries, pineapple, dried fruit, plums, apricots, and mangos, however this is not an exclusive listing.

If you have been eating more fruit than usual (including drinking fruit smoothies), and your stools are loose, try eating none for a couple days and see if that creates better-formed stools.

(Just the other day I spoke to a new client whose son is autistic. She told me that he couldn't eat garlic, as when he ate a lot of it a while back, it made his stomach hurt and stools loose. I know that loose stools is not a possible reaction to garlic consumption, but I let it go, as sometimes, trying to convince someone that their "cause and effect" conclusions are wrong is difficult and exhausting, and I was saving this discussion for later in our work together. Later, as we discussed the cleansing effects of fruit, she brought it up again, and proclaimed that she now understood what had really caused his problems. Her son was on a super-strict diet from a nutritionist and she had added cantaloupe into this diet (not understanding, of course, the cleansing effect of fruit, but then again, most practitioners don't). She told me that at the same time he ate the garlic, he was eating a lot of cantaloupe. The cantaloupe caused his stomach problems, not the garlic. Garlic is a fabulous anti-bacterial anti-fungal agent, and these are especially helpful for autistic children, as they usually have numerous fungal and bacterial infections, so it was a shame that she unknowingly "blamed the wrong thing." It is a shame that many of you have done this too. One of my top goals in writing my books is to help you "blame the right thing," as you will never succeed in healing your bowel and body if you don't.)

## More loose stool triggers

If your stools are loose, avoid the following for the next few days and see if these are causing the problem: stress, fruit, tomatoes, spicy foods, beans, chocolate, dairy products (especially milk and ice cream), coffee, alcohol, sugar, and red meat. Also, be sure that you are eating the exact same amounts of protein and carbohydrates that you were eating at the start of this program.

## . . . and more loose stool triggers

If your bowel is unhealthy, the consumption of dairy and/or wheat/gluten can also make your bowel loose (and/or too frequent).

Fiber moves acids from your blood into your bowel and a high fiber diet can also trigger loose stools if your bowel is unhealthy (think beans, raw vegetables, salads, nuts, bran, etc.)

If you are menstruating, this can trigger loose stools as well. Blame this, and not the products you are taking, if this occurs to you.

Loose stools are a possible side effect of a number of medications, too. If you have recently started a new one and your stools become loose, check with your doctor to see if this is a possible side-effect and if so, find out if there is another medication that you can take that won't cause this to happen.

Finally, an increase in stress can also trigger loose stools if your bowel is unhealthy. This can be a hard variable to control, in which case, if you stop the supplements and your stools continue to be too loose, think about what is happening in your life. Is a relative ill, have you been worried about your job, did you lose a lot of money in the stock market, has your dog run away, or have any other unusually stressful conditions been going on?

## Avoid the following supplements if your stools are loose

Vitamin C, aloe, senna, mineral oil, cascara sagrada, rhubarb, and magnesium can trigger loose stools and need to be discontinued if you have them. (Then again, if you get loose stools or diarrhea after taking one of these, these items are simply the trigger and not the cause of it. If your stools were formed, these items would not trigger loose stools. I have proven this time and again with numerous clients. If you take one of these items and your stools become loose, it is a sure sign that you need to take more *Body Bentonite*, by the way.)

If you take a calcium supplement it may also contain magnesium. Check the label for the main ingredients, and if magnesium is included, stop the supplement for a few days and see if your bowels are less frequent and/or better formed off of it. Remember, it is better to have only one bowel movement a day than two if they are loose. If your stools are better and you still want to take calcium use *Unique Healing Calcium Citrate*, as it does not contain additional magnesium (for this reason). If your stools are not better off magnesium, then it is okay to add it back.

Other herbs and products, not listed above, can also have a laxative, and loose-stool triggering effect. These are commonly added to "colon cleansing," "bowel cleansing," and weight loss products, so if you have incorporated one of these into your daily routine, or any other new supplement, stop this for a few days to see if it is the culprit.

## *Unique Healing Colloidal Silver* cannot cause diarrhea!

The challenge at times of recommending a supplement crutch to a client with a symptom, which this supplement is designed to eliminate, is that sometimes the symptom is wrongly blamed on the usage of the supplement itself. The use of *Unique Healing Colloidal Silver* for diarrhea is a prime example. If a client calls me with diarrhea, I recommend the use of this supplement. Sometimes they tell me that one or two hours after taking it they had diarrhea, and therefore, they think the silver gave them diarrhea (of course, remember they originally called me because they *already had* diarrhea, before using this product).

> Sometimes you tend to look for an immediate cause and effect relationship with everything you put into your body, and coupled with some fear about this and other products, wrong conclusions can be made.

*Unique Healing Colloidal Silver* can in *no way* make your stools loose. Period. It also cannot immediately make them better. After taking it, you need to wait until the *following day* to see an improvement in the form of your stools. Sometimes this same client tells me that they stopped the silver after they had diarrhea and the next day their bowels were great (and they imply that this is the result of having stopped the silver), but what they miss is the fact that their bowels are great because they took the silver *the day before*!

Just the other day I had a challenge of enormous proportions trying to convince a client with tarry diarrhea who had been taking colloidal silver for a while that the silver was not the cause; that she had simply not taken enough for it to help, and that the increased amount I suggested could not immediately trigger diarrhea. She had a bad infection. Three times during our conversation I almost had her stop it just to prove to her it was not the culprit. She finally agreed to continue with it, and sure enough, as I emphatically stated to her, her diarrhea went away.

## And *Body Bentonite* cannot cause loose stools, either!

Likewise, *Body Bentonite* cannot cause loose stools or diarrhea either. This product sometimes gets wrongly blamed for this problem as well.

If you have a bacterial infection, or have eaten some contaminated food, and your stools become loose as a result, *Body Bentonite* cannot cause more loose stools, but it cannot eliminate them, either. *Body Bentonite* can eliminate loose stools caused by excess acids, but not diarrhea or loose stools caused by infections. (Pepto Bismol works the same as *Body Bentonite*. Today a client told me that her mom, who is a nurse and who has lived in third world countries, where there are a lot of diarrhea problems, has always said that if Pepto does not help loose stools, then you know you have a bacterial/fungal/parasitic infection. Just like I said.)

A client may increase their *Body Bentonite* when they have an infection and loose stools, expecting it to help. Because they are using the wrong crutch (they need to be taking *Unique Healing Colloidal Silver*), they wrongly assume the *Body Bentonite* is making things worse. Things are getting worse because they are using the wrong crutch.

If an increase in *Body Bentonite* does not help your loose stools within 24 hours of increasing it, you too probably have the wrong crutch. In this case, switch to *Unique Healing Colloidal Silver* and take as directed in Chapter 5.

## *Unique Healing Colloidal Silver* is a crutch, not a cure

If you take this for diarrhea and it goes away, but you are then exposed to another infection two weeks later, you will get diarrhea again (if you have stopped taking the colloidal silver). Your use of this product has no future protective effects. If you take colloidal silver for 500 days in a row, stop it, and are exposed to a bacterium one week later, you can end up with diarrhea.

Remember, crutches only work when you take them. The use of *Unique Healing Colloidal Silver* is no exception.

This same concept applies to the use of antibiotics for an infection as well, by the well. Do not expect different results. If you are constantly getting diarrhea, I know that is frustrating. Use this frustration to be even more motivated about healing your bowel with *Bowel Strength*, as when your bowel is healthy, and only then, will you stop being vulnerable to diarrhea from bacterial infections.

## Success With Diarrhea/Loose Stools

"Before this program, I had diarrhea 15 times a month. I was constantly concerned about leaving the house, and always had to be near a restroom. I have done this program for 18 months and for the past three months, I have only had two (versus 45) episodes of diarrhea."

"I used to have loose, frequent stools. Travelling abroad made things worse. I always ended up with diarrhea when I did. I recently got back from a trip to South America and not only did I not have loose stools, I was the only one, out of a large travel group, who did not have this problem!"

"As soon as I started taking the *Unique Healing Colloidal Silver* my loose stools, stomach cramping, bloating, and gas went away."

"Eating salads used to make my stools loose. Now I eat them regularly with no discomfort."

### Watch My Video,
### "Why THIS Program Eliminates Diarrhea/Loose Stools"
This video, and all of my videos, can be found at *www.UniqueHealing.com* or at *www.YouTube.com/UniqueHealing*.

## Difficulty Gaining Weight
See "Underweight"

## Diverticulitis
See "Bowel Conditions"

## Drug Addictions
See "Addictions"

## Dry Eyes
See "Eye Problems"

# Dry Skin
See "Skin Conditions"

# Ear Infections
See "Bacterial Infections" and "Viral Infections"

# Eating Disorders
## Anorexia, Bulimia, Overeating, Starvation, Obsessive Eating/Calorie and Fat Counting
(See also "Addictions," "Bloating and Gas," "Diabetes and Hypoglycemia," and "Underweight")

If you actively partake in anorexic or bulimic behaviors, you are labeled with an eating disorder. (And if you are extremely thin but not anorexic or bulimic, you may be wrongly labeled with an eating disorder. More on this later.)

While these conditions are extreme and can lead to serious complications, and they deserve attention, and are given much in this section, it is also true that many of you have an "eating disorder," one that is affecting the health and emotional quality of your life. This section is therefore relevant to you as well.

In other words, if you constantly worry about how much you have eaten; if you constantly count calories or grams of carbohydrates or fat you eat; if you exercise fanatically after overeating; and if you skip meals, for example, even if you are not extremely thin or do not subject yourself to vomiting, you have an eating disorder. If you are a slave to a diet or weight loss program, this is a disorder. I used to live in these shoes. It is a dreadful place to be.

You do not have to live this way. This program will help you get out of this jail.

Like popular treatments for addictions (see "Addictions" earlier), the popular approach (usually heavily psychologically-based) for those of you with eating disorders fails to address the underlying *physiological* imbalances that exist with these conditions. As a result, these approaches also have a very high failure rate. If you have one of these disorders, you *do* have emotional issues that have to be addressed, but when only these are addressed and not the underlying physiological ones, failure is high. Then,

213

as is true with addiction programs and weight loss programs that also fail to address and heal the underlying physiological conditions contributing to these problems, you are led to blame yourself, feel shameful and worthless that you could not "control yourself." This is horribly untrue. It is not your fault.

This program addresses, and heals, the physiological disorders underlying these problems and as a result, success is very high.

## Healing Your Body With This Program Eliminates Eating Disorders

There are several common physiological conditions that exist with eating disorders. Many of these are also addressed in other sections of this book, so refer to these as well.

For example, there is a high prevalence of gas and bloating and/or stomachaches (which are usually the result of this gas and bloating) after food consumption when you have an eating disorder. ("Bloating and Gas" were covered in an earlier section.) For some of you, this discomfort leads to the avoidance of food, fear of food, and/or elimination/vomiting of this food. Healing your body eliminates the acids that can trigger gas and bloating.

Healing your body eliminates the acids that cause water retention and fat production (i.e. weight gain). Ironically, perhaps, I encourage you to thoroughly read Chapter 4 regarding weight gain. When you understand how and why this program will prevent you from gaining weight and help you have complete control over your weight, this may, hopefully, be immensely helpful. Many of you are afraid to gain weight. This program leads you to a place where maintaining your weight is effortless; where the fear is eliminated.

When you heal your body with this program, you eliminate the acids that otherwise reduce your blood oxygen and glucose levels, which reduce the amount of these necessary nutrients to your brain, which can lead to anxiety and depression. This program eliminates the acids that trigger anxiety and depression.

When you eat little or no food, this too reduces the acids that cause these discomforts (when you "fast" there is little to no food entering your body that is acidic or cleansing, or that increases the acidity in your blood.

Also, when your body is not busy digesting food, it has more energy to eliminate the accumulated acids in your blood.)

In other words, another way to reduce the acids in your blood that trigger gas and bloating, weight gain, and anxiety and depression is to simply stop eating. Some of you have discovered this, and have turned to this to "look and feel better."

> When you heal your body with this program, you will be able to eat food without it causing gas and bloating, weight gain, or anxiety and depression.

In my experience, individuals with eating disorders have a less healthy body than average. You will need to be diligent and committed to this program.

## Healing Your Bowel With This Program Eliminates Eating Disorders

A healthy bowel manufactures an enormous supply of brain chemicals that help you feel happy. Happy people are much less control freaks than unhappy ones. A healthy bowel can digest fiber, meat, wheat, dairy and all other foods without creating gas and subsequent bloating and discomforts. A healthy bowel keeps fungal, bacterial, and other infections away; infections that can cause bloating and stomachaches.

The digestion of protein yields amino acids, and a healthy bowel helps your body absorb these needed nutrients. Amino acids are necessary for brain health and the formation of muscle, for example. When you heal your bowel, you will gain some "healthy and attractive" muscle weight. "This" is what you want. It is what everyone wants. You do not want to gain water and fat weight (as is often the case when you follow an eating disorder program). You want to look great. Muscle weight is healthy and it helps you look great. Healing your bowel helps this happen.

> When you eat and the food becomes muscle and energy—not fat, bloating, and water retention, you will be less scared of eating. The less healthy your bowel is, the stricter your diet needs to be to "maintain control."

215

In addition to its many other important functions, a healthy bacterial environment in your bowel is a necessity for the complete elimination of acids (toxins, heavy metals, pesticides, etc.) from your body. A healthy bowel eliminates acids from your body so that you can eat foods, all foods, without feelings of bloating, water retention, or any other discomforts.

In my experience, individuals with eating disorders have a less healthy bowel than average. You will need to be diligent and committed to this program.

## Why My Crutches Work for Eating Disorders

*Body Bentonite* binds to and eliminates acids (toxins, heavy metals, chemicals, etc.) from your body. It helps prevent them from becoming re-absorbed into your bloodstream, where they trigger a response by your body to protect you from them. It eliminates the acids that trigger the production of gas, water, and fat, and that reduce oxygenation.

*Unique Healing Calcium Citrate* is an alkalinizing mineral that helps neutralize the acids that your bowel does not eliminate. When these acids are neutralized, less gas is produced, and more oxygen is available to feed your brain and keep you happy, and the less fat and water that is retained.

*Unique Healing Methyl Vitamin B-12* provides your body with easy to assimilate levels of this nutrient, which can reduce anxiety, depression, sugar cravings, irritability, and other conditions that may otherwise be remedied by the avoidance of, or elimination of already eaten, food.

*Unique Healing Colloidal Silver* has natural anti-bacterial, anti-fungal, anti-parasitic properties. It eliminates the bloating and stomachaches, and resultant avoidance or discomfort with food that is caused by these infections.

### How much do I take?/Questions about using these

See Chapter 5 for information on using these crutches, including recommendations on the amount to use, as well as a discussion of the misunderstandings about the particular crutch that may, if not understood correctly, cause you to fail to look and feel better while you heal your bowel and body with this program.

### How long will I need to use crutches for my eating disorder?

Eating disorders occur at Levels 2, 3, and 4 of your pipe. They are the second, second to last, and last areas of your body to heal (assuming that other areas are unhealthy too). Refer to the diagram "Sequence of Healing" in Appendix A at the end of this book to better understand this concept, as well as to Chapter 1 under this subject heading.

The bacterial environment in your bowel also affects eating disorders. To better understand how long you may need crutches for this, refer to Chapter 1 under this subject heading.

## Misunderstandings About Eating Disorders and Other Information for Your Success

### Keep your stools well-formed

Because eating disorders are caused in part by un-eliminated acids, and because well-formed stools prevent the re-absorption of acids into your blood, you will be most successful in overcoming this disorder if you keep your stools well-formed while you are healing your bowel and body.

If you do not have a very good handle on how to define well-formed stools, review Chapter 6 of *Unique Healing* now. (And remember, when your stools are hard and slow you are eliminating more acids, and will therefore feel better, than when your stools are one or more times a day but they are not all extremely well-formed.)

If your stools are not well-formed, the following changes can help: increase your *Body Bentonite* intake; reduce your carbohydrate intake (pasta, breads, grains, cereals, yogurt, etc.); reduce your sugar intake (including natural healthy sugars such as agave, honey, raw sugar, cane juice, etc.); reduce your alcohol, salt, coffee, and/or soda intake; do not have a massage, chiropractic adjustment, or any other body work; drink a lot of water; rest; and keep your exercise aerobic (see Chapter 4 for more information on how to attain this, and why it is important.)

If these changes do not noticeably help the form of your stools in two days, take them further (i.e. take more *Body Bentonite*, reduce your carbohydrate intake more, etc.)

Out of all of these recommendations, increasing your *Body Bentonite* intake is one of the most productive and helpful. It heals your body, unlike many of the other recommendations. It will do the most to lead you to a place where looking and feeling good is effortless, and some of the other suggestions, such as reducing sugar intake, are simply "too hard to do when your blood is too acidic."

(Note: the exception to this information is when your poorly formed stools are caused by an infection, in which case *Unique Healing Colloidal Silver* is needed to reduce your symptoms. Refer to Chapter 5 for information on when and how to use this crutch.)

## Dietary and other crutches

When you have an eating disorder, it is extremely important that you use the crutches discussed earlier while you are healing your bowel and body. In extreme cases, medical care and psychological counseling, in addition to this program and this program's crutches, may be an absolute necessity.

Dietary crutches are equally important, and this may include eating foods that are low in fiber (i.e. avoiding beans, raw salads and other raw vegetables, nuts, and other high fiber foods), and eating protein foods that are very east to digest, like fish, nut butters, and protein powders. Amino acids supplements are also helpful.

Foods that are easy to digest reduce gas, bloating, and other digestive discomforts that can lead to vomiting or starvation. They also help to build a stronger, healthier body. Eating easy-to-digest proteins helps create muscle weight, and let's face it; everyone wants extra muscle weight, not extra fat weight, especially someone with an eating disorder.

See Chapter 9 of *Unique Healing* for a thorough discussion of dietary crutches to use while you are healing your bowel and body with this program.

## The psychological aspects of eating disorders

If you have an eating disorder, you likely have issues with self-esteem and control. These are largely psychological, but not entirely. Psychological counseling is very beneficial for you (but then again, *most people* would benefit from counseling).

Your "psychology" is heavily influenced by your physiological health. Balanced brain chemistry reduces depression. You can take medications for this, but in the long-term, this is unsafe, as these drugs are toxic and harmful to your body, like *all* drugs. It is also risky, as it requires that you take these drugs every day. Several years ago, I read that a well-known movie star was on anti-depressants, which he had *stopped, at which time he attempted suicide.* This points to the risky reality of not healing your bowel and body, and the deadly consequences that can happen if you only rely on crutches, like anti-depressants, for your emotional health.

When you eat food and feel energetic afterwards, with no bloating, gas, or other discomforts, food becomes your friend, not your enemy. Some people are more susceptible to react to this by not eating or vomiting the food up so it no longer triggers discomfort, while others simply learn other ways of dealing with it. I believe that people who are parented with unconditional love and who have higher self-esteems and are less likely to "dislike" getting heavy or bloated, but at the same time, many people with eating disorders have come from emotionally healthy parents who, I can only imagine, are especially distraught over their child's condition, and feel the most unable to help.

## Not all overly thin people have eating disorders, but they are all unhealthy

We've all heard the very thin model or actress defend their weight and claims of anorexia by saying that they eat but just don't gain weight. Many people view them suspiciously, as do I, but some of them *are* telling the truth. I can personally relate to those who are.

When I was very sick I also became very thin. At my lowest weight, I was eating three huge meals a day that consisted mostly of protein, vegetables, and whole grains. This was a diet plan that my nutritionist at the time had put me on. At the same time, I was in my least healthy, and most physically incapacitated, state. During this time I was accused of being anorexic. I wasn't. My sole focus and concern was on becoming healthy. I ate a lot of food, and I would have traded my thin, "dying" body for a fat and healthy one in a second. Emotionally, this is where I stood.

I believe and understand that some very thin people do not want to be that way and that they are eating, just not gaining weight. In my case, and perhaps yours if you are in these shoes, my bowel and body were too unhealthy to efficiently digest my food and create a healthy body/muscle weight.

Today, in my healthiest state, I eat at least half of what I did back then, but I have a lot more muscle weight, and no one accuses me of being anorexic anymore.

(For more information on how this program eliminates underweight conditions, see "Underweight" later in this chapter.)

## With a healthy body you will be in control

Therapists who work at eating disorder clinics say that when you have an eating disorder, you are "fighting for control." When areas of your life are out of control, you may resort to the only thing you *can* control, which is your food intake.

When you address underlying emotional issues and *also* heal your bowel and body, you will be in control.

Ironically, before I became ill, I remember telling a date one night that I like to be in control, only to proceed to get completely drunk and out of control later in the night. This happened all the time. Shortly after making this comment I became extremely ill, and my journey of healing brought me to a place of being in control that I had never before experienced. It's an amazingly empowering, confidence-building place to be. You can be here too.

## A low appetite is unhealthy

When I was starving myself in high school and college, this was very easy to do. I didn't get hungry. My bowel and body were so unhealthy, it couldn't handle food, and it didn't "ask" for more. (The same thing happens to people who are very ill, except we don't call them anorexic; we call them cancer victims, for example.)

It takes a healthy bowel and body to have a healthy appetite.

It also takes a healthy body to have a "normal" appetite, or one that does not crave a lot of food, and the resultant syndrome of overeating. Because we have a much greater fear in this country of being overweight than underweight, the perils of overeating have been consistently pushed on us, and many pills have been marketed to reduce our appetite.

We value a low appetite in this country, and this is very harmful. It causes a lot of problems, as the focus is on reducing appetite, and not on healing your bowel and body so that your appetite is neither too much nor too little. *It helps turn overeaters into under eaters, instead of into healthy eaters.*

Today, I eat a lot more than I did when I was in high school and college and constantly dieting, but less than the average American. I couldn't starve myself like I used to because I get too hungry and uncomfortable when I haven't eaten in a while.

People with eating disorders get uncomfortable when they eat; healthy people get uncomfortable when they don't.

## Forced eating—short-term gain, long-term failure

When you are forced to eat more food, as is a common approach in eating disorder programs, the result is usually excess bloating, discomfort, and water and fat gain—responses that, understandably, often result in your quitting the eating disorder program. This approach fails you; you who are following it are not the failure. And it fails because it fails to correct your underlying unhealthy bowel and body.

Modern treatments define success as the short-term ability to get you to eat and gain weight. Success needs to be defined as improving your health and creating a bowel and body that can eat food without becoming uncomfortable or vulnerable to excess weight gain. Success needs to be defined in the long-term, not just the short-term.

I do not pressure someone to gain weight right away because they cannot heal their body right away. Again, eating more food when your bowel and body are unhealthy can easily lead to bloating and fat and water weight gain, and who is going to be all right with this?

Sadly, I often feel the pressure of the well-intentioned parent of the eating disorder child to produce immediate results in weight gain with their child. To succeed, you *must* view this in the long-term.

The goal of an eating disorder program needs to be healthy weight gain, not just weight gain.

## An eating disorder *is* an addiction

When you have an eating disorder, you have an addiction, and you are faced with similar challenges as addicts. (Review "Addictions" earlier in this section.) For you, however, you do not use crutches like alcohol or nicotine to feel better or lose weight; your "crutch" is starvation, vomiting, excessive exercise, or maybe extreme laxative use (causing water loss and weight loss). A coffee addict uses coffee to function, just as an anorexic uses starvation to function.

Just as it is incredibly difficult to stop your other addiction crutches when no one has taught you how to heal your bowel and body and therefore eliminated your need for these crutches, it is incredibly difficult to stop your eating disorder crutches, until you heal your bowel and body.

Like an addict, you fail to succeed in eliminating your eating disorder because when your "crutch" is eliminated, you feel horrible. When you are forced to eat, you feel emotionally and physically horrible. Modern day treatments do nothing to heal your bowel and body so that the crutches, the eating disorders, are no longer desirable or needed.

Most (if not all) of you also have other addictions too, like a very strong craving and addiction for sugar or coffee. You may try to stop eating too much, which often happens because you fear becoming fat from doing so, but until you balance your blood and brain chemistry, this is hard, if not impossible, to achieve. It is a variable you cannot control very well, and the lack of control contributes to the attempt to exert control where you can with regard to your diet, which is to not eat at all, or to vomit after eating.

## Wheat-free, dairy-free, sugar-free, high protein and other "neurotic" diets

Some eating disorder clinics and programs have recognized the nutritional component of these disorders and the extremely high prevalence of food allergies/intolerances among these individuals. It is true that when these foods are eliminated there are often less gastrointestinal symptoms like gas and bloating. The problem, and inevitable failure, of this approach is that it is a crutch that does nothing to heal your bowel and body. It does nothing to strengthen your body and bowel, which cause these food allergies/intolerances. Once again, these diets are crutches with a high rate of long-term failure.

When you are advised to eat a low carbohydrate diet, and it is then concluded that this has helped eliminate your disorder, this is dangerous and wrong. If this diet helps it is because it is a crutch, and like all crutches, it will very likely fail you in the long run. This type of crutch is also very dangerous to your health and creates the very classic result of short-term improvement, yet *increased* problems and failure in the long-term.

These diets are especially harmful as they may at first appear to be desirable as you "get to" control your diet, but in the long run, you are actually working under precarious control, and it becomes very easy to eventually lose all control of your eating. You have simply traded one crutch—the eating disorder—with another—the strict diet, and this is no way to succeed.

## It's hard to let go of control

Ironically, when you have one of these disorders, you like to be given strict diets because you initially feel in control again; your diet choices have been controlled for you. In the long run, however, it backfires, and you keep failing. Nobody can control his or her dietary intake forever. When your bowel and body are healthy, you won't have to control it forever.

This is my greatest challenge with clients with these disorders. They don't trust their bodies, and I understand. A successful approach, and the one that I recommend, incorporates a gradual transition, in the absence of a medical crisis, to eating more food, as your body gets healthier.

## Hollywood is not to blame

Failing to take full responsibility for our problems is a recipe for ultimate failure in overcoming them. If you or someone you know has an eating disorder it is not caused by outside influences. Outside influences, like the pressure to be thin, can certainly *trigger* a disorder, but they are not the cause. This is a concept that we keep getting wrong; it is a concept that we accept and in doing so, keep going down the wrong road. If your roof did not have holes in it, a rainstorm would not "trigger" your house to become wet. The holes are the cause; the rain is a trigger. An unhealthy emotional and physiological body is the cause of these disorders; everything else is merely a trigger. Trying to control all of the triggers, or rain, is destined for long-term failure. It just can't be done forever. The act of trying to control all of this is stressful in and of itself.

You can't control all of the rain forever. What you can control is how strong your roof is. You can control how healthy your bowel and body are, and how they respond to these pressures/triggers. You can control your emotional health, too. You can get therapy to deal with your emotional issues.

## Stop blaming yourself

Like programs for addictions, where the addict is blamed for failing to conquer his addictions, we need to stop blaming the person with the eating disorder for failing, as well. The failure lies in the approach, or program, that is followed.

## Dehydration, electrolyte imbalances, and death

One of the most serious dangers of eating disorders is the depletion of electrolytes, like sodium and potassium, due to vomiting and diarrhea and the resultant risk of failure of your heart and death in this condition. This situation is a classic Catch-22. As electrolytes become depleted due to these disorders, your brain and blood chemistry becomes more unbalanced and you become more likely to engage in your bulimic or anorexic behaviors. This is true of anyone with an addiction as well. In the short run you feel better after vomiting, but the vomiting itself leads you even more physically vulnerable, and more likely to continue the behavior.

One way to help break this vicious cycle, and to help protect yourself while you are healing your bowel and body and working towards an elimination of these behaviors, is to ingest large amounts (3,000 mg/day) of alkalinizing minerals, like *Unique Healing Calcium Citrate*. This is a powerful alkalinizing crutch.

## Slip-ups in the behavior cannot be seen as failure

Success needs to be defined in the long-term, not short-term. When you heal your bowel and body, it is inevitable that there will be times when you fall back into your old behaviors. If you do, it does *not* mean that this program is not working; it means you are not healthy enough *yet* to avoid these behaviors. It means it rained and your house got wet because the holes on your roof are not fixed yet; it does not mean that these holes are not *getting* fixed.

If you have a slip up, keep going with this program. This slip up has not eliminated your progress to this point. It just means that you have more healing to do.

## You may lose a little weight before you gain it

During this program, you may even lose a little (toxic, unhealthy) weight before you gain healthy weight. This is scary I know. *But do not let it distract you.* (Read the section on "Underweight" later to better understand this.)

Put another way, you may eliminate toxic weight faster than you heal your bowel and are able to put on healthy muscle weight. (You may throw some old shoes out of you closet and have an empty closet, faster than you have time to buy new shoes and fill it up again). Ingesting protein powders and amino acids (from the health food or other stores) can help reduce this reaction.

If this reaction occurs and it still concerns you, contact me for an appointment. (Likely a loved one, who does not understand or support this program, will exert pressure on you if this happens. Have this person contact me for an appointment as well.)

## There is an end

This is one of the most amazing and empowering parts of this program, which contribute to its massive success. The fact that one-day, after you have healed your bowel and body, you will be in effortless control. You will not need crutches—like starvation, anorexia, counting calories, counting carbohydrates, anti-depressants—to look and feel good. You will not spend the rest of your life in fear of relapsing; you will not spend the rest of your life struggling to keep this under control.

## Help your child now

If you have young children who complain of stomachaches often, start healing their bowel and body now. My guess is that many of the teens and adults with these disorders did, too. And just because your child is not complaining daily does not mean it isn't happening. The other day my daughter had a friend sleep over and we discovered that her stomach hurt. She said that it happens all the time, so she is used to it, and has learned to ignore it.

Even if your child does not experience stomachaches, start healing his or her body now, anyway. Once they become teens, the pressure to be thin is overwhelming. Healing their bowel and body with this program eliminates difficulties with weight gain as they get older, and reach this vulnerable state.

My daughter, at age 13, is muscular but very healthy and slender, and she eats a lot of food. She describes her friends that eat no lunch (and it is the overwhelming majority of them), and are constantly struggling to stay thin. They are constantly remarking about her food intake, and are shocked she is thin. There is no chance my daughter will subject herself to eating disorder practices; she doesn't "need" to. Your daughter won't need to either when you heal her bowel and body with this program. But start now, so you have time to heal her *before* she reaches the difficult teenage years.

# Success With Eating Disorders

"When I was younger I struggled with bulimia. I eventually stopped this behavior, and I also eventually gained thirty-five extra pounds of weight. When I started this program I felt horrible and I hated this extra weight. I was always one step away form reverting to my behaviors of past, and I was always fragile and scared it would happen again. I have spent almost three years healing my bowel and body with this program and for the first time in my life I can honestly say that these fears are gone. I have lost weight and feel great, but most importantly, I am not afraid of gaining it."

"I could hardly eat because every time I did I had extreme bloating. I was afraid to eat because of this. Now I rarely get bloated and most of all, I am eating more food than I used to but am not gaining weight."

"When I started this program I was ten pounds underweight. I was constantly being pressured to gain weight, but no one understood that food was my enemy; it made me feel awful. Because of this program, I can now see that I was unable to see that I had a problem or was too thin. I felt like the thinner I became, the "more room for error" I had. Then if I gained a little weight, and I was very susceptible to gaining weight quickly, I would still not be too heavy. It spiraled out of control. As time went by, I gained weight more quickly than before and I tried to lose more weight to protect myself from this. I was always on the edge and every day I counted my calories obsessively. Only now, two years into this program, can I honestly say that I am no longer fearful."

## My story

In high school I became conscious of my weight and of calories and dieting. Back then it was all about calories. This calorie-counting thing, which is making a comeback, has been around a long time.

While I was very thin at the time, I easily became bloated, and it stressed me out. I felt out of control and always on the verge of gaining weight. My self-esteem was low and my looks gave me the attention I craved. So I dieted. This consisted of a daily assessment of how many calories I had eaten and a constant effort to reduce them. Very often I binged at night and spent the entire next day starving myself to make up for this. I was utterly and totally consumed with my diet. I spent at least six years, in high school and college, starving myself daily. I was obsessed with food and the highlight of my day was the time I allowed myself to eat a small slice of pizza, for example. The quality of my diet was atrocious. I mostly ate refined carbohydrates and alcohol. But I didn't think it was wrong to eat this way, as the "experts" told us that calories were all that mattered, and I was eating very few of them. I also lived on diet sodas, and for a while, I drank at least four to six of them a day. They reduced my appetite. I used other methods for helping me to eat less too, like diet pills, speed, and cocaine. Looking back, I ate very little food. And yet as I ate less and less, my weight remained the same. (Had it not been for all of the alcohol I drank I probably would have looked anorexic.) After college I discovered aerobics and became addicted to the gym. I lived in a jail of obsession about my weight and the constant need and desire to control it. It was awful.

Since healing my bowel and body with this program, I have cured myself of my eating disorder mentality. I have complete and effortless control over my eating and weight. I never think about or worry about calories, grams of carbohydrates, grams of fat, or my weight. I am no longer addicted to the gym. For me, this outcome alone is worth millions.

### Watch My Video,
### "Why THIS Program Eliminates Eating Disorders"

This video, and all of my videos, can be found at *www.UniqueHealing.com* or at *www.YouTube.com/UniqueHealing*.

# Eczema
See "Skin Conditions"

# Emphysema
See "Asthma/Lung Disorders"

# Endometrial Cancer
See "Breast Cancer"

# Endometriosis
See "Female Issues"

# Epilepsy
See "Neurological Disorders"

# Exercise Addictions
See "Addictions"

# Eye Problems
## Cataracts, Glaucoma, Macular Degeneration, Vision, Jaundice/Yellow in Eyes, Dry Eyes, and Others

Eye problems are one of the least common complaints that I encounter from clients. When I see few conditions, it usually results from the fact that either a) the condition is not a priority and/or b) there is little awareness that these conditions can be helped. My guess is that in this case, it is the latter. They can be helped.

# Healing Your Body With This Program Eliminates Eye Problems

A section of your lymphatic system is responsible for flushing toxins/acids away from your eyes. When these acids move into your bowel and are not eliminated (sometimes referred to as "lymphatic congestion), they recycle back to your eyes, reducing the oxygen and nutrients available to them, resulting in damage, like cataracts, macular degeneration, blurry vision, etc.

Yellow eyes/jaundice is the result of un-eliminated bilirubin. This program eliminates this waste product from your body, preventing yellow eyes/jaundice.

Eliminating acids from your body increases the hydration of all of your body's tissues, your eyes included. Un-eliminated acids cause your body to draw water from your tissues, like your eyes, to dilute these acids, protecting you from them. Unfortunately, this results in dry eyes. Healing your body with this program eliminates the acids that cause dehydration, and dry eyes.

Healing your body with this program heals your lymphatic system so that even if there are acids, your body is strong enough to handle them without a reaction (it fixes the holes on your roof so that even if it does rain, your house does not get wet).

# Healing Your Bowel With This Program Eliminates Eye Problems

In addition to its many other important functions, a healthy bacterial environment in your bowel is a necessity for the complete elimination of acids (toxins, heavy metals, pesticides, etc.) from your body. A healthy bowel prevents the re-absorption of acids into your blood that cause an unhealthy body, and trigger lymphatic congestion, reduced oxygen and nutrient availability to your eyes, dehydration, and the retention of bilirubin.

# Why My Crutches Work for Eye Problems

***Body Bentonite*** binds to and eliminates acids (toxins, heavy metals, chemicals, etc.) from your body. It helps prevent them from becoming re-absorbed into your bloodstream, where they trigger a response by your body to protect you from them. It eliminates the acids that congest your lymphatic system, reduce oxygen and nutrient levels to your eyes, and cause dehydration.

***Unique Healing Calcium Citrate*** is an alkalinizing mineral that helps neutralize the acids that your bowel does not eliminate. When these acids are neutralized, your body does not need to "use up" oxygen or nutrients, nor retain water, to buffer them.

### How much do I take?/Questions about using these

See Chapter 5 for information on using these crutches, including recommendations on the amount to use, as well as a discussion of the misunderstandings about the particular crutch that may, if not understood correctly, cause you to fail to look and feel better while you heal your bowel and body with this program.

There are no crutches for degenerative conditions, like vision problems, cataracts, and macular degeneration. Crutches can offset the effects of acids in your blood, or the effects of poor function of your bowel bacterial environment (as these can be quickly altered), but degeneration is caused by depletion and damage to your organs, and organs take time to heal.

## How long will I need to use crutches for my eye problems?

Eye problems like dry eyes occur at Level 3 of your pipe. It is the second to last area of your body to heal (assuming that other areas are unhealthy too). Refer to the diagram "Sequence of Healing" in Appendix A at the end of this book to better understand this concept, as well as to Chapter 1 under this subject heading.

Again, there are no crutches for degenerative conditions and accumulations of acidity in your organs like vision problems, cataracts, and macular degeneration; however, degenerative conditions are the first to become eliminated as you heal your bowel and body with this program.

# Misunderstandings About Eye Problems and Other Information for Your Success

### Keep your stools well-formed

Because un-eliminated acids cause eye problems, and because well-formed stools prevent the re-absorption of acids into your blood, you will suffer from the least amount of eye problems if you keep your stools well-formed while you are healing your bowel and body.

If you do not have a very good handle on how to define well-formed stools, review Chapter 6 of *Unique Healing* now. (And remember, when your stools are hard and slow you are eliminating more acids, and will therefore feel better, than when your stools are one or more times a day but not all extremely well-formed.)

If your stools are not well-formed, the following changes can help: increase your *Body Bentonite* intake; reduce your carbohydrate intake (pasta, breads, grains, cereals, yogurt, etc.); reduce your sugar intake (including natural healthy sugars such as agave, honey, raw sugar, cane juice, etc.); reduce your alcohol, salt, coffee, and/or soda intake; do not have a massage, chiropractic adjustment, or any other body work; drink a lot of water; rest; and keep your exercise aerobic (see Chapter 4 for more information on how to attain this, and why it is important.)

If these changes do not noticeably help the form of your stools in two days, take them further (i.e. take more *Body Bentonite*, reduce your carbohydrate intake more, etc.)

Out of all of these recommendations, increasing your *Body Bentonite* intake is one of the most productive and helpful. It heals your body, unlike many of the other recommendations. It will do the most to lead you to a place where looking and feeling good is effortless, and some of the other suggestions, such as reducing sugar intake, are simply "too hard to do when your blood is too acidic."

(Note: the exception to this information is when your poorly formed stools are caused by an infection, in which case *Unique Healing Colloidal Silver* is needed to reduce your symptoms. Refer to Chapter 5 for information on when and how to use this crutch.)

### Few misunderstandings, so far . . .

Daily I combat misunderstandings about the conditions I am helping clients eliminate. I have not come across any regarding eye problems, so I leave this blank for now (and hope it stays blank in the future, but should any misunderstandings arise that may prevent you from successfully healing your eye problems with this program, I will be sure to address them in a future book, blog, or video.)

## Success With Eye Problems

"Prior to doing this program, I was diagnosed with macular degeneration. At my last visit with my eye doctor I was told I no longer had this condition. Amazing!"

"My eye doctor was astonished with the changes he saw with my eyes yesterday: optical nerve relaxed; both retinas healed from the detachments and tear, and vitre-ectomy & repair; Pressure test normal. Visual Field test normal. He took a picture of each retina and you couldn't even see that there had been problems. Guess my body is repairing first things first!!!! I am elated! I was dreading this exam—after the last time, it didn't look good."

### Watch My Video, "Why THIS Program Eliminates Eye Problems"

This video, and all of my videos, can be found at *www.UniqueHealing. com* or at *www.YouTube.com/UniqueHealing*.

# Fatigue/Low Energy
(See also "Adrenal Disorders," "Anemia," and "Autoimmune Diseases,"
"Sleep Problems," and "Thyroid Problems")

Fatigue is a top complaint from the clients I see. It is an issue that is affecting the lives of many of you. Coffee, with its stimulating caffeine, is a top seller, and billions of dollars of "energy boosting" crutches are sold every year.

Fatigue is present with many of the other conditions described in this chapter. It occurs with anemia, insomnia, autoimmune disorders, bacterial infections, viral infections, addictions, allergies, cancer, and depression, for example. It is connected to dehydration, poor circulation, low nutrient levels, low oxygenation, and inflammation, as described in Chapter 3, as well.

## Healing Your Body With This Program Eliminates Fatigue

When acids are not eliminated from your body, your body may, in an attempt to protect you from them, "use up" oxygen to buffer them. Oxygen can attach to acids and reduce their danger. When this oxygen is used to buffer acids, less is available for your muscles and brain, and this can result in physical and mental low energy. Healing your body with this program eliminates the acids that deplete you of the oxygen you need to be energized.

Excess acids in your blood also disrupt blood sugar levels. When these levels are not stable, your brain and muscles may not get all of the energy/"sugar" they need to be energized. Healing your body with this program eliminates acids and stabilizes blood sugar levels.

Excess acids also disrupt the secretion of thyroid hormones. Low thyroid levels are also associated with fatigue.

Healing your body with this program heals your organs, like your thyroid, and blood-sugar regulating organs, so that even if there are acids, your body is strong enough to handle them without a reaction (it fixes the holes on your roof so that even if it does rain, your house does not get wet).

# Healing Your Bowel With This Program Eliminates Fatigue

The beneficial bacteria in your bowel are responsible for the production of vitamin B-12. Vitamin B-12 is a nutrient that is very much involved in energy production. Your beneficial bacteria are also responsible for the production of melatonin. Inadequate levels of melatonin can cause poor sleep/insomnia, and inadequate sleep is a contributing cause to fatigue. Bacterial, fungal, and parasitic infections can also cause fatigue, and a healthy bowel prevents these infections from occurring.

In addition to its many other important functions, a healthy bacterial environment in your bowel is a necessity for the complete elimination of acids (toxins, heavy metals, pesticides, etc.) from your body. A healthy bowel prevents the re-absorption of acids into your blood that cause an unhealthy body, and trigger low oxygen levels, low blood sugar, low thyroid levels, and fatigue.

## Why My Crutches Work for Fatigue

*Body Bentonite* binds to and eliminates acids (toxins, heavy metals, chemicals, etc.) from your body. It helps prevent them from becoming re-absorbed into your bloodstream, where they trigger a response by your body to protect you from them. It eliminates the acids that reduce oxygen, blood sugar, and thyroid levels.

*Unique Healing Calcium Citrate* is an alkalinizing mineral that helps neutralize the acids that your bowel does not eliminate. When these acids are neutralized, your body does not need to "use up" oxygen to buffer them. Buffering these acids also improves blood sugar and thyroid levels.

*Unique Healing Methyl Vitamin B-12* provides your body with easy to assimilate levels of this nutrient, which can increase energy production and reduces fatigue.

**Unique Healing Colloidal Silver** has natural anti-bacterial, anti-fungal, anti-parasitic properties. It eliminates the fatigue associated with these infections.

**Melatonin** helps regulate your sleep cycles, which can help you sleep through the night without waking up. A good night's sleep can make you less tired during the day.

## How much do I take?/Questions about using these

See Chapter 5 for information on using these crutches, including recommendations on the amount to use, as well as a discussion of the misunderstandings about the particular crutch that may, if not understood correctly, cause you to fail to look and feel better while you heal your bowel and body with this program.

## How long will I need to use crutches for my fatigue?

Fatigue occurs at Levels 1,2, 3, and 4 of your pipe. They are the first, second, second to last, and last areas of your body to heal (assuming that other areas are unhealthy too). Refer to the diagram "Sequence of Healing" in Appendix A at the end of this book to better understand this concept, as well as to Chapter 1 under this subject heading.

The bacterial environment in your bowel also affects fatigue. To better understand how long you may need crutches for this, refer to Chapter 1 under this subject heading.

# Misunderstandings About Fatigue and Other Information for Your Success

## Keep your stools well-formed

Because fatigue is caused in part by un-eliminated acids, and because well-formed stools prevent the re-absorption of acids into your blood, you will suffer from the least amount of fatigue if you keep your stools well-formed while you are healing your bowel and body.

If you do not have a very good handle on how to define well-formed stools, review Chapter 6 of *Unique Healing* now. (And remember, when your stools are hard and slow you are eliminating more acids, and will therefore feel better, than when your stools are one or more times a day but not all extremely well-formed.)

If your stools are not well-formed, the following changes can help: increase your *Body Bentonite* intake; reduce your carbohydrate intake (pasta, breads, grains, cereals, yogurt, etc.); reduce your sugar intake (including natural healthy sugars such as agave, honey, raw sugar, cane juice, etc.); reduce your alcohol, salt, coffee, and/or soda intake; do not have a massage, chiropractic adjustment, or any other body work; drink a lot of water; rest; and keep your exercise aerobic (see Chapter 4 for more information on how to attain this, and why it is important.)

If these changes do not noticeably help the form of your stools in two days, take them further (i.e. take more *Body Bentonite*, reduce your carbohydrate intake more, etc.)

Out of all of these recommendations, increasing your *Body Bentonite* intake is one of the most productive and helpful. It heals your body, unlike many of the other recommendations. It will do the most to lead you to a place where looking and feeling good is effortless, and some of the other suggestions, such as reducing sugar intake, are simply "too hard to do when your blood is too acidic."

(Note: the exception to this information is when your poorly formed stools are caused by an infection, in which case *Unique Healing Colloidal Silver* is needed to reduce your symptoms. Refer to Chapter 5 for information on when and how to use this crutch.)

## Fatigue is not always caused by adrenal disorders

Over twenty-five years ago I was diagnosed with "Chronic Fatigue," and was subsequently diagnosed with adrenal fatigue by numerous alternative health practitioners. At the time I did have very unhealthy adrenal glands, but fatigue is not always caused by stressed out adrenal glands (and if it is, this program heals your adrenal glands, anyway).

Some of you with fatigue do not have unhealthy adrenal glands, and therefore the traditional adrenal gland crutches recommended by the many practitioners who often automatically diagnosis adrenal disorders when you present yourself with fatigue, won't work. This may leave you wrongly believing that your fatigue can't be improved.

Low levels of vitamin B-12 and an unhealthy immune system may also cause fatigue, and they may be your only cause of fatigue. It is always important that you use the right crutch for your symptoms, and this is no exception.

## Or thyroid disorders

Thyroid problems are another commonly assumed diagnosis of fatigue. While this does cause fatigue in many cases, for some of you, this is not the cause of your fatigue, either.

For some of you, your fatigue is solely the result of low levels of vitamin B-12, and not only will adrenal gland supplement crutches not work, but neither will thyroid gland supplement crutches help, either.

In this program, you are given crutches to address *all* of the possible triggers of your fatigue. More importantly, you are healing your bowel and body, which addresses all of the underlying *causes* of your fatigue in the first place. As a result, your experience with eliminating fatigue with this program is complete, permanent, and remarkable.

## Fatigue is not caused by a low protein diets; an unhealthy bowel and body cause it

Fatigue is often the result of low blood sugar (glucose) and low oxygen levels. When these are low, your brain and muscles do not get the fuel they need to function optimally, and this leaves you feeling less energized, as a result. The more acidic your blood is, the lower your blood sugar and oxygen levels will be.

One reason low carbohydrate, or high protein, diets help with fatigue is because they prevent acidity from moving out of your organs, where it cannot trigger low blood sugar and low oxygen levels (but can eventually trigger disease and death), into your blood, where it *can* trigger low blood sugar and low oxygen levels. If you do not yet understand this concept, re-read this book, and *Unique Healing*, and watch my videos at *www.YouTube.com/UniqueHealing*, until you do. Your understanding of this is critical to your success.

By eliminating acids from your bowel, as this program does, you eliminate them from your blood too, causing your blood sugar and oxygen levels, and your energy, to rise, without having to "shove" these acids into your organs, as these diets do; you do not have to trade "more energy for more disease and death," in other words.

As I have repeated numerous times in *Unique Healing*, as well as in this book, it is dangerous to use a low carbohydrate or high protein diet to treat *any* of your problems, fatigue included.

## Coffee is not just a habit; it is a crutch you depend on for energy

Caffeine is a stimulant that energizes your brain. As much as I hear clients tell me on day one of this program that their coffee drinking is a habit, and/or that they just love the taste of coffee, it never fails that as they heal their bowel and body with this program, their coffee consumption goes down.

Coffee is acidic, so desiring/needing less of it is beneficial to your health.

On the other hand, if you try to reduce your coffee consumption at the start of this program, it may backfire (the only exception to this is if you replace coffee with caffeinated tea, which I recommend, if possible, as tea is alkalinizing/good for your health, and caffeinated tea will give you the "energy boost" you need). If you try to cut out caffeine altogether, you may end up eating more sugar, drinking more alcohol, or simply just feeling more tired (and depressed), and none of these reactions will help you look or feel better while you are healing. In fact, sugar and alcohol create *more* weight, and symptoms, than coffee, so be careful about reducing this too quickly, if you decide to do this at all.

Be careful of coffee and tea that is anything other than black (coffee or tea) or green (tea). Many "designer" coffee and tea beverages contain enormous amounts of sugar, and this will do nothing but make you more addicted, heavier, and more symptomatic and fatigued, over time. Stick to coffee and tea with less than seven grams of sugar/serving. Check your labels and/or ask your coffee shop for nutrition facts on the beverages you purchase from them. Low calorie coffee and tea are often deceptively very high in sugar, too.

Likewise, be careful of "energy" boosters. Ones that contain caffeine but little (less than seven grams/serving) of sugar, or no sugar, are great crutches to use while you are healing, but energy "boosters" that contain larger amounts of sugar, and many do, can "backfire" on you, too.

As always, the best way to make dietary changes on this program is to let them happen naturally. When your bowel and body are healthier, you won't "need" to replace your coffee with sugar or alcohol to feel better. As you become healthier, you will feel better consuming *less* of all of these energy-stimulating items.

## The vicious cycle of sugar consumption

Sugar is added to many products as an energy booster, too. Sugar consumption immediately increases your blood sugar levels, giving you quick energy, but because it is acidic and cleansing, hours after consuming it, it makes your blood more acidic, which causes your blood sugar to drop even more (causing your brain and muscles to be fatigued), resulting in a desire for *more* sugar. This works out great for the companies who sell you sugary items, but it does not work out great for you.

You would be better off consuming a low-sugar caffeine-containing drink or supplement, or better yet, using *Body Bentonite* and *Unique Healing Methyl Vitamin B-12*, to give you the energy you need while you are healing your bowel and body, and "waiting" for this energy to occur naturally.

In fact, if you ever get into a rut/vicious cycle where you "can't stop eating sugar," consider doubling your *Body Bentonite* and *Unique Healing Methyl Vitamin B-12* for a couple of days. It often works wonders to stabilize your blood sugar and help you break this uncontrollable sugar eating cycle.

## Melatonin does not cause fatigue

Melatonin helps regulate your body's circadian rhythm, and it can help you sleep through the night (as this is part of a normal "body clock."). Melatonin is *not* a tranquilizer or narcotic. If you are fatigued immediately, or soon after, taking it, do not blame it for your fatigue. Likely you are tired because the night before, when you didn't take melatonin, you didn't sleep well, and your fatigue is a result of this. Or perhaps you are fatigued because your blood is overly acidic; you ate too much fruit or sugar or alcohol the day before.

The point is, fatigue is not a side-effect of melatonin (and it is a crutch I highly recommend. See Chapter 5 for information on the benefits of using this crutch).

# Success With Fatigue

"When I came to Donna I had been disabled for several years with an autoimmune disease, and horrible fatigue (among many other symptoms). I was not able to work or go out much. Now, I am back to work and I can't believe how much I can do!"

"Prior to this program, I was dependent on 10 cups of coffee of day to get through my day. Donna told me that one day I would not need coffee, and I really didn't believe it until it happened. Now I drink one cup a day. What a difference."

"I can't believe how much more energy I have. I sleep great, I can work out again, I am feeling great, and my life has changed dramatically."

## My story

I was diagnosed with Chronic Fatigue when I was very ill 25 years ago. I was told there was no cure. This condition disabled me. After healing my bowel and body, I got my life back. Now, I have enormous amounts of energy, I accomplish a lot, and I do this *without* stimulants, sugar, caffeine, or any other crutch.

## Watch My Video, "Why THIS Program Eliminates Fatigue"

This video, and all of my videos, can be found at *www.UniqueHealing. com* or at *www.YouTube.com/UniqueHealing*.

# Female Issues
## PMS, Menopause, Cysts, Fibroids, Endometriosis, and Others

Female problems include PMS, symptoms of menopause, cysts, and fibroids, early onset of menopause or menstruation, irregular periods, endometriosis, cysts, and female cancers like breast, ovarian, and uterine cancers. Female cancers are covered in the section, "Breast/Female Cancers." See also "Infertility" for additional information on them.

While I have helped women with all of the female issues listed above, uncomfortable, and often unbearable, symptoms of PMS (premenstrual syndrome) are the most common complaints that I encounter with my female clients. This includes, but is not limited to: disabling migraines, emotional issues like depression, pain, sugar cravings, diarrhea, and breast and ovarian tenderness and pain.

In 2002, studies estimated that up to 40% of women age 35 and older already have or will develop uterine fibroids. So many women have PMS and menopausal symptoms that they have come to expect this as normal, and healthy. And many other issues, including irregular periods and endometriosis, are not only potentially uncomfortable, but potentially disruptive to your fertility, as well.

These conditions do not have to be accepted as normal, and they do not have to occur. In fact, when I was sick and healing my body, I expected to get better, but I never expected my horribly heavy and uncomfortable periods to go away as I became healthier. I too had accepted these problems as normal. It was when they went away as I followed this program that I really thought, "Wow, I've got to become a nutritionist and tell every women that their suffering is not inevitable." While my results in healing my body were extremely remarkable, this result was truly the "final catalyst" that inspired me to do this work.

# Healing Your Body With This
# Program Eliminates Female Issues

Many of your symptoms of PMS are not hormonal, but rather the result of excess acidity that is present at this time (read more on this later). Your body reacts to excess acidity in numerous ways, which includes the secretion of inflammatory chemicals (pain, like cramps and migraines), reduced oxygen and glucose to your brain (emotional issues), lymphatic congestion (tender breasts), and an increase of water drawn into your bowel (loose stools), for example.

Likewise, many menopausal symptoms are also the result of excess acidity (not just hormonal imbalances), and your body reacts to this in many ways that contribute to the symptoms of menopause, too. For example, your body may sweat more productively in an attempt to eliminate these acids (hot flashes), and draw water out of your vaginal area to buffer them (vaginal dryness).

Endometriosis is the result of normal tissue from the lining of your uterus which has been shed during your menstrual cycle but not expelled (i.e. eliminated by your bowel), reattaching itself elsewhere and growing, often forming cysts which can cause pain and cramping. Healing your body eliminates this tissue.

Some cysts and fibroids are also the result of great accumulations of toxicity/acidity in your body. Healing your body, which eliminates this toxicity, helps eliminate these conditions as well.

Healing your body with this program eliminates the acids that trigger the symptoms associated with the above-mentioned female problems. Healing your body with this program heals your organs so that even if there are acids, your body is strong enough to handle them without a reaction (it fixes the holes on your roof so that even if it does rain, your house does not get wet).

# Healing Your Bowel With This
# Program Eliminates Female Issues

Women make estrogen in their ovaries, a few other organs, and body fat. Estrogen flows through your body one time, stimulating your breasts, uterus, ovaries, and skin. After one passage through your bloodstream it goes to your liver, where it is attached to another substance and conjugated, or "bound." Conjugated estrogen, which is not absorbable, is excreted into your bowel to be eliminated through your stools.

Unfriendly bacteria deconjugate estrogen, or free it up, and allow it to pass through the body again, contributing to disease. Excess re-absorption of estrogen is implicated in the majority of cases of endometriosis, PMS, fibroids, and cysts. Excess estrogen causes your uterus to gorge with blood, which can lead to heavy menstrual bleeding. Hormonal imbalances are also implicated in many cases of decreased sex drive, early onset of menstruation, and irregular periods.

A healthy bowel regulates your hormone levels by excreting excess estrogen, preventing these conditions and diseases.

In addition to its many other important functions, a healthy bacterial environment in your bowel is a necessity for the complete elimination of acids (toxins, heavy metals, pesticides, etc.) from your body. A healthy bowel prevents the re-absorption of acids into your blood that cause an unhealthy body, and trigger many of your symptoms, weight problems, addictions, and disease.

## Why My Crutches Eliminate Female Issues

*Body Bentonite* binds to and eliminates acids (toxins, heavy metals, chemicals, etc.) from your body. It helps prevent them from becoming re-absorbed into your bloodstream, where they trigger a response by your body to protect you from them. It eliminates the acids that trigger the release of inflammatory chemicals (cramps and migraines), that reduce oxygenation and blood sugar levels (emotional issues), congest your lymph nodes (tender breasts), cause dehydration (vaginal dryness), instigate sweat (hot flashes), and cause build-ups of toxicity in your uterine lining (endometriosis), for example.

*Unique Healing Calcium Citrate* is an alkalinizing mineral that helps neutralize the acids that your bowel does not eliminate. When these acids are neutralized, your body does not react to them in the ways mentioned above.

**Natural Progesterone cream** provides a safe source of natural progesterone, which *balances* hormone levels and eliminates the problems associated with an excess or deficiency of them. It eliminates the menopausal and PMS symptoms caused by hormonal imbalances, as well as the cysts and fibroids that may be caused by hormonal imbalances as well.

### How much do I take?/Questions about using these

See Chapter 5 for information on using these crutches, including recommendations on the amount to use, as well as a discussion of the misunderstandings about the particular crutch that may, if not understood correctly, cause you to fail to look and feel better while you heal your bowel and body with this program.

### How long will I need to use crutches for my female issues?

This condition occurs at Level 3 of your pipe. It is the second to last area of your body to heal (assuming that other areas are unhealthy too). Refer to the diagram "Sequence of Healing" in Appendix A at the end of this book to better understand this concept, as well as to Chapter 1 under this subject heading.

The bacterial environment in your bowel also affects female issues. To better understand how long you may need crutches for this, refer to Chapter 1 under this subject heading.

Again, there are no crutches for degenerative conditions and accumulations of acidity in your organs like cysts, fibroids, and endometriosis, which can represent an accumulation of acidity/toxicity in your body, and there are no crutches that can immediately eliminate accumulations of acidity in your tissues/organs; however, degenerative conditions are the first to become eliminated as you heal your bowel and body with this program.

## Misunderstandings About Female Issues and Other Information for Your Success

### Keep your stools well-formed

Because female issues are caused in part by un-eliminated acids, and because well-formed stools prevent the re-absorption of acids into your blood, you will suffer from the least amount of female issues if you keep your stools well-formed while you are healing your bowel and body.

If you do not have a very good handle on how to define well-formed stools, review Chapter 6 of *Unique Healing* now. (And remember, when your stools are hard and slow you are eliminating more acids, and will

therefore feel better, than when your stools are one or more times a day but not all extremely well-formed.)

If your stools are not well-formed, the following changes can help: increase your *Body Bentonite* intake; reduce your carbohydrate intake (pasta, breads, grains, cereals, yogurt, etc.); reduce your sugar intake (including natural healthy sugars such as agave, honey, raw sugar, cane juice, etc.); reduce your alcohol, salt, coffee, and/or soda intake; do not have a massage, chiropractic adjustment, or any other body work; drink a lot of water; rest; and keep your exercise aerobic (see Chapter 4 for more information on how to attain this, and why it is important.)

If these changes do not noticeably help the form of your stools in two days, take them further (i.e. take more *Body Bentonite*, reduce your carbohydrate intake more, etc.)

Out of all of these recommendations, increasing your *Body Bentonite* intake is one of the most productive and helpful. It heals your body, unlike many of the other recommendations. It will do the most to lead you to a place where looking and feeling good is effortless, and some of the other suggestions, such as reducing sugar intake, are simply "too hard to do when your blood is too acidic."

(Note: the exception to this information is when your poorly formed stools are caused by an infection, in which case *Unique Healing Colloidal Silver* is needed to reduce your symptoms. Refer to Chapter 5 for information on when and how to use this crutch.)

## Many symptoms of PMS and menopause are due to cleansing, *not* hormonal imbalances

While unbalanced hormones (i.e. an unhealthy bowel) cause many of your female issues, many of these issues are the result of "something else," or excess acidity.

During your period, your body automatically cleanses. This happens during menopause, too. There is an automatic release of stored acidity out of your female organs when your hormones change at this time. This cleansing occurs even if your hormones are healthy and balanced.

This cleansing often causes more acids to be dumped into your blood and bowel than you can eliminate, triggering many symptoms as a result (as discussed earlier).

The reason that it is important that you understand that these cleansing symptoms cause many of your female issues is because one, it means that if you take hormones, natural or synthetic, and your female issues are not completely eliminated, you may think that these "leftover" symptoms are inevitable. They are not. They simply have a different cause, one that these hormones do not address. Two, if you are taking natural progesterone cream, a crutch I *highly* recommend that all females use, and you have symptoms of PMS due to cleansing, for example, and you do not understand this, you may wrongly blame this valuable cream for your symptoms, and perhaps be concerned about my recommendations.

If you are using natural progesterone cream and you have female issues, try doubling your progesterone cream for a month. If this provides no help, double your intake of *Body Bentonite* for a month. One of these changes should reduce your symptoms. (See *Unique Healing* for more information on reducing the acids in your blood while you heal.)

## Loose stools during your period are not healthy

It is common for women to have loose stools with their periods; it is not healthy, however, if this happens to you.

Looser, or "worse" stools, during your period, occur when your body cleanses at this time, as described above, and this cleansing occurs at a rate faster than your bowel can handle. Loose stools can reflect a large amount of toxins/acids in your bowel that are aggravating it. Remember, when you have loose stools, you also have a large amount of acidity being re-absorbed into your blood and body, triggering many uncomfortable symptoms as well.

As you heal your bowel and body with this program, loose stools will not occur during your period, as your bowel will be better able to eliminate these acids, and as a result, you will feel better at this time too.

## Bad PMS signals trouble ahead for menopause

In 2004, University of Pennsylvania researchers discovered that PMS sufferers were up to twice as likely to experience troublesome hot flashes, depression, and poor sleep during menopause.

This makes sense, as hormonal imbalances and ill health/excess acidity cause many of your symptoms of PMS, just as they cause many of your symptoms of menopause. It make sense because if you are younger and not eliminating acidity, and/or your bowel is unhealthy and not regulating your hormones properly, you are likely to be even more acidic as you get older and reach menopause, and more likely to have an unhealthier bowel then too, and you are more likely to experience the symptoms of menopause caused by these.

In other words, if you currently suffer from PMS, you are likely going to suffer during menopause, unless you heal your bowel and body with this program.

## Soy foods and menopause

In Asia and other countries, symptoms of menopause, like hot flashes and vaginal dryness, are insignificant compared to what American women experience.

Many years ago, the soy content of the Asian diet was targeted as the sole factor responsible for their improved hormonal health status. As a result, many of you rushed to the store and loaded up on soy powders, soy nuts, soy energy bars, soymilk, and many other soy-based products. Food companies added soy to just about anything they could, as they capitalized on this craze.

Because there are components of soy that act naturally to help stabilize estrogen levels in women, many responded with an "if a little is good, more must be better" attitude.

Before long, you found yourselves faced with articles about the risk of soy, and many of you became understandably confused. With nutrition matters, confusion often leads to frustration, and this often results in people quitting what they are doing. This happened with the soy craze, too. Not long after it started, it came to an abrupt halt. Very few of the women I see eat soy products. And this is very unfortunate. Their estrogen-balancing effects aside, soy foods are great for the health of your bowel and body.

The great fear and misunderstanding about the benefits of soy likely arose out of the fact that soy is much lower in protein than animal protein foods. Many of you replaced your hamburgers with soy burgers; your sausage with soy shakes; and your eggs with soymilk.

*By making these healthy substitutions, many of you moved towards a cleansing diet.* By eating less animal protein, you found your body cleansing faster than you could handle. Compared to eating an equivalent amount of animal protein, soy products contain less protein and cause many more of the acids that are in your organs to dump into your blood. When these acids dump into your blood faster than your bowel can eliminate them, they trigger numerous symptoms, weight problems, and bad blood tests. Some practitioners claimed that soy caused thyroid problems, when in reality, the acids that the soy dumped into your blood too quickly triggered high TSH levels in some of you, but to conclude that soy was therefore unhealthy or hurtful was wrong. Dumping acids out of your organs into your blood is not unhealthy or hurtful. But it is scary and uncomfortable when you don't understand what is happening. And it is preventable, too. I have told you numerous times that cleansing diets, like higher soy, lower animal protein ones, can cause a cleansing affect that is not harmful, but often uncomfortable, You have been warned time and again that, ideally, you are not to eat a cleansing diet (lower in animal protein and higher in soy protein) unless your bowels can handle it; unless your stools remain well-formed while you are doing so.

When you heal your bowel and body with this program, you will be able to replace your animal protein foods with soy foods and not experience any cleansing reactions from doing so. Eating soy will not trigger symptoms or bad blood tests, leading you to wrongly believe that this diet is wrong. You will be able to eat a healthy diet consisting of some soy products, and therefore, you will be able to take advantage of the estrogen-balancing effects of soy, too.

## Normal periods on the pill do not mean that you are healthy

One sign of a healthy hormonal system is regular periods that occur approximately every 28 days. Your bleeding should be light and last only 3-4 days. If neither of these occur for you, they are signs that your hormonal system is not as healthy as it could be, and that you are at risk for more serious hormonal problems, like cysts, or breast cancer, if you do not correct this imbalance (ideally, by healing your bowel and body with this program.)

When you take the birth control pill you no longer have this feedback about your hormonal health. More so, be careful that you do not conclude that your hormonal health is good simply because you have regular and short periods, but are taking the pill.

## Bone loss and estrogen

The vast majority of women around the world do not take hormones during menopause, and they experience much less bone loss than American women do.

Americans are ranked low among the industrialized nations as far as health goes, and it is your overall health that determines how strong your bones will be as you age, not a lack of synthetic hormones in your body.

Estrogen has dangerous side effects. Healing your bowel and body with this program, which prevents bone loss (see "Osteoporosis/Osteopenia" later on), has no risky side effects.

## Estrogen is dangerous

A wealth of knowledge and research points to the increased risk of breast, ovarian, uterine, and endometrial cancer when you take estrogen. Estrogen is also implicated in many cases of fibroids, cysts, endometriosis, and other female issues.

Estrogen continues to be prescribed because many doctors have been convinced that the benefits outweigh the risk. When you heal your bowel and body with this program, you won't need to make this choice. It is "all benefit" when you follow this program.

If possible, avoid estrogen at all costs. On the other hand, I support its use in a birth control pill to avoid an unwanted pregnancy, if the pill is your only option for birth control. If you must use it, then it is especially important that you heal your bowel and create a system that can help eliminate harmful excess estrogen from your body (which is not to be confused with eliminating the "birth control" effectiveness of the pill.)

## Dietary and other sources of estrogen

Vegan women, who eat no animal protein, have four times as much estrogen in their stool as women who eat the typical Western diet (i.e. less absorbed estrogen to trigger breast, uterine, endometrial cancer, cysts, fibroids, etc.).

A study published in "Obstetrics and Gynecology" compared women hospitalized for fibroid surgery with women hospitalized for non-gynecological reasons, and found that women with fibroids regularly ate a lot of beef and other red meat. Eating green vegetables was associated with a decreased risk.

When you heal your bowel and body with this program, one day you will desire very little animal protein, and you will look and feel great eating this hormonally healthy low protein diet.

Dairy products, meats, and plastic products have also been found to contain estrogen, or compounds that cause estrogen production in your body. Buying organic dairy and meats is therefore valuable, as is avoiding the use of plastic containers. Do not rely on these alone to protect you from excess estrogen and cysts, fibroids, or breast cancer, however. This action may reduce the estrogen in your body, but just as your body's production of cholesterol, and not the cholesterol-containing foods you eat, has the greatest impact on your cholesterol levels, so it is true for your estrogen levels. The majority of estrogen in your body is what your organs have produced, and the majority of the excess estrogen comes from here, too. You are safest healing your bowel and body with this program so that *all* sources of excess estrogen can be eliminated.

## Early onset of menstruation is a warning

Menstruation that occurs too early, or before age twelve, is unhealthy. If it happened to you long ago, it is another warning that you need to heal your bowel and body.

If you have a daughter who is younger than twelve who has begun to menstruate, I strongly encourage you to place her on this program now. Consider this a warning that if her bowel is not healed, as she grows older, she may be faced with more serious hormonal problems.

Early menstruation is a relevant sign that the medical profession often ignores, but you shouldn't. When a woman gets breast cancer, for example, there have always been warning signs, like this one, for years prior to this.

## In fact, you are given lots of warnings

Heavy periods, cramps, tender breasts, irregular periods, and other symptoms of PMS, as well as symptoms of menopause, are warnings that your bowel and body are not as healthy as they could be. You may have an unhealthy bowel and body and never get breast or ovarian cancer; but I have never seen someone with breast or ovarian cancer who had a healthy bowel and body.

I have not had a Pap smear in over twenty years. Ironically, but understandably, this concerns some people, but it doesn't concern me. (This is my personal decision, and respectfully, it might not ever be yours.) I mention it because when I was younger, I was at great risk of breast cancer and other hormonal diseases. I had horrible symptoms of PMS and my body and bowel were very unhealthy. I got Pap smears back then. Ironically, back then, when I was very unhealthy and had these symptoms, no one was worried about my hormonal health. But they should have been!

Since healing my bowel and body with this program I have no PMS (see "My story" at the end of this section). What I know and believe is that in this state, my hormonal system is very healthy, and I know and believe that hormonal diseases are not the result of genetics, bad luck, or old age, but of an unhealthy bowel and body. I feel extremely safe about my hormonal health.

## Hormonal crutches will not save your life, however

Estrogen, bio-identical hormones, chaste tree, wild yam, saw palmetto, Viagra, and testosterone treat some of the symptoms of hormonal imbalances, but all of them ignore the cause of the problem. This is true of natural progesterone cream as well.

When you only use crutches for your hormonal imbalances and do not heal your bowel, you get "unstable and risky" results. These hormonal symptoms are a warning that your bowel is unhealthy, and if you simply take a crutch and do not heal your bowel, you are ignoring the fact that you have an unhealthy bowel, which not only can cause additional symptoms and disease as time goes on, but which allows for the rapid accumulation of acidity in your body, which leads to premature diseases like cancer and heart attacks.

When I recommend natural progesterone cream to my clients I make it very clear that it is a valuable crutch for their symptoms, but that it is just a crutch and that it does nothing to extend their life (although it may do this to some degree indirectly, because my clients who use this cream are not being diagnosed with breast and other hormonal cancers, and as a result, they are not being subjected to toxic chemotherapy and radiation treatments, or the stress of this diagnosis.)

## Post-partum depression

While I have helped many pregnant clients through healthy pregnancies and births with this program, I must again defer you to contacting me for a personal consultation if you are pregnant.

However, I do want to mention post-partum depression here because by this time, your baby has been born, and at this time, your following this program without my personal direction is not only okay, but highly recommended.

Like all of the other female issues, post-partum depression has two main physiological causes. One, after your baby is born, your body cleanses once again, this time, as it attempts to eliminate the (acidic) materials that accumulated during your pregnancy that are not longer needed. This is especially prevalent in the first 4-6 weeks after giving birth. When this acidity is not completely eliminated, they are re-absorbed, and your body may protect you from them by binding them to oxygen. They can cause your blood sugar levels to go down. Low oxygen and low blood sugar are implicated in depression, as your brain needs these two ingredients to function optimally. In this case, extra *Body Bentonite* is extremely helpful in reducing post-partum depression,

Two, if your bowel is unhealthy, your body may not be able to regulate your hormones effectively at this time, and in this case, natural progesterone cream is extremely helpful in reducing post-partum depression.

## Nothing has the potential to balance your hormones as perfectly or as safely as your bowel itself

By the time most women reach their menopausal years, their organs are unhealthy to such an extent that this natural internal balancing mechanism fails.

For example, in addition to the important role your bowel plays in regulating your hormone levels, your adrenal glands produce some of the estrogen that your ovaries used to make before menopause started, but only as long as your adrenal glands are healthy enough to do so. Your lymphatic system plays a key role in regulating your hormonal levels too. Again, this regulation will be done efficiently only as long as these organs are strong.

Some of your organs help produce extra hormones, and others play a role in regulating their levels to the exact amount needed at a given time, something a synthetic or natural hormone replacement can never do.

When you heal these organs with this program, you get the best results as menopause approaches. When your adrenal glands, lymphatic system, and bowel are healthy, you will not only breeze through menopause, you will also benefit from the improved function of these organs in many other ways as well, such as with weight loss, an elimination of aches and pains, and lots of energy, for example.

When you experience menopausal symptoms and you take a hormone, synthetic or natural, you are missing out on a warning from your body that something needs to be healed; you are missing an opportunity to help improve your health and lose weight naturally. When you take a hormone replacement product, you may feel better, which may wrongly lead you to think that you are healthier than you really are.

Many of my female clients have eased through menopause without the use of hormones.

# Success With Female Issues

"I had horrible hot flashes when I came to see Donna. I also had a history of breast cancer and could not and would not take synthetic hormones. I am using the natural progesterone cream and my hot flashes are 90% better."

"My periods were horrible. They were completely irregular. Some months they were 24 days, and some they came every 35 days. They were long and heavy and very uncomfortable I had horrible breast tenderness and I lived on Advil during this time. It made my life miserable. I did not want to take hormones, so I tried a lot of natural remedies, but they only helped a little and they only helped some of my symptoms. Now, my PMS symptoms are completely gone. My periods are regular and they only last a few days and they are light, too. I am able to do things during this time that I couldn't before, like ride my bike and work out. I am a new woman."

"I had an ultrasound which showed a large uterine cyst. My last ultrasound showed that it was completely gone."

"Prior to beginning this program I had three bad Pap smears in a row. I followed this program for 6 months and had another pap smear, and this one was normal!"

"I suffered from monthly endometrial pain, and a lot of other problems, when I started this program. I can't believe how much better it is, as are all of the other problems I had before I did this program."

"My daughter began showing signs of early puberty, and this concerned me. She started this program and her development has slowed down, which is a good thing."

## My story

When my periods first began at age 12 ½ they were debilitating, painful, and incredibly heavy. A super tampon would be soaked and leaking within one hour. At age 12 ½ I was not very healthy, and the pain and bleeding were accepted as "what some women experience." Gradually the amount of blood became manageable, but my periods continued to be very painful. Eventually I started using the birth control pill and this helped reduce the pain and blood flow. After I became very ill and healed my bowel and body, I stopped taking the pill and my periods became unusually comfortable, and the blood flow became very light. My period is over within three days, and during this time I usually go through only seven or eight tampons, a world of difference compared to my teens and twenties. I have also been pregnant twice and nursed two babies for a total of 4 ½ years. I experienced tremendous hormonal changes at this time. These experiences were positive, as the symptoms I experienced during those hormonal changes were minimal.

## Watch My Video, "Why THIS Program Eliminates Female Issues"

This video, and all of my videos, can be found at *www.UniqueHealing.com* or at *www.YouTube.com/UniqueHealing*.

## Fibromyalgia
See "Autoimmune Diseases"

## Food Allergies
See "Allergies (Food)"

## Fungal Infections
### Candida/Yeast, Parasites

When I first re-located my practice to Boulder many years ago, I gave a number of local talks on a variety of subjects. The topic that received the largest attendance was Candida. (Candida is a term often used to describe the overgrowth of fungus or yeast in your intestinal tract.)

For several years after, I saw a large number of clients who had been diagnosed with Candida (usually by a chiropractor, nutritionist or naturopath) and had tried numerous approaches to rid themselves of it. As the years went by, the Candida craze diminished, but it occasionally finds renewed popularity.

Likewise, I read about parasites and fungal infections many years ago, and I have long discussed these in my practice (in fact, *Bowel Strength* contains anti-parasitic and anti-fungal herb crutches, because this is a much more common problem than most people realize. Parasites can be picked up from water, food, insects, pets, the soil, and other people, for example.) These conditions have found an audience lately, especially in relation to the treatment of disorders like autism, Lyme's, PANDAS, and other neurological conditions.

(Here forward, as I use the term "fungal infections," it is used broadly to include Candida, yeast, and parasites as well.)

Fungal infections often make their home throughout your entire digestive system. Symptoms of these may include acne, athlete's foot, dandruff, psoriasis, itchy skin, allergies, bloating, diarrhea, green or yellow stools, difficulty sleeping, fatigue, nausea, neurological disorders, behavioral problems, and many others.

There is a fine line between bacterial and fungal infections, and a great similarity between the two of them. Therefore, the information under "Bacterial Infections," described earlier, is valuable for you to read as well.

## Healing Your Body With This Program Eliminates Fungal Infections

While an unhealthy bowel cause these infections, many symptoms that are due to an unhealthy body (i.e. un-eliminated acids) are *wrongly attributed to these infections*, and because you will feel better when you have eliminated these acids, healing your body with this program is invaluable when you have one. (See a lengthier discussion on this topic later.)

## Healing Your Bowel With This Program Eliminates Fungal Infections

It is the responsibility of your bowel bacteria to fight fungal infections in your body. Healing your bowel with this program, therefore, eliminates these infections.

## Why My Crutches Eliminate Fungal Infections

*Unique Healing Colloidal Silver* has natural anti-bacterial, anti-fungal, anti-parasitic properties.

Note: *Bowel Strength* contains anti-fungal and anti-parasitic crutches, too. It is for this reason, as well as the fact that its is far less expensive than a similar strength of probiotics, that I strongly encourage you to use this product over probiotics, whenever possible.

## How much do I take?/Questions about using these

See Chapter 5 for information on using these crutches, including recommendations on the amount to use, as well as a discussion of the misunderstandings about the particular crutch that may, if not understood correctly, cause you to fail to look and feel better while you heal your bowel and body with this program.

## How long will I need to use crutches for my fungal infections?

The bacterial environment in your bowel affects fungal infections. To better understand how long you may need crutches for this, refer to Chapter 1 under this subject heading.

# Misunderstandings About Fungal Infections and Other Information for Your Success

## Many symptoms are wrongly blamed on these infections

Acids that are not eliminated from your body, which are then reabsorbed into your blood and tissues, cause *many* symptoms, and many practitioners automatically call this a Candida, parasitic, or fungal infection.

In truth, many of the symptoms attributed to these infections are merely symptoms of un-eliminated acids, and not true Candida, parasitic, or fungal infections. You may have one of these infections, as well as a lot of un-eliminated acidity causing symptoms, but wrongly, all of your symptoms may be blamed on an infection.

You need to understand how to differentiate between true Candida, fungal, and parasitic infections and acidity symptoms, because products that treat these infections do nothing to eliminate acids from your body, which means they do nothing to eliminate the vast array of your symptoms that are caused by these un-eliminated acids.

## You likely have one if your bowels meet the following criteria

In my experience, it is very easy to determine if you have a Candida, fungal, or parasitic infection (other practitioners may request elaborate and/or expensive tests but I find this to be completely unnecessary).

If your bowels are more than two times a day, and/or your stools are green or yellow, you probably have some type of Candida, fungal, and/or parasitic infection. (Note: to correctly determine the frequency of your elimination you must count every time you eliminate, even if this only produces a very small piece of stool.)

*You can have well-formed stools yet still have one of these infections (if your stools are green, yellow, or more than two times a day).*

Because a healthy bowel eliminates fungal, Candida, and parasitic infections, and you are healing your bowel with this program it is not important to determine *which* type of infection you have. Likewise, because *Unique Healing Colloidal Silver* fights fungal, Candida, *and* parasitic infections, again, you do not need to determine exactly what type of infection you have. (If you seek medical care and are looking for a medication for your infection, then this is more important, as medications are more specific and generally need to be prescribed to match the infection you are trying to treat.)

## Nystatin, Diflucan, caprylic acid, anti-fungals, and other crutches

Doctors and alternative practitioners prescribe a number of crutches to kill fungus, Candida, and/or parasites. When these are used and your bowel is not healed (and most of you are not doing this, as the average practitioners' recommendations for bowel-healing products is usually completely inadequate to accomplish this, as is their knowledge and experience in healing your bowel), you will need to take these intermittently for decades to keep these infections away, a situation that is highly profitable for the people/companies who sell them.

I have found *Unique Healing Colloidal Silver* to be the most effective crutch for these, but there are some other adequate crutches too. It is just important that you recognize that they are just that; you must understand that these are just crutches for these infections and that you must concurrently heal you bowel.

You must also understand that these crutches, *Unique Healing Colloidal Silver* included, do not and cannot permanently eliminate these infections from your body (that can only happen once your bowel has been healed.) In the meantime, you may need to use *Unique Healing Colloidal Silver* repetitively, and sometimes daily, until your bowel is healthier in order to keep these infections away. One treatment with these, in other words, does not make you immune to their return.

Should you decide to treat your fungal, Candida, and/or parasitic infections with a product other than *Unique Healing Colloidal Silver*, I urge you to stay away from Nystatin, Diflucan, and all other medications, as much as possible. They are toxic/acidic, and contribute to a less healthy bowel (which means that your use of them makes you *more* vulnerable to an infection in the future.) There may be a short-term period when you feel better because the "bad guys" have been killed, but they eventually return, and often at a higher level than before, because of the damaging effect of the drug on your bowel health.

In other words, if you have holes in your trashcan, trash will leak out onto the ground, which will attract bugs. Killing the bugs gets rid of them for a while, but they will eventually come back, because killing them did nothing to fix the holes in the trashcan. The leaky trashcan will continue to leak, and the bugs will eventually find their way back. This happens all the time. To completely eliminate these bugs, the holes in the trashcan must be fixed, as this program does.

This "kill the Candida or fungal infection" approach is popular however, and continues to be prescribed, because everyone likes a quick fix. There is often an initial immediate improvement in your weight and/ or symptoms, and when in the long run your weight or symptoms come back, many of you wrongly think you are to blame.

## No "die-off" with my program

Programs that recommend products that kill fungal, Candida and parasitic infections describe a side effect they term "die-off." You are told you might experience uncomfortable symptoms while using these products, but that these symptoms are a valuable result of the product "killing off" the unwanted fungal, Candida, and/or parasitic organisms.

If you take a product and feel worse, there is nothing valuable or productive about this. If you feel bad, something is wrong.

When I was ill and diagnosed with Candida, I was prescribed Nystatin. I vividly remember the experience. I remember exactly where I was, whom I was with, and what I was doing at the time, because the use of this medication made me feel extraordinarily toxic. I felt as though I had swallowed a bottle of poison. My blood was stinging. It was one of the most horrible experiences of my illness. I too was wrongly told this was a valuable side effect, but I stopped the Nystatin after two days because my symptoms were unbearable. And it just felt wrong.

What is called "die off" is simply a toxic reaction to the medication you are using. This is not only invaluable, but it is harmful.

You will not experience "die-off" with *Bowel Strength* or *Unique Healing Probiotics* (or *any* of the *Unique Healing* products), because these products are not toxic.

## The high-protein, sugar-free, wheat-free, dairy-free dietary crutch approach to these infections

Commonly, advice given for these infections includes a dietary approach that includes high protein, low sugar, and wheat-free, dairy-free food recommendations. (So what really helped you feel better—the diet, or the mediation or anti-fungal or anti-parasitic herb or drug? If you follow both at the same time, you won't know, and you will sometimes be wrongly led to believe that because you felt better, this is proof that the recommended anti-fungal helped. This is definitely not an assumption that can be made.)

A high protein diet temporarily reduces the symptoms that often get blamed on these infections (see this discussion earlier); in the short run, it stops the movement of acids from your organs into your blood and bowel, which creates numerous symptoms when they are not eliminated. But in the long run, this approach is dangerous and causes your symptoms to worsen

This concept is one of the most important ones for you to understand, and it has been repeated numerous times throughout this book, as well as in *Unique Healing*, and in many of my videos at *www.UniqueHealing. com* or *www.YouTube.com/UniqueHealing*. If it still confuses you, call me for a brief visit. It is imperative that you are not confused by it.

### Also called "leaky gut"

Leaky gut is a term that is often used to describe the conditions of fungal infections. I thoroughly discussed the problems with using this terminology in Chapter 3 of *Unique Healing*. Refer to this chapter for a better understanding of why I choose not to use this term in my practice, yet why this program eliminates the condition that is called "leaky gut."

# Success With Fungal Infections

"*Unique Healing Colloidal Silver* eliminated my dandruff."

"My five year old son was diagnosed with autism. He had frequent stools that were frequently green. We had tried many anti-fungal programs prior to this one. None of them helped. When he began this program and his stools became brown—for the first time in years—we immediately observed that he slept all night long, his OCD was dramatically improved, and his behavior was remarkably improved, as noticed by many others."

"I struggled with allergies constantly and within one week of using *Unique Healing Colloidal Silver* they went away."

"My seven year old daughter had horrible psoriasis, which cleared up quickly on the *Unique Healing Colloidal Silver*."

"I was prescribed Nystatin by my doctor and soon after taking it, I had blurry vision, headaches, insomnia, anxiety, and nausea. I stopped it soon after and instead added in colloidal silver and none of those symptoms occurred. I will never take anything like that drug again."

## My story

Twenty-five years ago, when I was incredibly ill, I was diagnosed with Candida. At the time I didn't know anything about nutrition and the physiology of the human body, so I too thought it made sense to attack the Candida, and attack it I did. I tried every Candida-killing drug and supplement available. I know of nothing that is used today to treat this condition that did not exist back then. When I failed to respond, I was told that I was the "hopeless case" and led to feel privileged that my nutritionist had some connections and could smuggle an illegal Candida drug in from France for me. This didn't work either. In fact, there was great concern about the function of my kidneys after I used it, one of the known dangers of the drug. Sure enough, I landed in the emergency room with kidney problems.

Following this fiasco, I went to a homeopath, and at the time, white spores of Candida were flying out of my mouth. He immediately sent me for an AIDS test. My test came back negative, thank goodness, but my white tongue and symptoms continued for years.

I no longer have symptoms of Candida, and I do not take supplements, or have to follow a strict diet, to keep these infections away. My healthy bowel and body do this for me, and yours will too, once you heal them with this program.

## Watch My Video, "Why THIS Program Eliminates Fungal Infections"

This video, and all of my videos, can be found at *www.UniqueHealing. com* or at *www.YouTube.com/UniqueHealing*.

# Gallstones/Gallbladder Problems
## Kidney Stones

Your gallbladder is responsible for secreting a substance called bile into your small intestines. Bile is used to digest the fat in your diet. It also transports toxins into your bowel. When this goes awry, you may experience a gallbladder attack. Gallbladder attacks are also often the product of clogged bile ducts, inflammation, and/or gallstones, as these can all occur at the same time/have the same cause (a gallstone can cause inflammation, and it can cause a bile duct to become blocked, for example.)

Gallbladder problems are largely confined to problems with gallstones, hence the following discussion, which focuses on these.

Kidney stones, gallstones, and plaque are very similar problems. All exist when there is an accumulation of acidity, and a build-up of cholesterol as a result. Gallstones exist when you have an excess build-up of cholesterol and bilirubin, a bile waste product, and inadequate bile salts (i.e. alkalinity). Over 90% of stones (gallstones, kidney stones) contain cholesterol, *not* calcium, as is commonly thought. See the discussion on this misunderstanding later.

Kidney stones occur at the bottom of your pipe, gallstones in the middle, and plaque at the top (plaque is the most dangerous, then gallstones, then kidney stones, in other words). Also, if you have or have had gallstones, and you do not heal your bowel and body, this can lead to plaque later on, so if you have had stones, respect this warning, and heal your bowel and body now.

(Note: The information in the following section is relevant to kidney stones as well, and in the majority of places where you see "gallstones" or "gallbladder," you can simply replace it with "kidney stones" or "kidneys.")

## Healing Your Body With This Program Eliminates Gallstones/Gallbladder Problems

Cholesterol is manufactured by your liver and used to buffer un-eliminated acids, but this can lead to gallstones. Inflammation is another response to un-eliminated acids. Bilirubin is a toxin/acid that should be eliminated by your body.

Healing your body with this program eliminates the acids that cause excess cholesterol production and inflammation. Healing your body with this program heals your gallbladder (and kidneys).

## Healing Your Bowel With This Program Eliminates Gallstones/Gallbladder Problems

In addition to its other many important functions, a healthy bacterial environment in your bowel is a necessity for the complete elimination of acids (toxins, heavy metals, pesticides, etc.) from your body. A healthy bowel prevents the re-absorption of acids into your blood that cause an unhealthy gallbladder, and trigger cholesterol/gallstone production and inflammation.

## Why My Crutches Work for Gallstones/Gallbladder Problems

**Body Bentonite** binds to and eliminates acids (toxins, heavy metals, chemicals, etc.) from your body. It helps prevent them from becoming re-absorbed into your bloodstream, where they trigger a response by your body to protect you from them. It eliminates the acids that trigger the release of inflammatory chemicals, and gallbladder pain and discomfort.

**Unique Healing Calcium Citrate** is an alkalinizing mineral that helps neutralize the acids that your bowel does not eliminate. When these acids are neutralized, your body does not need to produce inflammatory chemicals to buffer them.

There are no crutches for degenerative conditions and large accumulations of acidity in your organs, like gallstones. Crutches can offset the effects of acids in your blood, or the effects of poor function of your bowel bacterial environment (as these can be quickly altered), but degeneration is caused by depletion and damage to your organs, and organs take time to heal.

On the other hand, *Body Bentonite* and *Unique Healing Calcium Citrate* can help prevent *future* stones from occurring.

## How long will I need to use crutches for my gallstones/ gallbladder problems?

Again, there are no crutches for great accumulations of acidity, like gallstones. This takes time to eliminate. However, your gallbladder is in the "middle of your pipe" and the second level of your body that heals, assuming your first level needs to heal as well.

# Misunderstandings About Gallstones/Gallbladder Problems and Other Information for Your Success

## Calcium reduces stones; it does not increase them!

I commonly have doctors warn my clients to be careful about the amounts of calcium I recommend, because, they state, it may cause kidney stones. These comments are made even though *medical* research shows the opposite to be true (that extra calcium *reduces* stone formation). It is very frustrating!

In a systematic review of studies investigating the relationship between calcium intake and risk of kidney stones, it was concluded that calcium intake (dietary and supplements) is not associated with an increased risk of kidney stones in postmenopausal women. On the contrary, the reviewers point out that, "there is a substantial body of evidence, both from controlled trials and from observational studies, indicating that there is an inverse relationship between calcium intake and stone risk."

In other words, the *more* calcium someone took (dietary and supplements) the *fewer* stones they had.

This study observed kidney stones, but it would surely apply to all stones, gallstones included, should this variable be observed and measured as well.

Also, this review looked at postmenopausal women, but that should not be implied to be limited to you, if you are not postmenopausal, or if you are a male. Likely, postmenopausal women were studied because as a group, they are the most likely to consume large quantities of calcium (in an attempt to prevent osteoporosis.)

Finally, notice that this is not a study, but rather a review of *many* studies, which makes it even that more credible and powerful. ("Calcium supplementation and incident kidney stone risk: a systemic review" Heaney RP, J Am Coll Nutr, 2008; 27(5): 519-27.)

## Take extra *Unique Healing Calcium Citrate*

Continuing with the above theme, if you have or have had stones (kidney, gallbladder, etc.) and/or are worried about them, take extra *Unique Healing Calcium Citrate* while you are healing your bowel and body with this program. When your bowel and body are healed you will not get these stones, but in the meantime, extra calcium is a great crutch to prevent or reduce their occurrence. Take an extra 1,500 mg/day (in addition to the 2,500 mg/day recommended in Chapter 5).

## So why the confusion with calcium?

The medical doctors who warn my clients about extra calcium consumption and kidney stone production likely make this warning due to the fact that stones (kidney and gallbladder) often contain calcium. The conclusion that calcium is therefore the cause of these stones is yet another example of medicine seeing two variables coexisting, and concluding, "one must cause the other."

Calcium is an alkalinizing mineral that your body may use to buffer the un-eliminated acids that cause these stones, hence their presence in them. But it is wrong to imply that calcium is the cause, or that it is harmful, or that taking calcium increases stone formation. Calcium is the good guy. It is trying to protect you. Taking more calcium is, again, not only not going to cause stone production, but by buffering the acids that *do* cause stone production, it can help reduce the formation of stones in your body.

## Removing an organ removes the symptom, not the problem

Think of your gallbladder as a home for excess waste products/acids (cholesterol and bile), and if it is removed, your body will find another home, like your arteries perhaps, to store these. This is a much more dangerous and deadly place to store waste products.

If you were in the emergency room in the midst of a severe gallbladder attack, I would certainly understand your decision to have it removed. Once this has been removed, and if this applies to you reading this and it was removed years ago, I strongly warn you to see this as a sign that acids have accumulated to the "middle of your pipe," and will likely soon find their way to the top, which is eventually life threatening. Healing your bowel and body with this program stops this from happening.

## Fats don't cause gallbladder problems, excess un-eliminated acids do

Just as excess fat is not the cause of high cholesterol, it is not the cause of gallbladder problems, either. Acids are the cause, so avoid acidic fats—like chicken fat, beef fat, pork fat and other animal meat fats, and margarine—but do eat a lot of non-acidic fats, like olive oil, avocadoes, even butter, as these help *reduce* the acidity in your blood that leads to gallstones and gallbladder problems in the first place.

And just as excess sugar, soda, alcohol, and even fruit and carbohydrates—which cleanse your organs and release acids into your blood that are not eliminated when your bowel is unhealthy—can increase cholesterol levels, so too can these items increase gallstone production and gallbladder problems. Minimize your intake of these until your bowel and body are healthy enough to handle them.

## Success With Gallstones/Gallbladder Problems

"I was diagnosed with gallstones but I was not in pain so I decided to wait and see if they would go away with this program. They did."

"I had my gallbladder removed and was told I had to forever be careful about eating fat. Donna had me slowly healthy fats back into my diet, and along with the other dietary advice, and this program, I have remained symptom-free."

## Watch My Video, "Why THIS Program Eliminates Gallstones/ Gallbladder Problems"

This video, and all of my videos, can be found at *www.UniqueHealing. com* or at *www.YouTube.com/UniqueHealing*.

## Gas
See "Bloating and Gas"

# Glaucoma
See "Eye Problems"

# Gluten Allergies
See "Allergies (Food)"

# Hay Fever
See "Allergies (Environmental)"

# Headaches
See "Aches and Pains"

# Heart Attack
See "Cholesterol/Heart Disease"

# Heartburn
See "Reflux"

# Heart Disease
See "Cholesterol/Heart Disease"

# Heavy Metal Toxicity
**Aluminum, Cadmium, Copper, Lead, Nickel, Mercury, and Others**

I was exposed to the dangers of heavy metal toxicity twenty-five years ago when I was very ill, and I am glad to see that a much larger percentage of you are now being informed of the dangers of this as well.

Heavy metals, like all acids/toxins, can damage every organ in your body, and like all acids, they contribute to a myriad of problems, including weight problems, addictions, symptoms, and disease.

# Healing Your Body With This Program Eliminates Heavy Metal Toxicity

Like other acids, heavy metals are acids that are eliminated from your body with this program.

# Healing Your Bowel With This Program Eliminates Heavy Metal Toxicity

In addition to its many other important functions, a healthy bacterial environment in your bowel is a necessity for the complete elimination of acids (like heavy metals) from your body. A healthy bowel prevents the re-absorption of metals into your blood that cause an unhealthy body, and trigger many of your symptoms, weight problems, addictions, and disease.

# Why My Crutches Work for Heavy Metal Toxicity

*Body Bentonite* binds to and eliminates acids (toxins, heavy metals, chemicals, etc.) from your body. It helps prevent them from becoming re-absorbed into your bloodstream, where they trigger a response by your body to protect you from them, and damage to your organs and overall health.

*Unique Healing Calcium Citrate* is an alkalinizing mineral that helps neutralize the acids, like heavy metals, that your bowel does not eliminate. It buffers the acidity of metals in your blood so they do not trigger uncomfortable symptoms.

## How much do I take?/Questions about using these

See Chapter 5 for information on using these crutches, including recommendations on the amount to use, as well as a discussion of the misunderstandings about the particular crutch that may, if not understood correctly, cause you to fail to look and feel better while you heal your bowel and body with this program.

## How long will I need to use crutches for my heavy metal toxicity?

Heavy metal toxicity occurs at Levels 1, 2, 3, and 4 of your pipe. How long you will need crutches to offset this depends on the condition you are most concerned about. Refer to the other sections in this chapter to understand how long you will need to use crutches for that particular condition. Refer to the diagram "Sequence of Healing" in Appendix A at the end of this book to better understand this concept, as well as to Chapter 1 under this subject heading.

# Misunderstandings About Heavy Metal Toxicity and Other Information for Your Success

### Keep your stools well-formed

Because heavy metal toxicity is caused by the incomplete elimination of these from your body, and because well-formed stools prevent the re-absorption of heavy metals into your blood, you will suffer from the least amount of heavy metal toxicity symptoms, and blood test imbalances, if you keep your stools well-formed while you are healing your bowel and body.

If you do not have a very good handle on how to define well-formed stools, review Chapter 6 of *Unique Healing* now. (And remember, when your stools are hard and slow you are eliminating more acids, and will therefore feel better, than when your stools are one or more times a day but not all extremely well-formed.)

If your stools are not well-formed, the following changes can help: increase your *Body Bentoni*te intake; reduce your carbohydrate intake (pasta, breads, grains, cereals, yogurt, etc.); reduce your sugar intake (including natural healthy sugars such as agave, honey, raw sugar, cane juice, etc.); reduce your alcohol, salt, coffee, and/or soda intake; do not have a massage, chiropractic adjustment, or any other body work; drink a lot of water; rest; and keep your exercise aerobic (see Chapter 4 for more information on how to attain this, and why it is important.)

If these changes do not noticeably help the form of your stools in two days, take them further (i.e. take more *Body Bentonite*, reduce your carbohydrate intake more, etc.)

Out of all of these recommendations, increasing your *Body Bentonite* intake is one of the most productive and helpful. It heals your body, unlike many of the other recommendations. It will do the most to lead you to a place where looking and feeling good is effortless, and some of the other suggestions, such as reducing sugar intake, are simply "too hard to do when your blood is too acidic."

(Note: the exception to this information is when your poorly formed stools are caused by an infection, in which case *Unique Healing Colloidal Silver* is needed to reduce your symptoms. Refer to Chapter 5 for information on when and how to use this crutch.)

## Chelation therapy, iodine, methionine, and other "metal detoxifiers" are crutches that do not eliminate metals from your body . . .

. . . and therefore, they are much less valuable than you are led to believe.

Chelation, methionine, iodine and other nutrients, do not eliminate toxic metals from your body. They may buffer them, making them less visible in your blood, and less symptom-producing, leading to the declaration from the practitioners who recommend them that this means they have exited your body, but this is not true. If I spray my trash with perfume I may not notice that the trash is there anymore, but this perfume only masked the ill effects of the trash, it did nothing to eliminate it from my house. Just because you can no longer smell the odor from this trash does not mean that it is gone.

Ninety percent of mercury is excreted in bile (attached to glutathione and cysteine), creating a waste product that needs to be excreted by your bowel. When your bowel is unhealthy, this waste is not eliminated, and like all un-eliminated acids, these heavy metals become re-absorbed into your blood and tissues.

In other words, just because the mercury is attached to these nutrients and formed into bile does *not* mean that it has been excreted from your body. Researchers have stated that they believe that over 70% of mercury goes through "enterohepatic cycling" which is a fancy way of saying that it is returned to your liver; that it is not eliminated from your body. I believe this amount is much higher, because it takes a healthy bowel to eliminate mercury (and all metals), and my experience is that the vast majority of you do not have a healthy bowel.

Glutathione, cysteine, chelating agents, and other "metal-eliminating" supplements only bind to mercury and other heavy metals in your blood and reduce the uncomfortable symptoms associated with their presence there, but this *does not* mean that they have been eliminated from your body. It takes a healthy bowel, as created in this program, to *eliminate* heavy metals from your body.

Remember, there are only four ways to eliminate acids, or toxins, like heavy metals, from your body, which is by way of your breath, sweat, urine, and stool. Deep breathing, drinking more water, and saunas eliminate toxins like metals through your breath, sweat, and urine; "heavy metal detoxifiers" do not. *Body Bentonite* binds to toxins like metals in your bowel so that they exit your body through your stool; "heavy metal detoxifiers" do not.

## Blood tests for heavy metal levels can be very wrong and misleading

Blood tests are a horrible way to measure the health of your organs. This includes blood tests that measure heavy metals, as well. If you have a large storage of these metals in your organs, which pose a threat to your longevity, this will not necessarily show up in your blood, and on a blood test.

If you are ever temped to follow a protocol that promises to eliminate heavy metals from your body, you must demand a test that measures these metals on the *tissue* (i.e. organ) level. Additionally, if it is claimed that this protocol has eliminated heavy metals from your blood and body, then a blood test needs to be followed up three months later, when you are taking no supplements (crutches), *and* you are eating a high carbohydrate diet (as this diet dumps metals from your organs into your blood, and if you really eliminated all of the metals from your body, as is often claimed, this diet would not cause metals to show up in your blood).

Likewise, if you are following this program and will be having a blood test done of your heavy metal levels, you may improve these by following the instructions on "manipulating blood tests" found in Chapter 8 of *Unique Healing*. It is important that you try to manipulate these, otherwise you may be tempted to fall for a quick-fix crutch program, and the dangers of these approaches are many.

## How *do* you accurately test your metal levels?

I know of no accurate and simple test that measures the amount of metals in your organs/tissues, yet again, numerous programs claim to eliminate metals from your organs. Without accurate testing, these claims can't and should not be made.

If you Google this question you will find numerous sights that advertise hair analysis testing as a tool to measure tissue levels of heavy metals.

I recently went back to the hair analysis tests that I had done almost twenty years ago. I too was convinced these might have some validity (although I have never recommended that a client pay to have one done).

When my test results came back they also came back with a long list of supplement crutches that I was to take to "improve my health." At this time, I had already been down this road many times, and had seen it get me nowhere, but I drove down it again, anyway (to some degree, that is). I took many of the supplements they recommended but not all of them, and I did not take them consistently throughout the eighteen months that I did these tests (I did a total of four tests over this time).

I looked at these results, and some variables, including the heavy metals, minerals and other nutrients they tested, were not consistent. They did not consistently improve. Once they did get better, but got worse again in the following test, about five months later. If these tests accurately measured the storage of toxins in my tissues, and if the supplements they gave me actually eliminated them, these results could not occur. (Unless you are exposed to an enormous amount of metals, or toxins, which is very rare, and not the situation in my case, metals and toxins take many years to accumulate in your body, not just five months). This was done a long time ago but my guess is that when I took a test without all of the crutches (i.e. supplements) they advised, the test came back worse.

In other words, this test did not measure the health of my organs; it was another measurement of the un-eliminated acids in my blood, and if you only measure these while following a program, you will be led astray.

I no longer support the use of hair analysis testing as a viable way to measure organ health.

When your organs are healthy and free of heavy metals, you will be able to eat a very cleansing, high fruit and carbohydrate diet, and not gain weight or feel horrible doing so.

That's the most accurate, and only, test for heavy metal toxicity that you need (and it is very inexpensive, too).

## We can't control the rain, just the strength of our roof

Heavy metals are just one of hundreds of possible toxins that you may be exposed to, and that can cause symptoms, illness, addictions, and weight problems. It is just one of the many rocks on the scale. It is just one possible "rain storm." These storms can be avoided to some degree, but not completely. Think of the recent disaster in Japan and the outpouring of radiation, which was not under our control. What we *can* control is how our body reacts to this and other toxins; we can control the health of our bowel and body so that when we are exposed to heavy metals, and all other toxins, our body can effectively eliminate them, and therefore prevent them from harming us.

## *Body Bentonite* does *not* contain heavy metals

Some very wrong, and dangerous, comments have been made online, and by medical and alternative health practitioners, about the "dangers" of bentonite due to "its aluminum content."

These claims and concerns are unfounded. They are *not* based on experience or studies. Beware of everything you read and hear. People are allowed to make any claim they want. Before you give these any credibility, ask the questions that you deserve to get the answers to. Where are the studies that show it is dangerous? What experience does the person who is writing these claims, or repeating them (which is usually the case), has to make such a statement?

There are no valid studies that show bentonite is dangerous, and the people who I have seen make these false claims have zero personal experience using large amounts, for long periods of time, with a large group of clients, as I do, and are therefore not qualified to make them.

For the last 19 years I have used bentonite and similar products with my clients. I have had hundreds of clients take amounts that are considered "massive" by the alternative and medical field. *Unlike these people making negative claims about bentonite, I am qualified to comment about the safety of this product.*

*Body Bentonite* does not contain aluminum. There *might* be extremely small amounts of aluminum in some other bentonite products. I cannot attest to their contents. Still, in my experience, bentonite removes *far* many more toxins, including heavy metals like aluminum, from your body than it adds. However, if you are concerned, use *Body Bentonite* as your source of bentonite.

My experience has revealed that bentonite does *not* add aluminum to your body. On the contrary, it *eliminates* it from your body (and the symptoms and diseases associated with excess aluminum stores). In fact, the larger the ingestion of bentonite, the faster heavy metal tests improve. The more bentonite you take, the more toxins, aluminum included, that are eliminated from your body.

I have never seen any harm done by the ingestion of large amounts of bentonite. On the contrary, I have seen people lose weight and keep it off, eliminate polyps, cysts, many diseases, congested arteries, high cholesterol, headaches, bloating, blood sugar problems, ADD, alcoholism, etc. I have seen it heal one's organs and greatly extend the quality and quantity of one's life.

It is sad that some of you are being led to be afraid of a product that can dramatically improve the quality *and* longevity of your life; something that modern *and* alternative medicine is failing to do.

So why are these inaccurate, fear-mongering comments made? I can only guess at this. Maybe it is because if everyone took large quantities of bentonite, many *billions* of dollars of profit would be lost yearly in the medical and alternative field? Maybe it is because bentonite is a major threat to the many people and industries that earn a very good living treating your symptoms with crutches? (I just read that the drug companies sold $20 billion dollars worth of cancer drugs alone in the year 2009–wow.)

*In nature, as with humans, there is a natural tendency to react to a threat——to our safety, financial stability, etc.——with an attack. So you decide what is more important to you—their profit, or your longevity and health?*

## Unique Healing Colloidal Silver is not a toxic heavy metal

I understand this concern, and misunderstanding, and I hear it sometimes, mostly with parents of children with neurological disorders like autism and A.D.D. Most of these children have moderate to severe fungal/bacterial infections and the recommendation to give them colloidal silver is one I often make.

*Unique Healing Colloidal Silver* is not a heavy metal, however, and there is no known harm that can come from using it. I have recommended very large amounts to a large number of clients, and I have seen not only safety after its use, but effectiveness and benefit from doing so, as well.

A complete discussion on the misunderstandings and fears of using this product can be found in Chapter 5.

## Mercury in vaccinations and dental fillings

Excess mercury re-absorption is said to be the primary risk of vaccinations containing mercury, and neurological disorders, like Autism, are being blamed for this (although I disagree that mercury is the cause of these disorders. For more information, see "Neurological Disorders" later in this chapter.)

For a discussion on the dangers of mercury in dental fillings, and my recommendations for dealing with existing ones, refer to "Dental Problems" earlier in this section.

# Success With Heavy Metal Toxicity

I have seen a number of clients who have presented themselves to me with a diagnosis of heavy metal toxicity who were on a "heavy metal detox" program; on an aggressive and strict regimen of diet and supplements that they were told were eliminating metals from their body. The story below mirrors that of almost everyone I have seen in this situation.

"I was extremely fatigued, anxious, irritable, and in pain, and I found a very highly educated specialist in the area of heavy metal toxicity who encouraged me that he had developed a protocol for the elimination of metals from my body, and that he had all the answers to my symptoms and ill health. I ingested an enormous handful of supplements every day and I did feel better, about 50% better than I had before. I was thrilled to have these metals out of my body. His test showed they were no longer in my body. After a few months on the protocol, and a lot of money, I stopped these supplements, and all of my symptoms returned. When I found Donna she told me that the supplements I had ingested were only crutches that masked the symptoms produced by the metals but did not actually eliminate them from my system. I was angry at first and I really didn't want to believe this either. I wanted/needed to believe that the thousands of dollars I had spent on the other protocol was worth my money and had actually benefitted me. I was skeptical, but deep down I knew she was right. Eventually I embraced this program and its concepts and have taken very large amounts of *Body Bentonite*, and *Bowel Strength*, and my symptoms have improved to a level beyond which I achieved with the approach I followed earlier. More importantly, they remain improved even if I do not take my supplements. I have let go of my anger over my past attempts and failures and am actively working to help others understand this process too."

## My story

I was diagnosed with heavy metal toxicity via live cell analysis and hair analysis twenty-five years ago when I was ill, as described earlier. I was told that these metals were a significant contributor to my symptoms, and I ingested numerous supplements that I was told would eliminate these metals from my body, as well as spent a lot of money having all of my old amalgam dental fillings removed. I never felt better on these regimens. I figured out long ago that these crutches (methionine, glutathione, etc.) were just that, crutches. Now I have zero symptoms of heavy metal toxicity and I do not need to take supplements to feel better/maintain these results.

### Watch My Video, "Why THIS Program Eliminates Heavy Metal Toxicity"

This video, and all of my videos, can be found at *www.UniqueHealing.com* or at *www.YouTube.com/UniqueHealing*.

# Hemorrhoids
See "Bowel Conditions"

# Hepatitis
See "Liver Disease" and "Viral Infections"

# Herpes
See "Viral Infections"

# Hypertension
See "Blood Pressure"

# Hypoglycemia
See "Diabetes and Hypoglycemia"

# Hypotension
See "Blood Pressure"

# Indigestion
See "Reflux"

# Impotence
See "Sexual Health"

# Indigestion
See "Reflux"

# Infertility
(See also "Female Issues")

The incidence of infertility in this country is staggering, and heartbreaking.

In the United States, infertility affects a very large percentage of the reproductive-age population, or about one in every seven or eight couples. Fertility treatments tripled from 1996 to 2008, and yet the overall IVF success rate is only about 30% (which drops substantially the older you are; it is only about 10% successful if you are in your early 40's, for example).

I predict that in the near future, girls and women will return to early pregnancies, as their parents who struggled with fertility issues in their thirties encourage them "not to wait." This may last a while and improve fertility rates, but then that may even stop "working" one day. Fertility is a product of health, and our health is rapidly declining to the point that one day soon, even young women may struggle to reproduce.

Is greater technology the answer? Personally, I think this is something we should be extremely concerned about. I think that one day we will learn the dire consequences of it. The long-term safety of modern day methods of improving fertility, like hormone therapy, in vitro fertilization, etc., has not been adequately tested. Never in the history of mankind have we had such a large percentage of the population who are the product of these methods. We have yet to witness the long-term health consequences of the children born as a result of them.

Healing your bowel and body is very effective at reversing infertility. It also dramatically reduces your chance of miscarriage, premature birth, and difficulties during pregnancy. And most importantly, it dramatically improves not only your health, but the health of your child as well.

If you have tried everything to get pregnant without success, I am certain you have not yet healed your bowel and body.

This works. If you want to get pregnant, do this program. Do it for yourself, but more importantly, do it for your child.

## A Healthy Body Eliminates Infertility

Conception is half of the equation to having a baby. After conception, conditions must be right for your baby to "stick around." The prevention of miscarriage is dependent on a number of variables that reflect the health of your body. In my office, I over-simplify this statement by saying that your baby wants to live in a "clean home." You wouldn't want to live in a dirty house, either! (I believe that this half of the equation may be more of a problem than women realize; many women have likely become pregnant and very shortly thereafter miscarried without ever having known that their egg was fertilized.)

A more complex explanation describing conditions that have been proven to cause, or are believed to cause, miscarriage include: Antiphospholipid Syndrome (APS), a condition where your immune system blocks the molecules that prevent *blood clots*, causing clots to form in the placenta, damaging it and leading to a miscarriage; Hereditary thrombophilias, genetic mutations that cause *blood to clot* in the placenta; Abnormal blood flow to the uterus, which occurs when one or more of the uterine arteries constrict, robbing the fetus of *oxygen* and vital *nutrients*; An overabundance of NKCs (natural killer cells), which cause *blood clots* to form in the placenta, or produce "bad" proteins called TH1 cytokines that are toxic to the embryo.

Healing your body with this program eliminates the acids that cause low oxygen levels in your blood, and a subsequent risk for blood clots. It eliminates the acids that cause low oxygen and nutrient levels, which are two major issues that affect your ability to carry a baby to term. Healing your body with this program eliminates the toxins/waste/acids that cause a "dirty home."

# A Healthy Bowel Eliminates Infertility

Conception, and the prevention of miscarriage, depends on proper hormonal regulation, and a healthy bowel balances the hormones in your body.

When your egg is fertilized a number of physiological changes take place to help your baby grow. One of them is the increased production of progesterone. High levels of this hormone are needed to maintain the viability of the embryo. Once your egg is fertilized, your progesterone levels need to rise sharply in order for the fetus to develop. (An additional medical explanation given for miscarriage is a condition called "luteal phase defect," which is a progesterone defect that, as they explain it, keeps the uterine lining from developing properly, which prevents the uterus from supporting a pregnancy.)

A healthy bowel bacterial environment, as created with this program, keeps these progesterone levels balanced.

As for conception, a certain level of estrogen triggers the onset of your monthly menstruation. If you have high levels of estrogen, your periods will come sooner than the ideal every 28 days. If you have insufficient levels, your periods will be late. When your periods are regular (defined as every 28 days), it is easy to predict when you are ovulating, and therefore fertile. Having sex when you are fertile is a necessity to become pregnant, hence the promotion of ovulation kits that can measure this for you. Having sex very frequently helps if your periods are irregular, hence the stories you often hear of women getting pregnant in the "honeymoon" stage of their relationship.

A healthy bowel regulates all of your hormone levels, estrogen included.

Infertility specialists focus primarily on the administration of synthetic hormones to improve a woman's chance of conceiving. By healing your bowel with this program, you create a system that regulates your hormones naturally and perfectly. No synthetic drug could ever match the perfect regulation of a complex matter like hormones.

In addition to its many other important functions, a healthy bacterial environment in your bowel is a necessity for the complete elimination of acids (toxins, heavy metals, pesticides, etc.) from your body. A healthy bowel prevents the re-absorption of acids into your blood that causes an unhealthy body, and causes a build up of acidity/toxicity in your uterus, and that reduce the vital oxygen and nutrients that your growing fetus needs to survive. It eliminates the acids that cause blood clots.

# Why My Crutches Work for Infertility

*Body Bentonite* binds to and eliminates acids (toxins, heavy metals, chemicals, etc.) from your body. It helps prevent them from becoming re-absorbed into your bloodstream, where they trigger a response by your body to protect you from them. It eliminates the acids that reduce oxygen and nutrient levels, improving the delivery of these vital elements to your developing fetus. It eliminates the acids that make for a "dirty house that your baby will not live in." (I have also seen this product eliminate morning sickness, fatigue, premature births, edema, and diabetes during pregnancy.)

**Natural progesterone cream** provides a safe source of natural progesterone, so that once your egg is fertilized, there is sufficient levels of this hormone to sustain the pregnancy. It can reduce the chance of miscarriage. It can also help ensure that your baby is not born prematurely, and it is extremely valuable for reducing post-partum depression.

## How much do I take?/Questions about using these

See Chapter 5 for information on using these crutches, including recommendations on the amount to use, as well as a discussion of the misunderstandings about the particular crutch that may, if not understood correctly, cause you to fail to look and feel better while you heal your bowel and body with this program.

If you get pregnant while doing this program, or are currently pregnant, I strongly suggest you contact me for an appointment before starting this program.

## How long will I need to use crutches for my infertility?

Infertility occurs at Level 3 of your pipe. It is the second to last area of your body to heal (assuming that other areas are unhealthy too). Refer to the diagram "Sequence of Healing" in Appendix A at the end of this book to better understand this concept, as well as to Chapter 1 under this subject heading.

The bacterial environment in your bowel also affects infertility. To better understand how long you may need crutches for this, refer to Chapter 1 under this subject heading.

# Misunderstandings about infertility and other information for your success

## Keep your stools well-formed

Because infertility is caused in part by un-eliminated acids, and because well-formed stools prevent the re-absorption of acids into your blood, you will suffer from the least amount of infertility issues if you keep your stools well-formed while you are healing your bowel and body.

If you do not have a very good handle on how to define well-formed stools, review Chapter 6 of *Unique Healing* now. (And remember, when your stools are hard and slow you are eliminating more acids, and will therefore feel better, than when your stools are one or more times a day but not all extremely well-formed.)

If your stools are not well-formed, the following changes can help: increase your *Body Bentonite* intake; reduce your carbohydrate intake (pasta, breads, grains, cereals, yogurt, etc.); reduce your sugar intake (including natural healthy sugars such as agave, honey, raw sugar, cane juice, etc.); reduce your alcohol, salt, coffee, and/or soda intake; do not have a massage, chiropractic adjustment, or any other body work; drink a lot of water; rest; and keep your exercise aerobic (see Chapter 4 for more information on how to attain this, and why it is important.)

If these changes do not noticeably help the form of your stools in two days, take them further (i.e. take more *Body Bentonite*, reduce your carbohydrate intake more, etc.)

Out of all of these recommendations, increasing your *Body Bentonite* intake is one of the most productive and helpful. It heals your body, unlike many of the other recommendations. It will do the most to lead you to a place where looking and feeling good is effortless, and some of the other suggestions, such as reducing sugar intake, are simply "too hard to do when your blood is too acidic."

(Note: the exception to this information is when your poorly formed stools are caused by an infection, in which case *Unique Healing Colloidal*

*Silver* is needed to reduce your symptoms. Refer to Chapter 5 for information on when and how to use this crutch.)

## Be careful when using crutches for infertility

If you have headaches and take a crutch to get rid of them, and forget the crutch for a few days, your headaches may return. This may be uncomfortable, but that is the worst of it.

On the other hand, if you are pregnant and take a crutch to prevent a miscarriage, for example, but forget that crutch for a few days, you could lose your baby. This is one risk of using crutches to become pregnant. If you understand this risk and are willing to accept it, try the crutches above. It is preferable, when possible, that you work aggressively to heal your bowel and body *prior* to trying to conceive, because the healthier they are, the fewer crutches you will need, and this risk is subsequently reduced or eliminated.

In my experience, clients who suffer from loose bowels during the first three months of pregnancy have a much higher likelihood of miscarrying than clients who do not. (Among the many ideas I have for studies, this is one I would like to see done on a much larger scale.)

Follow the instructions in Chapter 5 for using the above-mentioned crutches very carefully, and contact me for an appointment as soon as you become pregnant while following this program.

## Get your man on this program too

According to some statistics, male infertility accounts for up to 40% of all infertility problems. While the majority of my clients become pregnant, regardless of their male partner's fertility (i.e. health), you might not want to take that chance.

You have a better chance of becoming pregnant if your male partner is healthy, too. (And even if his health would not have prevented you from becoming pregnant, once your child is born, you surely want him around a long time. Healing his bowel and body with this program reduces early mortality from heart attack, stroke, cancer, etc.).

The health of your partner's fertility is affected by the acidity in his body, and his hormone levels, just as yours are. The health of his sperm, and the production if it, depend on these variables. A healthy bacterial environment in a man's bowel is necessary to prevent the excessive re-accumulation of testosterone into his body, and excess levels of testosterone have been implicated in low sperm counts, for example.

Ideally, get your male partner to do this program, too, including the use of natural progesterone cream. This hormone is made by women *and* men alike to balance hormone levels, and your man will benefit from its use too. He will not "become more feminine." Estrogen is the "feminine hormone," not progesterone. On the contrary, just as progesterone balances a female's hormone levels, and increases her sexual health (see "Sexual Health" later on), so too does it balance a man's hormones and increase his sexual health as well.

## Your odds are better

You may not immediately conceive when you start this program (as that requires the right crutches while you are healing your bowel and body, and you may not use your crutches at the correct amounts), but with infertility treatments, there isn't much chance of conceiving immediately either. However, a very high percentage of my clients have been very successful in becoming pregnant, and carrying their child to full term.

Also, with this program, you are at least healing your bowel and body while you are "waiting to conceive" and this is priceless—for you, and your future children.

## The risks of using low carbohydrate/high protein diets for infertility

These diets are a risk for all aspects of your health, your fertility included.

One study found that mice fed a high-protein diet had more fertility problems than mice on a lower-protein diet. High-protein diets are unhealthy and therefore I would expect to find greater fertility problems because of it.

I have seen a number of clients who have had fertility problems who were following these diets; a large percentage of overweight, non-high-protein dieters have not. Have you ever wondered why the "unhealthy" overweight woman next door could get pregnant when you, the thin fit one, could not? Did that seem unfair? Maybe your high-protein diet is partly to blame.

## The risk of infertility treatments for your child

Improving the health of your bowel and body with this program has significant benefits beyond helping you to conceive and deliver. By improving your bowel and body health, you dramatically improve the bowel and body health of your child as well, and reduce future symptoms, weight problems, addictions, and disease in your child. Infertility treatments cannot deliver this outcome, and it is an outcome that *should* be a priority when you decide to have a family.

There are very serious problems with modern day fertility methods. When a baby will not grow inside a woman's womb, it is because the conditions are not right for the baby to thrive there. It is nature's way of creating and ensuring a healthy, vibrant human species. We interfere with this process when modern medicine manipulates conditions with medications so that a baby will grow in an otherwise less than desirable environment. As your baby is growing and developing inside your womb, its development depends on your health. Your child's organ development and bowel health are dependent upon you being healthy. This is really what much of that genetic weakness stuff is all about: if a mother carries a fetus and has an unhealthy bowel and/or body, her baby likely will, too.

We *need* to talk about this situation so that women know the risks associated with fertility methods, and the risks of having a child whose health is not what it could and should be. "Infertility children" have been shown to have a 25% to 30% chance of developing severe handicaps such as cerebral palsy and blindness. But what about the chance of less severe handicaps, like asthma or A.D.D.? What about later in life? Do they suffer from higher rates of cancer and heart disease? This has not been studied, but it needs to be. I think this correlation would be found. Finally, mothers who are not healthy enough to reproduce naturally may not live as long to nurture these children, and the consequences of mother-less children is a social dilemma that we may face one day.

The health of the mother not only affects the health of the child, but it also affects the experience of pregnancy and delivery. An unhealthy mother often will not be able to conceive naturally, and therefore conception achieved through fertility methods also results in more complications both during pregnancy and delivery.

## . . . not to mention the risks to the mother of these treatments

There are no long-term studies that show that fertility treatments are safe. My knowledge of the human body and health leads me to conclude with confidence that one day, they will be found to have increased your risk of cancer and other diseases.

You are gambling with your life when you do infertility treatments, but I respect that *up until now*, you did not know there was a better solution.

Perhaps even now you feel it is worth the gamble. If infertility treatments were your only option in becoming pregnant, I would agree that it might be worth the risk. But they are not your only option for treating infertility, and therefore, the risk is not "worth it."

(If you have already had infertility treatments, the potential damage done by this process, to you and your child, can now be un-done by healing your bowels and bodies with this program.)

## Manipulating the sex of your child

When your periods are regular, as created with this program, you can predict when you are ovulating, and perhaps even affect the sex of your child.

It is known that male sperm swim faster than female sperm, but that they also die sooner. It is also known that a released egg will last a few days. It has been suggested that if you have sex before an egg is released, before ovulation, you have a higher chance of conceiving a girl, as by the time the egg makes its way down your tubes and is ready to be fertilized, the male sperm, that would swim faster and beat the female ones to the egg, have died. On the contrary, sex after ovulation might result in more boys, as the egg is already ripe to become fertilized, and the fast male swimmers will beat the female swimmers to it.

I had sex prior to ovulation and gave birth to my daughter nine months later. This does not prove that this works, but it doesn't hurt to know this and try, if desired. Keep in mind, however, that this is an option only if your periods are very regular and ovulation is very predictable. Also, of course, there are some moral considerations to this advice and I do not claim to support this entirely.

## It's not about bad luck

In *People* (August 30, 2002) there was an article about a baby born three months early, weighing only one pound. The mother had spent four years trying to get pregnant. She miscarried, then got pregnant, and delivered her baby three months too early. The doctor commented, "Jennifer (the mom) had no bad habits, she was just unlucky!" This comment makes my blood boil!

A woman who suffers from difficulty to conceive, and then has a miscarriage is unhealthy, and a severely premature baby is not unlucky; it is a product of that mother's sub-health. When you heal your bowel and improve your health, you greatly reduce your risk of delivering prematurely. The vast majority of my pregnant clients deliver within the week they are due.

## And you had plenty of "warnings you might struggle with fertility"

In an article I just read on a woman struggling with infertility, she mentions her history of endometriosis. An unhealthy bowel and body causes female issues like endometriosis, and an unhealthy bowel and body cause infertility.

Do you have a history of fibroids, cysts, PMS, irregular periods, heavy periods, and/or loose stools during your periods? If yes, then you are "at risk" of having fertility problems. Likely no one has warned you of this, but I am warning you now.

## A change of mind

The decision to have children or not is a very personal one, and one that I respect very much. There are many wonderful reasons to choose not to have children, but I have found that some of these are health-related.

I have worked with clients who told me that they did not want to have children—because of the environment, overpopulation, you name it, who then changed their mind when they became healthier. Because our population and environment problems had not improved, clearly there was a deeper, unspoken concern. Quite simply, many of these women admitted that they did not feel strong enough to deal with pregnancy and child care and/or were concerned about disease and not being able to raise their children. Many of them felt like they wouldn't be able to get pregnant even if they tried, and they masked this concern with the statement that children were not a desire.

I think this is an unspoken dilemma, and I share it in case you too have these feelings, in the hope that this book will offer some support, and comfort, to you.

## This program creates a healthier pregnancy, and birthing experience, too

The health of your bowel and body also has a profound effect on your pregnancy and birthing experience. When they are healthy, you do not experience morning sickness, headaches, high blood pressure, high blood sugar, anemia, toxemia, early labor, and/or prolonged labor, for example. Your chance of delivering vaginally is extremely high.

Positively affecting these experiences has a positive effect on your baby, too. Your baby needs large amounts of oxygen and nutrients to grow normally and healthfully. The less acidic you are, the more of these that are available. Your baby depends on you for a large part of his or her bacterial environment health. In fact, 100 species of microorganisms are transferred to your baby during birth/passage through the birth canal. You don't "get this" when you have a c-section (which are very common, and occurred in 32% of U.S. births in 2007, according to the C.D.C.).

Post-partum depression is eliminated when your hormones are balanced, as created when you heal your bowel, and when your blood and brain are rich in glucose and oxygen, which again, this program delivers.

If you get pregnant while doing this program, it is my legal requirement to advise you to stop this program and contact me for personalized instruction. If you are pregnant now, likewise, you should not begin this program unless you contact me personally.

In the ideal case, you will heal your bowel and body with this program for two years before you attempt to become pregnant. Many of you may not have "that time." But if you are a younger woman, and there is any possibility of your having children in the future, get on board now. If you have a young daughter, healing her bowel and body now will help her become pregnant, have an easy pregnancy, and deliver a healthy beautiful baby, with a strong foundation of bowel health, which will provide her with advantages in life that are boundlessly invaluable.

## This program can save you tens of thousands of dollars

I just finished reading an article from a woman who spent $70,000 last year on fertility treatments. She has "been at it" for 32 months, so her total cost may be adjusted to $115,000.

My average infertile client spends $6,000 to become pregnant, or $109,000 less.

Not only is this treatment dramatically less expensive, but with this program, *you and your baby* also get a much healthier body, less symptoms, fewer weight problems and addictions, and less disease and death, too. In my opinion, these outcomes are priceless.

# Success with Infertility

"After surgery for my endometriosis my doctor told me that due to damage and scarring, I would never have kids. Ha!! I have two sons, thanks to this program."

"I have never been fertile. After doing this program, I got pregnant on my first try!"

"My periods were very unpredictable. Once they became regular with this program, I got pregnant within two months of trying."

"When I came to Donna I was considered old and told my chance of getting pregnant was low. With this program I became pregnant and now have a beautiful baby girl."

"I tried infertility treatments with no luck. I also did a lot of other things, like acupuncture, a lot of supplements, and changed my diet. This program got me pregnant!"

## My story

Prior to embarking on this program, my periods were regulated by the birth control pill. Off the pill, they were late, very uncomfortable, and very heavy. When I became very sick and needed to take every ounce of stress off my body, I stopped the pill. During this time, I was very careless with using other forms of birth control, and yet over the course of many years, I never once got pregnant.

After healing my bowel and my body, my periods became very regular—every 28 days. (I experienced a great reduction in cramping and my flow became much lighter as well.) When my son was conceived at the age of 31, it was by accident, and the result of *one* mistake. When my daughter was conceived at the age of 34, it was a planned event, and once again it took *one* try for me to become pregnant: two tries, two babies. I worked at my job up until a few days before giving birth, and I had no "abnormal symptoms" of pregnancy like high blood pressure, early contractions, or toxemia. I never experienced morning sickness, either. I worked with a midwife and both of my children were born at home, naturally, without complication and with rather short periods of labor (eight hours with my first, and then four hours with my second child).

Many of my clients have experienced an improvement in the regularity of their periods and increased fertility. They also rarely miscarry. I will never forget the first year that I was in practice and a forty year old female client who was sexually active and did not use birth control (because she found she *never* became pregnant), got pregnant and called me up on the phone and yelled at me. A few months later she called again and was very pleased and excited about the impending birth. And yet even to this day I forget to "warn" many of my female clients: this program *will* make you more fertile. This is great news for those of you who are seeking to become pregnant, but it is a warning for those of you who don't, especially if you have become careless because of previous difficulty in conceiving.

### Watch my video, "Why THIS Program Works for Infertility."

This video, and all of my videos, can be found at ***www.UniqueHealing. com*** or at ***www.YouTube.com/UniqueHealing***.

## Inflammation
See "Aches and Pains" and Chapter 3

## Inflammatory Bowel Syndrome (I.B.S.)
See "Bowel Conditions"

## Insomnia
See "Sleep Disorders"

## Itchy Skin
See "Skin Conditions"

## Jaundice/Yellow in Eyes
See "Eye Problems"

## Kidney Stones
See "Gallstones"

## Lactose Allergies
See "Allergies (food)"

# Lead Toxicity
See "Heavy Metal Toxicity"

# Liver Problems
## Cirrhosis/Damage, Hepatitis

Your liver is in the "middle of your pipe," and many of you have an unhealthy one. Blood tests are not very good at detecting liver problems, and it is well known that the symptoms of liver problems are generally not very obvious, until there is a *major* problem. Many of you only become aware that there is a problem if a blood test shows elevated liver enzyme levels (like ALT/SGPT, AST/SGOT, or alkaline phosphatase). But like *all* blood test measurements, normal blood tests/liver function tests do not guarantee that you have a healthy liver.

Cirrhosis of your liver means that it has been damaged, and hepatitis is generally a condition of inflammation in your liver. (For information on liver cancer, see "Cancer" earlier in this chapter.)

Healing your bowel and body with this program heals your liver.

## Healing Your Body With This Program Eliminates Liver Disease

Healing your body with this program eliminates the acids that trigger inflammation and cause your liver to increase enzyme production to protect you from these acids. It eliminates the acids that damage your liver. This program heals your liver so that even if there are acids, your liver is strong enough to handle them without a reaction (it fixes the holes on your roof so that even if it does rain, your house does not get wet).

## Healing Your Bowel With This Program Eliminates Liver Problems

In addition to its many other important functions, a healthy bacterial environment in your bowel is a necessity for the complete elimination of acids (toxins, heavy metals, pesticides, etc.) from your body. A healthy bowel prevents the re-absorption of acids into your blood that trigger inflammation, elevated liver enzyme levels, and that damage your liver.

# Why My Crutches Eliminate Liver Problems

**Body Bentonite** binds to and eliminates acids (toxins, heavy metals, chemicals, etc.) from your body. It helps prevent them from becoming re-absorbed into your bloodstream, where they trigger a response by your body to protect you from them. It eliminates the acids that trigger the release of liver enzymes and inflammatory chemicals.

*Unique Healing Calcium Citrate* is an alkalinizing mineral that helps neutralize the acids that your bowel does not eliminate. When these acids are neutralized, your body does not need to produce enzymes or inflammatory chemicals to buffer them.

## How much do I take?/Questions about using these

See Chapter 5 for information on using these crutches, including recommendations on the amount to use, as well as a discussion of the misunderstandings about the particular crutch that may, if not understood correctly, cause you to fail to look and feel better while you heal your bowel and body with this program.

There are no crutches for degenerative conditions and accumulations of acidity in your organs, like liver damage, cirrhosis, and liver cancer. Crutches can offset the effects of acids in your blood, or the effects of poor function of your bowel bacterial environment (as these can be quickly altered), but degeneration is caused by depletion and damage to your organs, and organs take time to heal.

## How long will I need to use crutches for my liver problems?

Elevated liver enzyme levels occur at Level 2 of your pipe. They are the second area of your body to heal (assuming that other areas are unhealthy too). Refer to the diagram "Sequence of Healing" in Appendix A at the end of this book to better understand this concept, as well as to Chapter 1 under this subject heading.

Again, there are no crutches for degenerative conditions like liver damage, cirrhosis, and liver cancer; however, degenerative conditions are the first to become eliminated as you heal your bowel and body with this program.

# Misunderstandings About Liver Problems and Other Information for Your Success

## Keep your stools well-formed

Because liver problems are caused in part by un-eliminated acids, and because well-formed stools prevent the re-absorption of acids into your blood, you will suffer from the least amount of liver problems if you keep your stools well-formed while you are healing your bowel and body.

If you do not have a very good handle on how to define well-formed stools, review Chapter 6 of *Unique Healing* now. (And remember, when your stools are hard and slow you are eliminating more acids, and will therefore feel better, than when your stools are one or more times a day but not all extremely well-formed.)

If your stools are not well-formed, the following changes can help: increase your *Body Bentonite* intake; reduce your carbohydrate intake (pasta, breads, grains, cereals, yogurt, etc.); reduce your sugar intake (including natural healthy sugars such as agave, honey, raw sugar, cane juice, etc.); reduce your alcohol, salt, coffee, and/or soda intake; do not have a massage, chiropractic adjustment, or any other body work; drink a lot of water; rest; and keep your exercise aerobic (see Chapter 4 for more information on how to attain this, and why it is important.)

If these changes do not noticeably help the form of your stools in two days, take them further (i.e. take more *Body Bentonite*, reduce your carbohydrate intake more, etc.)

Out of all of these recommendations, increasing your *Body Bentonite* intake is one of the most productive and helpful. It heals your body, unlike many of the other recommendations. It will do the most to lead you to a place where looking and feeling good is effortless, and some of the other suggestions, such as reducing sugar intake, are simply "too hard to do when your blood is too acidic."

(Note: the exception to this information is when your poorly formed stools are caused by an infection, in which case *Unique Healing Colloidal Silver* is needed to reduce your symptoms. Refer to Chapter 5 for information on when and how to use this crutch.)

## Milk thistle and other liver "cleansers" or liver "support" products do not heal your liver

Millions, maybe billions, of dollars of "liver cleansing" supplements have been sold over the last few decades with the implied promise that they heal your liver. It is very appealing to think that you can do this simply by ingesting a few herbs and other nutrients.

The problem is, these liver cleanses don't really cleanse your liver. To better understand this concept, refer to my video, "Cleanses Don't Cleanse" at *www.UniqueHealing.com* or at *www.YouTube,.com/UniqueHealing*. The herbs and nutrients in liver cleansers, or liver detoxifiers, are merely crutches that can *buffer* the acids in your blood that cause liver symptoms and liver enzyme levels to be high, but crutches do not heal. These supplements do nothing to eliminate the acids that *damage* your liver. They do not heal it. This program does.

## Ultrasounds, CT scans, and biopsies of your liver are much more accurate than blood tests in measuring its health

You can have high elevated liver enzyme levels and a moderately unhealthy liver, and you can have normal liver enzyme levels but a very unhealthy liver. *Blood tests do not accurately reflect the health of any of your organs, your liver included.*

CT scans and ultrasounds of your organs, your liver included, are much more accurate for assessing the health of your organs like your liver. Even still, these tests can only detect a very unhealthy liver, and you deserve better than that. A moderately unhealthy liver will likely not be detected with these tests, and this can harmfully lead you to believe that yours is healthier than it really is.

One way to measure your liver health is to eat a very cleansing diet of only fruit and bread and sugar for five days and then have your cholesterol checked. If it is normal, your liver is probably in pretty good health. If it is high, it is not so healthy (and the higher the cholesterol reading, the less healthy it is. A reading above 250 indicates a less healthy liver than a reading of 210, for example.) To better understand why this "test" can help you more accurately determine the health of your liver, read the following section.

## High cholesterol levels indicate an unhealthy liver

While your blood test may only show elevated cholesterol levels (and not elevated liver enzyme levels), your liver produces cholesterol, and in most cases when it is too high it is because your liver is unhealthy. Cholesterol levels are not regulated by homeostasis, which means they can become elevated much easier than liver enzyme levels, which are regulated by homeostasis (your body tries to correct liver enzyme levels, while there is no "correction" for cholesterol levels.).

## Excess body fat indicates an unhealthy liver

Likewise, your liver has many other functions as well, such as the production of fat, so if you are overweight and your body fat percentage is high, your liver is not healthy. (Extra weight can also be caused by water retention. To make the differentiation, you can buy a scale that measures body fat. Also, health clubs and/or personal trainers often offer body fat analysis.)

## High protein diet crutches may help your blood liver enzyme tests, but they are damaging to your liver

Like *all* blood tests, liver enzyme tests reflect un-eliminated acids in your blood, and these can be manipulated by a high protein diet (which "shoves these acids back into your organs.") It is much more dangerous when this occurs, both from the perspective of your health as well as from the perspective that you can dangerously think you are much healthier, and safer, than you really are when you manipulate your liver enzyme levels with one of these diets.

If you are ever tempted to follow one of these diets for your elevated liver enzyme levels, make sure you have an ultrasound or CT scan before you do, and frequently during this diet, so you can accurately assess the health of your liver and the effect on it with this diet.

## You liver can be unhealthy even if you have never drank one sip of alcohol

Some of you have wrongly been led to believe that only alcohol can damage your liver, and therefore, if you have not drank much, you may think your liver is healthy, and safe from disease. It is not.

Your liver, like all of your organs, becomes damaged/unhealthy from too many un-eliminated acids. Coffee, sugar, soda, steak, turkey, chicken, salt, vinegar, pesticides, chemicals, and heavy metals are some of the many acid-producing items that can damage your liver.

## Success With Liver Problems

"At the age of 38, my blood tests showed elevated liver enzyme levels. These were tested for 4 years, and they continued to be high, even though I changed my diet and took supplements. After following this program for 9 months, I had them re-checked, and they were normal!"

"A liver biopsy showed that my liver was damaged. A couple of years after following this program I had it re-done and I was told it was the healthiest liver they had ever seen."

"I was diagnosed with liver cancer, and after following this program for about nine months, I was told it was gone. It has not returned within the last three years."

### Watch My Video, Why THIS Program Eliminates Liver Problems"

This video, and all of my videos, can be found at *www.UniqueHealing. com* or at *www.YouTube.com/UniqueHealing*.

## Low Energy
See "Fatigue"

## Lupus
See "Autoimmune Diseases"

## Lyme Disease
See "Bacterial Infections"

## Macular Degeneration
See "Eye Problems"

## Malaria
See "Bacterial Infections"

## Menopause
See "Female Issues"

# Mental Health Problems
## Depression, Anxiety, Bipolar Disorder, Dementia, Schizophrenia, Phobias, and Others
(See also "Neurological Conditions")

In general, the majority of mental disorders are the result of chemical imbalances in your brain and/or irritation to your nervous system. These physiological conditions can be alleviated by medication, proving that there is a physiological connection to them. Medications do not alter your emotional health and they are not therapy; they alter your neurochemical health, just as healing your bowel and body with this program does.

As for dementia and bipolar, these too are the result of neurochemical imbalances. They are simply more complex, much more profound, and require an incredibly aggressive approach (which is best undertaken with my personal assistance).

Mental health problems are very different from emotional health problems. Healing your bowel can eliminate the former; the latter requires a different approach.

# Healing Your Body With This Program Eliminates Mental Health Problems

Un-eliminated acids in your body reduce oxygen and blood glucose levels. Oxygen and glucose are much-needed sources of fuel for proper brain function. Inadequate levels of oxygen and glucose can trigger irritability, depression, anxiety, and/or fear. Healing your body with this program eliminates the acids that cause low oxygen and glucose levels, and poor brain function.

Your liver and adrenal glands are responsible for the production of neurotransmitters, which are brain chemicals that reduce depression, anxiety, etc. Healing your body with this program eliminates the acids that damage your liver and adrenal glands and negatively affect their ability to produce these brain chemicals.

There are more nerves in your bowel than in your brain. Some scientists have labeled your bowel your "second brain." Un-eliminated acids in your bowel irritate these nerve endings. Even researchers have found that excess acidity in your bowel creates fermented by-products that trigger depression. Healing your body with this program eliminates the acids that irritate your nervous system, and you.

Healing your body with this program eliminates the acids that trigger nervous system irritability. Healing your body with this program heals your nervous system so that even if there *are* acids, your body is strong enough to handle them without a reaction (it fixes the holes on your roof so that even if it does rain, your house does not get wet).

## Healing Your Bowel With This Program Eliminates Mental Health Problems

One of the jobs of your bowel bacteria is to produce neurotransmitters, which are chemicals that make you feel good. Drugs that are commonly prescribed for mental conditions, like Prozac, simply provide neurotransmitters for your brain. They do not fix an underlying emotional problem; you feel better with these drugs because they alter your body's chemistry. Altering your body chemistry is exactly what happens when you heal your bowel.

Poor intestinal bacterial health causes low levels of vitamin B-12 production. Low levels of B-12 have been implicated in cases of depression. When there is insufficient B-12, the sheath surrounding the delicate nerves of your brain and spine suffer. Vitamin B-12 is also needed for the production of the neurotransmitter serotonin and benzodiazepines. Valium and Xanax are pharmaceutical benzodiazepines. Without enough B-12, your body does not formulate enough SAMe (S-adenosylmethionine), an important mood regulator that boosts serotonin levels in your brain.

Studies show that up to 30% of people hospitalized for depression have low blood levels of B-12. A study published in the December 2003 issue of *BioMed Central Psychiatry* found that after six months of studying 115 Finnish patients with major depressive disorder, those who experienced a greater than 50% reduction in symptoms had the highest blood levels of vitamin B-12. (You can find a number of studies that have measured the connection between low vitamin B-12 levels and depression. One recently article appeared in the *New York Times*.)

John Cryan, a pharmacologist with the Alimentary Pharmabiotic Center at University College Cork in Ireland, and his colleagues, have found that probiotics have a direct impact on mood neurotransmitters in mice. The findings further support the idea that one of the ways to heal problems of the mind might be through the bowel.

As always, studies that look at the long-term connection between a healthy bowel and mental health are practically non-existent. The only somewhat relevant one that I have found was a recent study from the Mayo clinic showing a link between dementia and celiac disease. Researchers identified 13 patients from the Mayo clinic who showed mental decline within the two years of developing celiac. The adults were between the ages of 45 and 79. After switching to a gluten-free diet two individuals improved, reversing their dementia, and one stabilized. When you have a healthy bowel, you will not have gluten sensitivities or celiac, either, and as this study suggests, a reduced chance of experiencing dementia.

In addition to its many other important functions, a healthy bacterial environment in your bowel is a necessity for the complete elimination of acids (toxins, heavy metals, pesticides, etc.) from your body. A healthy bowel prevents the re-absorption of acids into your blood that trigger low oxygen and blood sugar levels, and that cause an unhealthy nervous system.

## Why My Crutches Eliminate Mental Health Problems

***Body Bentonite*** binds to and eliminates acids (toxins, heavy metals, chemicals, etc.) from your body. It helps prevent them from becoming re-absorbed into your bloodstream, where they trigger a response by your body to protect you from them. It eliminates the acids that reduce the oxygen and glucose that reach your brain, and that irritate your nervous system.

***Unique Healing Calcium Citrate*** is an alkalinizing mineral that helps neutralize the acids that your bowel does not eliminate. When these acids are neutralized, your nervous system is not aggravated and you blood glucose and oxygen levels remain in balance.

***Unique Healing Methyl Vitamin B-12*** provides your body with easy to assimilate levels of this nutrient, which can reduce anxiety, depression, irritability, and other nervous system conditions.

### How much do I take?/Questions about using these

See Chapter 5 for information on using these crutches, including recommendations on the amount to use, as well as a discussion of the misunderstandings about the particular crutch that may, if not understood correctly, cause you to fail to look and feel better while you heal your bowel and body with this program.

## How long will I need to use crutches for my mental health problems?

Mental health problems occur at Levels 2 and 3 of your pipe. They are the second, and second to last, areas of your body to heal (assuming that other areas are unhealthy too). Refer to the diagram "Sequence of Healing" in Appendix A at the end of this book to better understand this concept, as well as to Chapter 1 under this subject heading.

The bacterial environment in your bowel also affects mental health problems. To better understand how long you may need crutches for this, refer to Chapter 1 under this subject heading.

# Misunderstandings About Mental Health Problems and Other Information for Your Success

## Keep your stools well-formed

Because mental health problems are caused in part by un-eliminated acids, and because well-formed stools prevent the re-absorption of acids into your blood, you will suffer from the least amount of these issues if you keep your stools well-formed while you are healing your bowel and body.

If you do not have a very good handle on how to define well-formed stools, review Chapter 6 of *Unique Healing* now. (And remember, when your stools are hard and slow you are eliminating more acids, and will therefore feel better, than when your stools are one or more times a day but not all extremely well-formed.)

If your stools are not well-formed, the following changes can help: increase your *Body Bentoni*te intake; reduce your carbohydrate intake (pasta, breads, grains, cereals, yogurt, etc.); reduce your sugar intake (including natural healthy sugars such as agave, honey, raw sugar, cane juice, etc.); reduce your alcohol, salt, coffee, and/or soda intake; do not have a massage, chiropractic adjustment, or any other body work; drink a lot of water; rest; and keep your exercise aerobic (see Chapter 4 for more information on how to attain this, and why it is important.)

If these changes do not noticeably help the form of your stools in two days, take them further (i.e. take more *Body Bentonite*, reduce your carbohydrate intake more, etc.)

Out of all of these recommendations, increasing your *Body Bentonite* intake is one of the most productive and helpful. It heals your body, unlike many of the other recommendations. It will do the most to lead you to a place where looking and feeling good is effortless, and some of the other suggestions, such as reducing sugar intake, are simply "too hard to do when your blood is too acidic."

(Note: the exception to this information is when your poorly formed stools are caused by an infection, in which case *Unique Healing Colloidal Silver* is needed to reduce your symptoms. Refer to Chapter 5 for information on when and how to use this crutch.)

## Drug/medication crutches

It has been shown that people who use medications to treat their psychological problems end up with worse psychological problems in the long run, versus people who don't. (This is another classic example of short-term gain, long-term pain.) The drug that quickly eases your depression is at the same time toxic to your bowel and body, which are responsible for keeping you happy in the first place! As your bowel and body slowly become less healthy, in part from the drugs you are taking, your body's ability to produce brain chemicals suffers even more, and an eventual worsening of your psychiatric problem is almost inevitable.

I often support the short-term use of a psychiatric drug. At times it is valuable and necessary in order to keep someone focused enough to heal their bowel and body. I am all for that. (Especially considering that when the use of these drugs is coupled with this program, the ill-effects of these drugs are greatly diminished, and the benefit often outweighs the risk of using them.)

Additionally, if you are dealing with bipolar disorder, suicidal thoughts, schizophrenia, or any other complex, serious condition, my crutches may not be strong enough to help. In these cases a medication crutch from your doctor is usually in order (and a visit to your doctor for his advice on this is in order as well.). You will also need a very aggressive, individualized approach to healing your bowel and body, and I suggest you contact me for this.

But many of you who are taking these drugs are getting more harm than benefit from them. And you have to be especially careful about the drugs we give to your children for treating mental health issues.

## Additional, safer, non-toxic crutches

Numerous supplements exist for anxiety, depression, stress, etc. Some of these, like GABA, L-Theanine, SAMe, Kava, and 5-HTP may be helpful to you. All of these are completely safe, and like all crutches, you should feel better with a few days of using them.

Of these, the one I prefer is GABA. Buy GABA with 750 mg/capsule and take two a few hours before bed and again when you awake in the morning. If this does not reduce your symptoms of stress, anxiety, etc. in a couple of days, double the dosage, and if that does not help in a couple of days, consider that you may still be taking too few (in which you may need an individualized program with myself), or that you are taking the wrong crutch.

Even medical crutches should help quickly. It should not take two or three months to feel better with a medication. If you have been taking one longer than a week and are not functioning better, seek a doctor who is willing to adjust your prescription sooner so that you get the relief you deserve.

## A low acid diet can reduce symptoms

As is true of a number of your symptoms weight problems, and addictions, reducing your consumption of refined sugar, refined salt, refined carbohydrates, alcohol, and soda is helpful for reducing mental health symptoms because these highly acidic foods create acids, and un-eliminated acids reduce oxygen and glucose delivery to your brain.

A interesting study published in the *American Journal of Public Health* found that teens that drink one or more glasses of soda a day have higher rates of mental distress, behavior problems, hyperactivity, depression, anxiety, and lethargy.

Healing your bowel and body with this program balances your blood sugar levels, making it easy for you to reduce or eliminate these highly acidic substances from your diet.

## Electricity for mental illness

There is a growing consensus from neuroscientists that psychiatric illnesses stem from problems in your brain's electrical circuits

(*WSJ*—1/11/11). A crop of new devices that send microcurrents into your brain are being tested, and there are claims that this has helped people who are severely depressed and have been unresponsive to traditional antidepressants (which are found to help only about 35% of the people who use them).

Body electricity is regulated by pH; it is disrupted when your blood is overly acidic (largely because the alkaline minerals, like sodium and potassium, help regulate nerve signals, and these minerals can become depleted when they are used to buffer un-eliminated acids in your blood). Healing your bowel and body with this program improves your alkaline mineral levels and improves your brain's electrical circuits.

## Emotional issues require counseling and/or self-help work

Healing your bowel and body will dramatically improve your mental health, but it will not improve your emotional health. Mental health issues are a function of an unhealthy bowel and body; emotional health issues are the function of an unhealthy upbringing, scary or stressful experiences in life, etc. Medications can help with mental health issues, but not with emotional health issues, for this same reason.

Excessive stress often has an emotional basis, and if you are constantly battling with anger, fear, worry, and/or similar problems, you need help with your emotional health. Emotional health issues also include relationship problems, problems with self-esteem and self-respect, and fear of failure and abandonment. If you were raised with parents who were insecure, controlling, manipulative, critical, jealous, disrespectful, and/or self-absorbed, you likely have some emotional issues as a result. These need to be addressed in order for you to live a happy life. Sometimes they need to be addressed prior to healing your bowel and body, and sometimes only after one's bowel and body are healed do I find that clients are ready, and able, to address these.

If you struggled as a child to get your parents' attention and love, the pressure to be perfect in order to please them will be never-ending. Trying to please someone else is doomed for failure. If your parents approve of your superficial monetary and/or physical accomplishments over your accomplishments in character, if they are proud of how you look and or perform versus how you behave, you are in for trouble as an adult. If you are not respected as a child, you will grow up into an adult who does not respect yourself. A lack of self-respect can easily lead to abuse of one's body in the ways that I abused mine. When your parents are self-absorbed, you do not feel unconditionally loved. This is very painful and as a child, you take it personally. As an adult, you feel that you do not deserve to be happy.

*How can you possibly believe that you can eliminate all of your health and weight problems with this healing program if you don't feel like you deserve it?*

Healing your emotional issues takes a lot of commitment, time and energy, but it is well worth it. There are no crutches for these problems. Avoidance and denial may seem like crutches that help you cope, but one day, as with all crutches, you will likely fall down and crash with these. Find a great therapist to help you with your emotional health issues, if needed, and commit to this work for a while. You will be inordinately more successful with this program if you do.

## Emotional health and healing are interconnected

At age twenty-two my life came crashing down on me. This was the year I was diagnosed with an autoimmune disease. This was the year that my "new life" began. As my physical health slowly improved, so did my emotional health. My better physical health allowed me to separate out, and understand, the feelings and unhealthy actions I had experienced up to that point. It allowed me to understand my feelings of worthlessness and let them go, for example. It allowed me to become aware of the criticism and selfishness of some of the people in my life and to not take it personally. It allowed me to stop being a victim to their actions.

My physical improvements helped me have the clarity and energy to sort through all of the negative emotions I grew up with and reach a much healthier emotional state, as well.

Dealing with my dysfunctional and emotionally unhealthy upbringing was invaluable, but it did not completely eliminate my depression, anxiety, and phobias. Physically healing my bowel and body did.

## As with addictions, the physiological cause of these must be addressed for success

What a therapist cannot help you with are your physiological mental health issues. I did a lot of therapy when I was ill but it never eliminated my extreme feelings of anxiety, depression, lack of control, and fear. Alcoholics, people with eating disorders, sex addicts, and others with addictions fail to recover completely and often lead very difficult lives even after conventional psychotherapy has been in place for a long time if their physiological mental health has been ignored.

# Success With Mental Health Problems

"I suffered from terrible depression and was on anti-depressants for many years. I tried stopping them several times but always had to go back on them. I hated taking them and I needed them but they also made me feel bloated and the other side effects were annoying. And even on them, my depression was still not completely gone and my relationships were suffering as a result. I wanted to stop them right away when I started this program but Donna told me I shouldn't. I was also concerned that they would prevent me from healing my body and from helping me lose weight. I followed this program very aggressively for the last year and a half and I have had a remarkable response. I am not done yet, but I have lost a lot of weight and I have been able to stop my anti-depressants. My family thinks I am a new woman, and I am."

"I love the *Unique Healing Methyl Vitamin B-12*. Even though I had been getting B-12 shots prior to starting this program, they never made me feel even close to as happy as the daily B-12 does. It is amazing. I take very large amounts every day, but I know one day I will be able to stop it and for now, I am just very grateful to know about this crutch."

## My story

Prior to becoming ill I suffered from serious depression. I felt completely out of control in my life and was only happy when I was working or partying. Those two things temporarily numbed my pain and allowed me to ignore it. But it was always there. When I first became ill, I spiraled into a state of severe anxiety as well. "Panic attacks" was the first diagnosis I received when my body started crashing toward bottom. For years I woke up in the middle of the night feeling as though I were having a heart attack. A few times it was scary enough to send me to the emergency room. For years I felt like adrenaline was constantly coursing through my body. I could not calm my body down. Driving was terrifying. I thought I would crash. I always drove in the slow lane on the freeways of Los Angeles and would frequently pull off an exit so I could psych myself up for going farther. I had bizarre and scary fears too. I thought that if I got too close to a cliff or the edge of a bridge I might throw myself off. I thought I might intentionally run my car off the side of the road, even though mentally, I did not want to die.

When I healed my bowel and body, my depression and anxiety disappeared. Improving my mental health helped me heal my body; healing my body improved my mental health.

## Watch My Video, "Why THIS Program Eliminates Mental Health Problems"

This video, and all of my videos, can be found at *www. UniqueHealing. com* or at *www. YouTube.com/ UniqueHealing.*

## Mercury Toxicity
See "Heavy Metal Toxicity"

## Migraines
See "Aches and Pains"

## Mononucleosis
See "Viral Infections"

## Multiple Sclerosis
See "Autoimmune Diseases"

## Neurological Disorders
### ADD, ADHD, Alzheimer's, Autism, Parkinson's, Down's Syndrome, Tourettes, Epilepsy, Seizures, PANDAS, Schizophrenia, and Others

All of the above conditions are similar, both in the fact that they are defined as neurological conditions, as well as in the fact that underlying all of them, there is an unhealthy bowel and body.

The following information focuses on autism and young children, because this is the condition that has lately gained the greatest amount of interest, both in the area of the media, as well as in the area of people experimenting with alternative remedies to treat it. However, do not interpret my use of the word "autism" to mean that the following concepts apply only to this condition. These concepts, and the ability of this program to help, apply to *all* neurological conditions. If you are an adult who suffers from seizures, for example, replace "seizures" every time you see the word "autism," etc.

The incidence of these conditions has increased in the last decade. For example, in the past four years the rate of autism has doubled, and the CDC suggests that as many as one in every 166 children is now on the autism spectrum, while another one in six suffer from a neuro-developmental delay. The percentage of children age 5-17 who have been diagnosed with ADHD rose more than 30% in the last decade, and now affects roughly 4.7 million children.

Neurological disorders are multi-faceted, and many other sections in this book are relevant to this topic as well, and I encourage you to read them. This includes, "Diarrhea," "Allergies (Environmental and Food)," "Fungal Infections," "Heavy Metal Toxicity," "Liver Problems," "Mental Health Problems," and "Thyroid Problems" in this chapter, as well as the sections on "Inflammation," "Nutrient Levels," and "Oxygenation" in Chapter 3.

## Healing Your Body With This Program Eliminates Neurological Disorders

My experience, as well as that of researchers, is that children with autism have very high levels of acidity, stored both in their organs, and free-floating in their blood. Theses acids include, but are not limited to, heavy metals, preservatives, chemicals, and artificial food colorings. The high presence of these acids, or toxins, in children with these disorders has been strongly observed and documented by practitioners who specialize in this area.

An underlying cause of these disorders is often described as "poor liver detoxification." For example, Dr. Edelson, a physician doing innovative work with autistic children at his clinic in Atlanta, theorizes that a combination of increasing exposure to toxins (chemical and heavy metal) and an ill-functioning liver detoxification system is a primary cause of autism. Also, a study on autism published in a 1998 issue of *Toxicology and Industrial Health* found that 100% of the participants had abnormal liver detoxification function and 95% had abnormal blood levels of toxic chemicals. Another study found that mothers of 94 autistic children had statistically more amalgam (mercury) fillings during pregnancy than 49 mothers in the control group.

Excess acidity irritates your nervous system, and you, and reduces neurotransmitter production. Un-eliminated acids are dangerous, and your child's body reacts to protect him or her from these. One reaction to these acids is the utilization of oxygen to buffer them; oxygen can attach to un-eliminated acids and make them less harmful, but this results in lowered oxygen levels in your child's blood. When oxygen is used to protect your child from the imminent danger of an overly acidic bloodstream, the resultant lowered levels of oxygen deprive his or her brain of this element that is essential for proper brain function and development. Some studies have found that over 85% of children with autism have low blood oxygen levels. Dr. Daniel Rossignol of the International Child Development Resource Center has had success treating autistic children with hyperbaric oxygen. While this is indeed valuable, it is *much* more productive and effective (and permanent) to eliminate the acids that cause low oxygen levels in the first place. Healing your body with this program eliminates the acids that cause low oxygen, and low brain function levels, too.

Another response to un-eliminated acids is the release of inflammatory chemicals (which is an "immune response"). These too buffer acids and reduce the imminent danger of their presence. A neurologist at John's Hopkins found neurological inflammation in 100% of the patients he tested with autism. (As a result, some doctors are even testing the use of an anti-inflammatory antibiotic drug on these patients, a crutch I strongly caution you against using as your solution to these problems.) Inflammation reduces the amount of needed oxygen that reaches your brain. Healing your body with this program eliminates the acids that trigger inflammation.

It is also a common belief and finding that children with these disorders have low levels of antioxidants and other nutritional deficiencies. Your body "uses up" antioxidants and other nutrients to buffer, and protect you from, un-eliminated acids. Healing your body with this program eliminates the acids that cause low antioxidant and other nutrient levels.

Thyroid problems are also commonly present in children with neurological disorders. Dr. Peter Hauser conducted a study years ago and reported that 70% of the patients with ADD disorders had resistance to thyroid hormone, compared to only 20% of those who did not suffer from the disorder. When hyperactive patients were given thyroid resistance replacement hormone, 20 of the 104 patients showed an improvement in their symptoms. Thyroid replacement is a crutch. Healing your body with this program eliminates the acids that cause low thyroid levels.

Healing your body with this program eliminates the acids that trigger the symptoms associated with mental health problems. Healing your body with this program heals your nervous system (brain), thyroid, and immune systems so that even if there are acids, your body is strong enough to handle them without a reaction (it fixes the holes on your roof so that even if it does rain, your house does not get wet).

## A Healthy Bowel Eliminates Neurological Disorders

A common and emerging acceptable belief is that all behavioral disorders like autism and ADD are the result of intestinal dysfunction. "The answer to autism lies in the gut," say many scientists, researchers, and well-respected health care practitioners. But is it really that simple, and how, exactly, do you heal your child's gut? (As far back as 1943, a psychiatrist working with autistic children noted immune and digestive/bowel problems.) For 19 years I have "blamed the bowel." This connection has recently emerged as significant. I have 19 years of knowledge and experience addressing bowel issues. I am *way* "ahead of the gang."

For the last 19 years I have been studying gut, or bowel health. My entire nutritional practice has focused on healing the body by healing the bowel. I've been on "this bandwagon" for a very long time, and I have acquired an enormous amount of information and experience about how to heal the bowel, heal the body, and heal disease. The results have been remarkable.

My experience with children with autism is that they indeed *do* have *very* unhealthy bacterial environments in their bowel.

Scientists have called your bowel your "second brain." It contains millions of nerves and is responsible for the production of neurotransmitters that keep your brain "happy." A healthy bowel makes a lot of these chemicals; an unhealthy bowel does not.

A key area in the study of autism involves environmental toxicity and deficient detoxification, with one of the main bio-chemical pathways of interest being the methylation cycle. This pathway regenerates methionine from homocysteine via *vitamin B-12*-dependent methionine synthase. Methylation is a critical process for DNA synthesis and repair; protection of DNA and RNA against insertion of viral genes; neuronal myelination

305

and pruning; glutathione production; homocysteine regulation; control of gene expression; and metabolic detoxification.

One study found that when eight autistic children took key nutrients in this methylation pathway (including folic acid and methyl-B-12) there was a significant increase in important markers of methylation and glutathione synthesis, both of which reduce the manifestation of symptoms.

In more simplistic terms, vitamin B-12 is needed for neurotransmitter production and healthy neurological function. When there is insufficient B-12, the sheath surrounding the delicate nerves of your brain and spine suffer. Low levels of B-12 have been implicated in cases of *autism, A.D.D., Tourette's, multiple sclerosis, Lou Gehrig's disease, Alzheimer's, Parkinsons, seizures, and nerve damage.* An unhealthy bowel bacterial environment causes low levels of vitamin B-12 production, as your bowel is in part responsible for the manufacture and absorption of this vitamin. Healing your bowel with this program eventually increases your body's natural production and absorption of this needed nutrient.

There is a growing sense among autism researchers that infectious exposures may also be a major contributing factor to autism and its related disorders. A healthy bowel prevents infections such as yeast, parasites, fungal infections, and bacterial infections, such as staph, strep, Lyme's, etc., from invading your body and creating toxic, nerve-damaging side-effects.

Additionally, children with autism, ADD, and other similar disorders are more susceptible to heavy mal-absorption and food allergies. A healthy bowel digests lactose, gluten, and other foods without allergic reactions.

Professionals treating this disorder remark that these children frequently have severe intestinal disturbances, like diarrhea. An article in *Health* magazine (June 2004) described a family with an autistic son. In describing his physical condition the father said, "He had chronic abdominal pain and constant diarrhea." A few years back, someone whose child was autistic contacted me. This child had diarrhea six to seven times a day. I also had a client several years ago who worked at a children's hospital and she informed me that all of the children they saw with these disorders had intestinal problems, mostly diarrhea. Healing your bowel with this program eliminates the acids/toxins and bacterial, fungal, and parasitic infections that cause diarrhea.

The cover of the April 2007 issue of *Discover* magazine declared: "Understanding Autism: The Answer May Lie In The Gut, Not In The

Head" by Jill Neimark. According to this article, the connection between an unhealthy gut, or bowel, and autism is acknowledged and seen as highly relevant, but "no one quite knows what to do about it." *I do, and now that you have read my books, you do too.*

In addition to its many other important functions, a healthy bacterial environment in your bowel is a necessity for the complete elimination of acids (toxins, heavy metals, pesticides, etc.) from your body. A healthy bowel prevents the re-absorption of acids into your blood that trigger inflammation, low oxygen levels, low nutrient levels, nutritional deficiencies, poor thyroid function, and many other conditions associated with neurological disorders, as well as damage to your nervous system/brain and other organs.

## Why My Crutches Eliminate Neurological Disorders

***Body Bentonite*** binds to and eliminates acids (toxins, heavy metals, chemicals, etc.) from your body. It helps prevent them from becoming re-absorbed into your bloodstream, where they trigger a response by your body to protect you from them. It eliminates the acids that trigger the release of inflammatory chemicals, reduce blood flow/circulation and oxygenation to your nervous system and brain, reduce antioxidant and other nutrient levels, and upset the balance of your thyroid hormones.

***Unique Healing Calcium Citrate*** is an alkalinizing mineral that helps neutralize the acids that your bowel does not eliminate. When these acids are neutralized, your body does not need to produce inflammatory chemicals or bind to oxygen or nutrients to buffer them.

***Unique Healing Methyl Vitamin B-12*** provides your body with easy to assimilate levels of this nutrient, which has been shown to improve many neurological symptoms.

***Unique Healing Colloidal Silver*** has natural anti-bacterial, anti-fungal, anti-parasitic properties. It eliminates the infections that otherwise create toxic by-products that are aggravating and damaging to your nervous system/brain.

**Melatonin** Sleep disorders are also very common in children with neurological disorders. This makes sense, as a healthy bowel is needed for the production of melatonin, which helps regulate sleep cycles/your child's ability to "sleep through the night." A good night's sleep is important for healing your nervous system, and for everyone's sanity!

## How much do I take?/Questions about using these

See Chapter 5 for information on using these crutches, including recommendations on the amount to use, as well as a discussion of the misunderstandings about the particular crutch that may, if not understood correctly, cause you to fail to look and feel better while you heal your bowel and body with this program.

My experience with these disorders is that extremely large amounts of crutches are need and beneficial for quick reductions in symptoms. It is advisable that you contact me for a personal consultation if you (or your child) have one of these.

There are no crutches for degenerative conditions (i.e. damage to your organs) and accumulations of acidity in them, like your brain, which occur with Alzheimer's, M.S., autism, etc. Crutches can offset the effects of acids in your blood, or the effects of poor function of your bowel bacterial environment (as these can be quickly altered), but degeneration is caused by depletion and damage to your organs, and organs take time to heal.

## How long will I need to use crutches for my neurological disorders?

Neurological disorders occur at Level 3 of your pipe. It is the second to last area of your body to heal (assuming that other areas are unhealthy too). Refer to the diagram "Sequence of Healing" in Appendix A at the end of this book to better understand this concept, as well as to Chapter 1 under this subject heading.

The bacterial environment in your bowel also affects neurological disorders. To better understand how long you may need crutches for this, refer to Chapter 1 under this subject heading.

Again, there are no crutches for degenerative conditions like Alzheimer's, autism, M.S., etc; however, degenerative conditions are the first to become eliminated as you heal your bowel and body with this program.

# Misunderstandings About Neurological Disorders and Other Information for Your Success

## Keep your stools well-formed

Because neurological disorders are caused in part by un-eliminated acids, and because well-formed stools prevent the re-absorption of acids into your blood, you will suffer from the least amount of symptoms of these if you keep your stools well-formed while you are healing your bowel and body.

If you do not have a very good handle on how to define well-formed stools, review Chapter 6 of *Unique Healing* now. (And remember, when your stools are hard and slow you are eliminating more acids, and will therefore feel better, than when your stools are one or more times a day but not all extremely well-formed.)

If your stools are not well-formed, the following changes can help: increase your *Body Bentonite* intake; reduce your carbohydrate intake (pasta, breads, grains, cereals, yogurt, etc.); reduce your sugar intake (including natural healthy sugars such as agave, honey, raw sugar, cane juice, etc.); reduce your alcohol, salt, coffee, and/or soda intake; do not have a massage, chiropractic adjustment, or any other body work; drink a lot of water; rest; and keep your exercise aerobic (see Chapter 4 for more information on how to attain this, and why it is important.)

If these changes do not noticeably help the form of your stools in two days, take them further (i.e. take more *Body Bentonite*, reduce your carbohydrate intake more, etc.)

Out of all of these recommendations, increasing your *Body Bentonite* intake is one of the most productive and helpful. It heals your body, unlike many of the other recommendations. It will do the most to lead you to a place where looking and feeling good is effortless, and some of the other suggestions, such as reducing sugar intake, are simply "too hard to do when your blood is too acidic."

(Note: the exception to this information is when your poorly formed stools are caused by an infection, in which case *Unique Healing Colloidal Silver* is needed to reduce your symptoms. Refer to Chapter 5 for information on when and how to use this crutch.)

## Does autism cause diarrhea, or does the diarrhea cause the autism?

Diarrhea is highly prevalent among children with autism, which has led some to assume that autism causes diarrhea. I insist it is the latter—that diarrhea (i.e. an unhealthy bowel) causes autism.

Harvard pediatric neurologist Martha Herbert says "I no longer see autism as a disorder of the brain but as a disorder that affects the brain . . . It also affects the immune system and the gut." This assumption is wrong, and backwards. It is your gut, or bowel, that affects your immune system, which affects your brain.

## Alternative treatments are not really healing your bowel or body

The vast majority of alternative treatment programs for these disorders depend on crutches to treat the symptoms of them.

Vitamins, antioxidants, glutathione, selenium, and other supplements, drugs, exercise, food allergy diets, low carbohydrate diets, alkaline diets, fasting, organic/pesticide-free foods, detoxification programs, laxatives, enemas, chiropractic, and acupuncture are "crutches" that do *not* eliminate acids from your child's body (nor do they heal his or her bowel). You will get temporary and incomplete results if you only rely on crutches for your child's neurological problems. (You are also likely to give him or her much too few of these to make a remarkable difference in his or her symptoms, anyway. You may also give him or her these daily for many months, thinking that they will eventually improve his or her symptoms. That is not how crutches work. They either work right away/reduce symptoms immediately, or they do not work at all.)

While these crutches do not heal your child's bowel or body, many false claims are made that they do. (My experience is that practitioners who make these claims believe/want to believe that when the crutches they recommend reduce one's symptoms, that healing has also occurred.)

Again, crutches like antioxidants can neutralize un-eliminated acids, which may improve the oxygenation of your child's brain and reduces the inflammatory response, but to heal his or her body and get complete and permanent results, acids need to be *eliminated* from his or her body, and crutches do not eliminate acids.

## Essential fatty acids, like flax seed and black currant oil capsules

Essential fatty acids have anti-inflammatory effects and can reduce the inflammation to your child's brain. The downside to these is that if often takes an enormous amount of these pills to obtain this effect.

I prefer that clients "get their fill" of bowel and body healing supplements. Essential fatty acids are the *least* essential nutrient to take, since they are one of the few supplements that can be duplicated with diet. In other words, essential fatty acids can be obtained through one's diet, by consuming large amounts of "good" fats, like avocadoes, olive oil, flax oil, nuts, and seeds. (On the other hand, you could never come close to duplicating the strength of *Bowel Strength* that you need by diet alone.)

## Diet cannot heal your child's bowel or eliminate acids, either

When wheat, dairy, and other foods are avoided, and fewer carbohydrates are eaten, the effect of this diet is a gradual worsening of your child's bowel health (as is true with antibiotic usage as well). You have been led to believe this diet is "the answer" because these diets have the effect of reducing the movement of acids out of his or her organs (which causes damage, and *eventually*, greater disease) into his or her blood stream (where symptoms are triggered). In other words, the solution to a dirty kitchen is not to shove the trash into your cabinets, as these diets do, but to eliminate it from your house. My program accomplishes this.

## Wheat, gluten, dairy and other allergy-free diet crutches

Jenny McCarthy and other famous people with autistic children have played a key role in popularizing the treatment of autistic kids with wheat-free, dairy-free, allergy-free diets.

The fact that children who follow these diets see some improvements offers proof that the intestinal environment in them is very unhealthy, because a very unhealthy intestinal environment is what causes allergies to wheat and dairy.

As a crutch, these diets can be tried, but be careful that you understand that these diets are crutches (they are not healing your child's bowel or body), and be very careful that your child's gluten-free, dairy-free diet does not become a long-term high protein one. When this happens, you are trading one problem for another, more deadly one later on.

## Anti-fungals (and antibiotics) are crutches that do not heal, either

Using anti-fungals and antibiotics to treat children with these disorders has gained a lot of publicity in recent years, in part due to some very famous advocates of their use, and books written advising them.

Anti-fungals help kill fungal infections and reduce fungal-irritating toxins, but they do nothing to heal your child's bowel, which is responsible for fighting these infections on a consistent and daily basis.

When medical anti-fungals or antibiotics are used to do this job, you may see a greater immediate improvement in some of your child's symptoms (as these substances are generally much stronger than natural products), but they are also more dangerous, as they destroy some of the healthy bowel bacteria that are supposed to keep these infections away in the first place (leading to "short-term gain, long-term pain). They are also acidic (toxic) and can increase some of your child's symptoms that are due to excess toxicity/acidity, so that one of his or her symptoms improve but others worsen.

When you heal your child's body and bowel with this program, it is all "gain-gain."

The greatest value of the publicity of this approach (as well as the food-allergy approach which is also extremely popular) is that it has empowered many of you with children with neurological conditions, who had previously felt completely hopeless about improving his or her condition, to believe that these conditions can be changed.

## Yet, you must use crutches!

It can take several years of aggressive *Bowel Strength* or *Unique Healing Probiotic* usage before your child's bowel can eliminates acids effortlessly, produce adequate amounts of vitamin B-12, keep infectious conditions like strep and staph from invading his or her body, etc. During this process, my clients are given extremely large amounts of bentonite clay to grab these acids and excrete them from their body, as well as extremely high, and safe, levels of *Unique Healing Methyl Vitamin B-12* and *Colloidal Silver*, as needed (in addition to a couple other possible crutches, including some of the dietary crutches described in Chapter 4 of this book, and in Chapter 9 of *Unique Healing*.) If you are looking for a quicker reduction in your child's neurological symptoms, and are not willing to wait the time needed to heal his or her bowel at which time his or her symptoms will improve, contact me at ***donna@UniqueHealing.com*** for an appointment.

## Current protocols are failing to heal your child's bowel

A healthy bacterial environment can be created in your child, but my experience is that due to many misunderstandings, this is not happening (with other programs that discuss the importance of bowel health). Some of the most common misunderstandings are as follows.

One, probiotics, which are most commonly recommended for improving bowel health, cannot quickly heal your child's bowel. It takes time (two to three years or longer) to create a healthy bacterial environment in his or her bowel. *And this only occurs if very large amounts are administered.* (In my practice, we routinely use 5-10 times or more of the standard recommended amounts of these.)

Two, probiotics do not immediately improve symptoms of autism. Rather, they are a healing agent that *eventually* eliminates these symptoms.

Again, for immediate results, very large and aggressive amounts of crutches need to be taken daily until your child's bowel (and body) are healthier.

Finally, your child's stools should never be soft, mushy, loose, skinny, green, yellow, less than 1x/day, or worse, more than 2x/day. If this is not eventually improved, then your child's bowel health has not improved, either.

## Is autism caused by vaccinations?

It is claimed that thimerosal, a mercury-containing vaccine preservative, has caused some children to suffer from neurological damage and subsequently, conditions like autism.

This has caused a great debate and defensive action from the medical and pharmaceutical community. They claim that there is no proof that mercury can cause these disorders. On the other side of the fence are parents and alternative health practitioners who insist that vaccinations cause damage, so what is the real story?

In my opinion, there is one primary reason why the medical profession defends the mercury used in vaccinations (and it is a tough one to fight!). Saying that mercury causes autism is similar to saying that pesticides cause cancer. In both cases, the mercury and pesticides should more accurately be labeled as triggers, not a cause. Mercury is likely a contributing factor to autism, but by itself, it cannot be called a cause. Otherwise, all kids given these vaccinations would have developed autism.

When you call something a "cause" and you do studies to prove this correlation, you are very likely to find data that does not prove this. If something is called a cause, you need to find a very high correlation between that substance and the illness it is said to cause.

Mercury, plus other toxins, plus an unhealthy immune system, plus an unhealthy bowel—all of these need to exist in order to "get autism." Your child's bowel and/or body were not very healthy *before* he or she got vaccinated and got autism, or any other behavioral or neurological condition. (You may not have realized this, as you likely were led to judge your child's bowel and body health inadequately, as described in Chapters 2 and 6 of *Unique Healing*).

Think of mercury as the straw that broke your "camel's back."

But a study, by its nature, can only test one variable at a time. Because it takes more than one variable, or "straws," to cause autism or any other disease or condition, studies will always miss the correlation. The medical profession will, therefore, always be able to do, and find, studies that show questionable links between toxins, like mercury, and disease.

## More mercury controversy and misunderstandings

When the first case alleging that vaccinations caused autism reached the courts, the parents claimed that mercury weakened the immune system of their daughter and that because of it, she was then unable to clear the measles virus in the vaccine from her system. It is argued that the virus then traveled through her bloodstream and caused inflammation in her brain, causing autism. Attorneys said that chemicals, like thimerosal, which contain mercury, are typically flushed from the body within a week. Doctors say there is no evidence that the measles virus persists in the intestines of anyone.

There are problems with this argument. For one, mercury can weaken the bowel bacteria, and this in turn can reduce the elimination of *future* toxins, from *all* sources, and these reabsorbed toxins can travel to the brain and trigger inflammation and reduced brain function. Even if the mercury is excreted, the damaging effects to the bowel persist. Also, the virus might not persist, but again, the affect of the damage to the bowel by the mercury in the vaccine would.

Additionally, it is said that neurological problems such as autism typically show up in children between the ages of seven to ten. In 2002, the use of thimerosal in vaccines was discontinued in most vaccines, and since then, there has been no decline in the diagnosis of autism. Do the math. If this substance was eliminated nine years ago, but it takes, on average, seven to ten years for the affect of it to show up, we need to do a study now to measure whether or not it has made a difference. We need to wait until the kids who got vaccinations without thimerosal reach age seven or ten before we judge the affect this has had.

When I was ill over twenty-five years ago I learned about the dangers of mercury and vaccinations and chose to never vaccinate my children. Now ages thirteen and sixteen, they have still never been vaccinated. (I have fought a lot of fights to maintain this stance.)

There is a much better and safer way to protect your child from disease than vaccinations. Heal their bowel and body. Vaccinations carry a risk with the benefit; healing your child's bowel and body is 100% beneficial.

## The human brain shrinks as we get older, but not so with the chimpanzee

I read an interesting, albeit frustrating, as usual, article about how it was discovered that the human brain shrinks as it gets older, leading to depression, dementia, Alzheimer's, poor memory, and other neurological problems, but that the chimpanzee, our closest animal kin, does not experience this shrinkage (*Wall Street Journal*, 7/26/11).

The reason for my frustration was the fact that the researchers who discovered this concluded that we are "very weird animals" and therefore accepted this shrinkage as inevitable. It is not.

Your brain (your main neurological organ) is made up of many tissues, as all of your organs are. Like all of your organs, it needs oxygen and nutrients to be healthy. Sure, as you get older, you become less healthy, and your poor health deprives your brain of oxygen and nutrients, but this does not have to be the case.

You will get "younger" as you heal your bowel and body with this program. You will eliminate the acids that cause low oxygen and nutrient levels and you will "save your brain."

## Genetics can be changed

Many neurological and developmental disorders have been accepted as unchangeable genetic defects, but blaming a condition on genetics is an "easy out." It is an easy excuse for a health condition that one does not know how to alter.

When my clients are diagnosed with a disorder that is called "an inevitable life sentence," which is what one is usually saying when they blame it on genetics, I tell them that only if once their body and bowel are healed, and the condition still persists, would I accept it as genetic, or "a life sentence." My clients with brown eyes do not have them turn blue, for example, but many other "genetic" inheritances are changeable, and should more accurately be defined as "genetic weaknesses" rather than "genetic blueprints."

An article in *Alternative Medicine* (April 2005) described kids with Down's Syndrome (DS) who are being treated with a powerful blend of nutritional supplements and, as a result, experiencing fewer seizures, higher IQs, and an overall noticeable improvement in their health and reduction of disease symptoms. Lawrence Leichtman, a clinical geneticist and director of the Genetics and Disabilities Diagnostic Care Center in Virginia Beach, Virginia, explains why a genetic disorder like Down's can be helped by nutritional supplements. As he says, the extra chromosome seen in Down's causes several metabolic disorders that themselves may be prime causes of mental dysfunction, and these metabolic disorders can be helped with nutritional supplementation.

In other words, nutrition won't change the chromosome, but it can change some of the ill effects that the chromosome is causing. At this and other centers for children with these disorders, a treatment objective is to assist methylation, a fundamental biochemical process that helps regulate which genes are expressed. This process is affected by your nutritional status, a controllable variable, which again, means that gene expression can be controlled by nutrition.

In the April 2007 article on autism in *Discover*, author Jill Newmark comments that there is a "growing sense that low-dose, multiple toxic and infectious exposures may be a major contributing factor to autism and its related disorders," and that a vivid analogy is that "genes load the gun, but environment pulls the trigger."

And neuroscientist Pat Levitt says, "We're beginning to understand that genetics is really about vulnerability."

Researchers have found that a variant of a gene called "Met" doubles the risk of autism. This gene is important for the repair of the intestine and immune function. The activity of the gene is affected by oxidative stress, the kind of damage one sees with excessive exposure to acids/toxins.

*In other words, she is saying that exposure to acids/toxins can affect our genes. And an unhealthy bowel that cannot eliminate toxins leaves one much more "vulnerable," as she puts it, to genetic diseases.*

And anyway, which came first, the unhealthy intestines (bowel), or the Met gene? Has it been proven that the gene impairs intestinal and immune function? Maybe this gene is created by impaired intestinal and immune function? I think this bears research, don't you? Does the gene cause an unhealthy bowel, or does an unhealthy bowel cause the genetic mutation? An unhealthy bowel can be healed.

If it is the unhealthy bowel that causes the genetic variant that is seen in many autistic kids, then healing the bowel should eliminate this genetic manifestation.

## Premature babies have greater neurological problems

Researchers have found that babies born prematurely have a much higher rate of ADD later in life, and that babies with a low Apgar score at birth (between one and four) have a 75% greater chance of developing this condition.

The implication of this research is that the ill health of the mother (who has the largest impact on her child's organ health and bacterial environment health) plays a pivotal role in the development of these conditions, not the vaccinations, heavy metals, toxins, wheat, pesticides, etc. that a child is exposed to later in life.

Given the great increase in premature births, this is a concerning statistic. It is *extraordinarily* rare for one of my clients to give birth prematurely.

## Are neurological disorders curable?

A recent article described an extreme, "hopeless" case of a 17-year-old autistic child who is nonverbal and suffers with horrible erosive esophagitis *in spite of the fact that he works closely with a gastroenterologist,* who was described as unable to help. This comment is stated as though just because this *doctor* can't help, this condition is hopeless and incurable.

In another article, in *People* under the section "Is Autism Curable," a doctor commented: "I'm not sure we're curing it."

No, they are not curing autism, or any of these other disorders, because drugs do not cure things. They treat symptoms. "Curing" cancer eliminates the cancer but it does nothing to "cure" the unhealthy immune system that allowed it to occur in the first place. With autism, like all diseases, I don't understand how there can ever be a "medical cure."

Taking a bunch of antioxidants and eating a food allergy diet can't cure it, either.

Nothing is curable if you only treat the symptoms with crutches, and not the cause of the problem.

People use "cure" freely, but go back to Chapter Two of *Unique Healing* and review the definition of curable, and you will see that a crutch is not a cure.

Are autism, ADD, and other neurological conditions curable? I say absolutely, if you heal the bowel and body of the person suffering with these conditions.

## Similar ideas, but a whole new path, with a whole new set of potential

If you have been altering your child's diet, trying to heal your child's bowel, and/or have taken steps to treat bacterial/fungal and other infections; and if you are aware of the toxicity problems in your child and have been trying to address these, you have made great progress in finding the answer to your child's issues. I am offering a path beyond this, a different path, based on similar ideas, but on a whole new level, with a whole new level of results, as well.

## Success With Neurological Disorders

"Continuing the Dr. K appt and prep work . . . these include the data from Alpine for January and the first 15 days of Feb. Can't argue with the data. Going to be a VERY interesting appointment. In spontaneous manding (requesting) he has seen a 65% improvement since June and in spontaneous tacting a 48% improvement since June."

"We just returned form a visit with his grandparents. They were blown away by the improvement in his behavior since the last time we visited (one year ago). We knew he was doing better, but sometimes it takes someone who does not see him all the time to confirm it."

For many years I worked with very few of these children. I think this is largely because most parents were led to believe that there was nothing that could be done to help them.

Fortunately, things are changing. This is in part due to the publicity of some famous actresses, and others, who have tried alternative methods with their children and seen improvements with them. Wheat and dairy-free diets, for example, are beginning to be accepted as approaches that can help. These have been around for at least twenty years; I did them when I was ill. But they have recently made their way into mainstream thought, and this food allergy approach, while it treats symptoms only, is a positive step in the direction of knowing and believing that an answer exists.

My program often is only understood, and sought out, once these more mainstream alternative approaches fail. I am just beginning to see the tides turning in this direction, and I will post updates with success stories on my website, in time.

In the meantime, I have seen noticeable improvements in neurological symptoms in adults and kids with autism, A.D.D., and similar disorders. I have not been given the opportunity to aggressively heal these children, but I look forward to it, and am confident that success will be found. (Bear in mind that there are no practitioners—medical or alternative—who can provide you with long-term success stories in treating these disorders either. I suggest that one day, I will.)

## Watch My Video, "Why THIS Program Works for Autism (and other neurological disorders)"

This video, and all of my videos, can be found at *www.UniqueHealing.com* or at *www.YouTube.com/UniqueHealing*.

## Nervousness
See "Anxiety"

## Nicotine Addictions
See "Addictions"

## Nickel Toxicity
See "Heavy Metal Toxicity"

# Osteoporosis/Osteopenia

Your bones are largely comprised of the alkaline minerals calcium and magnesium. Twenty-three percent of them are made up of the alkaline mineral sodium, as well. All of your bones are replaced every ten years. They are made up of cells that are living and changing, and this means that if you have already lost bone, this condition is not permanent; it can be improved and corrected. This program can help you build new, stronger, healthier bones.

I think that all women "know" that taking calcium supplements is good for their bone health. This quick fix for bone health has not been successful, however, because like all other aspects of your health, there is not a quick and easy answer. But there *is* an answer, and I present it to you here.

(Osteopenia is a condition of bone loss that precedes osteoporosis; with osteoporosis, your loss of bone is more significant than with osteopenia).

## Healing Your Body With This Program Eliminates Osteoporosis/Osteopenia

Your body's first line of defense against excess un-eliminated acids in your blood are your four elimination channels—lungs, kidneys, skin, and especially, your bowel. After they become unhealthy, your liver, adrenal glands, stomach, pancreas, and small intestine are stimulated to protect you against these acids. It is after *they* become unhealthy that your body turns to its alkaline reserves—calcium, magnesium, sodium, and potassium—to neutralize this acidity.

Your bones contain a lot of these alkaline minerals, and when they are leached out of your bones to buffer un-eliminated acids, your bones degenerate, and eventually create the conditions of osteoporosis and osteopenia. (Review Chapter Three of *Unique Healing* for a description of this degenerative process in response to un-eliminated acids.)

Healing your body with this program eliminates the acids that cause your body to leach calcium and other minerals from your bones.

## Healing Your Bowel With This Program Eliminates Osteoporosis/Osteopenia

Dietary calcium helps create healthy bones, but in order to be of value, it has to be *absorbed*. Calcium mal-absorption is a significant cause of osteopenia and osteoporosis. Taking in more calcium, via your diet or supplements, does not always help your bone health, because the calcium does not always get absorbed effectively.

Your intestines ionize calcium so that it *can* be absorbed, and your bowel bacteria play a key role in this. It is not how much calcium that you ingest, but rather how much you absorb, that matters. Healing your bowel with this program improves your body's ability to absorb calcium (from your diet and from supplements) and create healthy bones.

A healthy bowel does not have lactose-intolerance problems, and when you heal it with this program, you will be able to drink milk and other dairy products and benefit from the calcium contained in them.

Also, people who tend to have higher homocysteine levels are 2-4 times more likely to suffer hip fractures. In a two-year study, half of the participants took 5 mg of folic acid and 1,500 mcg of vitamin B-12, and the others took a placebo. Even though both groups sustained roughly the same number of falls during that time, the treatment group suffered 80 percent fewer fractures. (It is unknown how exactly these two nutrients help bone health.) They also saw their homocysteine levels drop, whereas the patients taking the placebo saw their levels increase. The healthy bacteria in your bowel help with the manufacture of vitamin B-12, and therefore, help lower homocysteine levels and increase bone health.

In addition to its many other important functions, a healthy bacterial environment in your bowel is a necessity for the complete elimination of acids (toxins, heavy metals, pesticides, etc.) from your body. A healthy bowel prevents the re-absorption of acids into your blood that cause your body to eventually rob the minerals from your bones that they need to be healthy.

## Why My Crutches Eliminate Osteoporosis/Osteopenia

There are no crutches for degenerative conditions and great accumulations of acidity in your organs like osteoporosis/osteopenia. Crutches can offset the effects of acids in your blood, or the effects of poor function of your bowel bacterial environment (as these can be quickly altered), but degeneration is caused by depletion and damage to your organs, and organs, like your bones, take time to heal.

### How long will I need to use crutches for my osteoporosis/osteopenia?

Again, there are no crutches for degenerative conditions like osteoporosis/osteopenia; however, degenerative conditions are the first to become eliminated as you heal your bowel and body with this program.

Think of creating bone health as repairing the holes in your roof. This program (unlike programs that rely on crutches, as almost all of them do) repairs these holes; it repairs your organs, but you must invest some time into this program to get this result.

## Misunderstandings About Osteoporosis/Osteopenia and Other Information for Your Success

### Take *Unique Healing Calcium Citrate*

While there is no way to immediately improve your bone health, and while a healthy bowel and body will eventually improve yours, it is important that you take adequate amounts of an easy-to-absorb calcium, like *Unique Healing Calcium Citrate*, now. This will help prevent *future* bone loss, and it will give your body the minerals it needs to start re-building your bones *now*. (Use it to accelerate the repair of your bones, and rely on the healthy bowel and body that you create with this program to maintain their health.)

Women are typically advised to take an additional 1,200 mg of calcium a day in supplement form, although if your bowel is particularly unhealthy and/or you have accumulated a large degree of acidity, this amount will not be enough to improve your bones. The recommendation in this book of about 2,400 mg a day is much more helpful, and even larger amounts, up to 4,000 mg a day for 6-12 months, should be considered if you have been diagnosed with osteopenia or osteoporosis.

(I anticipate a reaction to this recommendation to be something along the lines of "watch out, we don't have studies showing that this amount is safe or helpful." My response to that is that it is dangerous to get osteoporosis, and the standard recommendations for preventing this are not working, and this should be your real concern. I have never had anyone hurt by my recommendations for larger amounts of calcium; on the contrary.)

For more information about using calcium, including common misunderstandings and fears, as well as support for the safety of taking large amounts of calcium, see Chapter 5.

## Drinking more milk is not the solution

Eating more dairy products does not necessarily help build strong bones. The calcium in the most commonly consumed dairy products, like regular milk, skim milk, and low fat milk, is often not utilizable, because many of you cannot digest dairy well (and it must be digested well for the calcium in it to be available to build strong bones).

A twelve-year study was conducted at Harvard University with over 75,000 nurses, aged 34-59. Researchers came to the *unbiased* conclusion that w*omen who drank two or more glasses of milk per day had a statistically significantly higher rate of osteoporosis than women who consumed one glass of milk or less per week.* (Feskanich, D., et al. Milk, dietary calcium, and bone fractures in women: a 12 year prospective study, Am J. Publ Health, 1997; 87:992-7.) This is a gigantic, long-term, unbiased study, and therefore, one that has great significance. Compare this to the majority of irrelevant scientific studies that get published in the medical journals, and subsequently announced on television, that last only 6-8 weeks and study only 20-100 people. Did you hear about *this* study on television? I wonder why not? Research has only ever proven that *calcium* can help prevent osteoporosis, not dairy products. We have been led to believe that since milk has calcium, milk prevents osteoporosis. This is the *assumption* that we have all been led to believe as *fact*. I have seen many commercials for milk that tout its high calcium content, and then comment that calcium intake helps to build strong bones. Note, they do not say that milk builds strong bones; they let you make this conclusion yourself. This is very clever of them.

The rate of osteoporosis in this country is significantly higher than in most other industrialized countries in the world, yet we consume more milk than the majority of them. For example, the Asian population, which consumes much less milk (and calcium) than us (an average of about 400 mg per day versus our recommendation of 1200 mg per day), yet they have much less osteoporosis than we do.

The point is, creating healthy bones is more complicated than simply drinking a lot of milk. On the other hand, milk certainly does have value in helping to build strong bones, but only when you can digest it effectively.

## The pros and cons of yogurt

Easier-to-digest dairy foods such as yogurt yield more calcium, and therefore may help to keep your calcium levels in balance. (Studies have shown that calcium is more readily absorbed in the presence of fermented lactic cultures, such as yogurt.)

Yogurt is very cleansing, however, especially when it is flavored (some contain up to 35 or more grams of sugar/serving and this is way "too much." Check your labels carefully. If it has over 10 grams of sugar/serving it will likely cause you "cleansing problems"). This means that even though it is healthy, and it is good for your bones, if you consume a lot of it in an effort to help your bones, you are likely to gain weight and/or feel bad and/or have bad blood test results. (Still don't understand this concept? Re-read *Unique Healing* and watch my videos until you do.)

## . . . and raw milk?

Raw milk is also easy to digest and may seem like the "solution;" unfortunately, in most states, raw milk is illegal and uncontaminated raw milk is hard to come by. Most of you have a relatively unhealthy bowel bacterial environment, and you risk diarrhea and other bacterial infections when you consume raw milk. I have a client whose daughter was in critical condition after consuming contaminated raw milk. It's risky. Healing your bowel and body are not risky.

## Another reason to eat cheese

Cheese is less acidic and much easier to digest than milk, due to the enzymes added to it during its production, which aid in its digestion, and your consumption of cheese is a great way to increase your bone health (assuming you are not allergic to it, of course).

Compared to yogurt, cheese is non-cleansing, so you will not feel lousy when you eat it, and it does not carry the risk of infection that raw milk does.

I am an advocate of cheese consumption, not only for your bone health, but also for overall health, symptom reduction, weight reduction, and addiction reduction. For more information on why cheese is so valuable, and why you should eat more, watch my video, "Eat a Lot of Cheese," available at ***www.UniqueHealing.com*** or ***www.YouTube.com/ UniqueHealing***.

## High protein diets increase osteoporosis and osteopenia

High protein diets are acidic, and they are damaging to your organs, your bones included. They reduce acids from entering your blood from your organs, and therefore these diets can help you look and feel better, but this is done at the expense of your organ health, like your bones, and your longevity.

Countries with the highest rate of hip fractures among the elderly—Norway, Denmark, and Sweden—also have the highest levels of animal protein consumption.

Positive changes in bone density have been reported amongst vegetarians because the less meat in your diet, the less acidic it generally is. The Seventh Day Adventist population, which is a large vegetarian group, shows lower rates of osteoporosis than other sub-populations in this country. In 1983, the *American Journal of Clinical Nutrition* published the largest study it had ever done on osteoporosis. Researchers found that by 65 years of age, female vegetarians had 18% bone loss compared to 35% bone loss (or approximately twice as much) as non-vegetarians. And in his article "Calcium: How Your Diet Affects Requirements," Robert Hearney, M.D., gives the following example: "A single fast-food hamburger, high in both protein and salt, can produce a negative calcium balance of 23 mg. Because net calcium absorption is only about 10% from most diets, eating this could increase calcium needs by as much as 230 mg."

A vegetarian diet is not a simple answer to improving bone health, however, as one can be a vegetarian and still consume way too many acidic foods, such as salt, sugar, alcohol, and soda. A vegetarian diet also cannot heal your bowel, which is involved in calcium absorption. Finally, when your bowel is unhealthy, a vegetarian diet can make you look and feel horrible, due to its cleansing effect, thus greatly minimizing the chance that you will stick to this bone-enhancing type of diet. Review my videos "Avoid Cleansing Diets for Now" at ***www.UniqueHealing.com*** or ***www.YouTube.com/UniqueHealing*** if you are still confused about this extremely important concept.

Here again is another reason why this program is desperately needed. Without it, many of you will fail to achieve bone health, as the diet that helps your bones, can also increase your symptoms and weight, and you are unlikely to stick with it long enough to benefit form the bone-health properties of it. This program heals your bones *and* reduces your symptoms and weight problems.

Additionally, when you heal your body, you will desire very little "calcium-leaching" animal protein.

## Coffee and other acidic foods increase osteoporosis and osteopenia

Acids eventually cause your bones to leach out calcium to buffer them and protect you from them. Eating a highly acidic diet is very strongly correlated with increased rates of osteoporosis and osteopenia. (Review Chapter 5 of *Unique Healing* for a listing of highly acidic foods.)

In 1990 the *American Journal of Epidemiology* reported that women who drink 2-3 cups of coffee a day, whether regular or decaffeinated, increase their risk of osteoporosis-related fractures by 69%; those who drink more than three cups per day increase their risk by 82%. One cup of coffee leaches 11 mg of calcium from your bones. (Note: coffee *is* acidic, whether it is caffeinated or not.)

In 1992, researchers at Brigham and Women's Hospital and Harvard Medical School in Boston found a significant correlation between osteoporosis and coffee consumption. In a long-term study of nearly 85,000 nurses between the ages of 34 and 59, scientists found that the women who drank the most coffee (four or more cups a day) had almost three times the incidence of hip fractures as women who drank little or no coffee.

Tea drinking did not appear to increase the risk of osteoporosis, researchers found. Tea is alkaline and coffee is acidic, and only acidic foods or beverages can cause calcium depletion, so this makes sense. (I highly recommend the consumption of unsweetened tea.)

Additionally, a 1995 study at the University of Western Australia found that women consuming more than 2,100 mg of sodium a day had greater bone loss than women consuming less. According to the study's head researcher, "If a woman cut her sodium intake from 4,000 mg to 2,000 mg a day, she would protect her bones as much as if she consumed about an extra 1,000 mg of calcium a day." (The sodium used in this study is regular, acidic, table salt. This is one more good reason to switch from regular refined salt to sea salt, which is alkalinizing and helps to keep your bones healthy.)

When you heal your bowel and body with this program, you will no longer desire much animal protein, sugar, coffee, alcohol, or other highly acidic, bone-damaging foods. It is one thing to tell someone "coffee is bad for him or her." This rarely "works." What does work is creating a body that does not desire it, as this program does. This works.

## Vitamin D and bone health

Vitamin D, and sometimes other nutrients, is commonly added to calcium/bone health supplements to aid in the absorption of calcium. When your bowel and body are healthy, extra vitamin D supplementation will not be needed to create bone health, but in the meantime, I have added vitamin D to *Unique Healing Calcium Citrate* to improve its value.

## Bone density tests vs. blood tests

A blood test typically includes a measurement of the amount of calcium in your blood. As is true regarding the use of blood tests to measure *any* nutrient level in your body, using a blood test to measure the health of your bones (and calcium levels) is harmfully inaccurate and misleading.

A normal blood calcium level does not mean that your bones are healthy and strong. Your body will leach calcium out of your bones and into your blood for a very long time before it becomes too deficient to do this, at which time a low blood calcium level may show up. By then, your bones are typically extremely depleted. Waiting for your blood test to show low calcium levels is very dangerous.

A valuable test for measuring your bone health is a bone density test. Numerous women have had this test done who have been found to have osteopenia (early stage osteoporosis) or osteoporosis, even though their blood test showed ideal calcium levels.

I recommend this test to anyone who can afford it or can get his or her insurance company to pay for it, regardless of age or sex. Currently, only older women are encouraged to have this done; yet younger women and men are also at risk of premature bone loss, especially with our ever-increasingly acidic lifestyles and unhealthy bowels.

When you get your test results, use this as a *baseline measure*. If your bones are strong at first, it is concerning if they become weaker in subsequent years, even if you still fall in the acceptable range. If your test is low the first time but stays there in the next couple of years, you may simply have a smaller frame than the standard that is used to assess bone health.

If your levels are low now, heal your bowel and body aggressively and have this test re-done in one year. These are baseline figures and it is the *continued lowering* of your bone density in subsequent tests that warrants concern.

## The controversy of using drugs to treat osteoporosis/osteopenia

Drugs for osteoporosis may slow further bone loss, but for the most part, they have not been shown to increase bone formation. Popular drugs used to treat osteoporosis have not been proven to be safe, or effective, in the long-term, either. (On 9/10/11 the *Wall Street Journal* reported that in one study, when the drug Fosomax, and similar drugs, were used for more than several years, there was an increased risk of fracture to the thighbone.)

Many of these drugs stop the leaching of calcium out of your bones (that is occurring to buffer un-eliminated acids in your blood). While this can improve bone health to some degree, it could lead to higher rates of heart attack, cancer, and other ailments. In other words, the calcium being leached out of your bones is your body's effort to buffer un-eliminated acids. If this calcium is forced, by a drug, to stop leaching out of your bones, these acids are *still* in your blood, and now they are un-buffered, so another part of your health will suffer to protect you from this acidity. You have simply shoved the trash from your bedroom to your living room, but is this really productive and beneficial overall, and does this add years to your life? I say "no."

With this program, these acids are eliminated so that not only will your bones stop leaching calcium, but none of your other organs will be damaged from these acids, either. Instead of one organ, your bones, being helped and another being harmed, as is the case with drug use, when you heal your bowel and body with this program, *all* of your organs are helped.

Also, drugs do nothing to improve the absorption of calcium in your diet, as building bowel health does.

## Unhealthy bones can occur with more serious conditions like cancer and heart disease

When your body turns to your bones for calcium to buffer excess un-eliminated acids in your blood, your cells and arteries are likely becoming unhealthy, too.

In other words, at this stage, you are at the "top of your pipe," which is a dangerous place to be. It is where deadly cancers and heart attacks occur. These conditions warrant a very aggressive approach to healing your bowel and body, as this program offers.

## High blood calcium levels indicate low levels in your bones

A high blood calcium reading does not mean that you are eating too much calcium, or taking too many calcium supplements. This can occur when your bones become extremely unhealthy and your body goes into crisis mode, dumping excess calcium into your blood to protect you from too much acidity in it. This condition warrants an immediate bone density test and attention. In this condition, the bone density test may show that your bones are very severely depleted, even cancerous.

If you have high blood calcium levels, increase your calcium intake (I know this goes against medical advice and "wisdom."). However, in the 19 years that I have done this work, I have consistently found that clients with high blood calcium levels experience a *reduction* in these levels (which also means less damage to their bones) when they take large amounts of calcium, as recommended by me. This improvement in calcium levels with an increase in calcium intake has occurred 100% of the time.

## Exercise is a crutch with very limited value

Exercise has been highly touted as a tool to improve bone health, but keep in mind that it is another crutch that has the same limitations in helping your bone health as all crutches do. In my old hometown of Boulder, Colorado, I saw a lot of athletic people who, despite this, had bone loss. It is much more protective and effective to create a healthy bowel and body.

Exercise does not eliminate the acids that leach calcium from your bones, and it does not heal your bowel, which should be helping you absorb adequate amounts of calcium from your diet.

If you have depended on the exercise crutch to prevent these osteoporosis and osteopenia, don't. And it you have depended on exercise to prevent these and your bone tests continue to worsen, do not think you have "done all you can" to prevent this. You have simply been led down the wrong road.

## Success with Osteoporosis/Osteopenia

"Eight years ago I had a bone density test and was diagnosed with osteopenia. I started this program and just had my test re-done (first time since the last one eight years ago). I am 62 years old and was just told that my bones are now 118% for my age. I am now SUPER BONE!"

"I am 63 years old and just had my first bone density test (I typically avoid medical doctors and tests.) I was told that I have the bone health of a 45 year old. I thank this program for my bone health."

"I was diagnosed with osteopenia at age 48 and it worried me. Extensive testing showed that I was not absorbing calcium. I have been doing this program for two years now and my recent bone density test showed that I now have healthy bones, and no more osteopenia."

"In April, before starting this program, my blood calcium levels were very high (126, and normal is 4-64), and I was diagnosed with osteoporosis. Now four months later, after doing this program, they are normal (43)." (By the way, this client is a doctor in town and I worked very hard to convince her to follow my very "controversial" approach.)

"I was put on drugs for osteoporosis, took extra calcium, and exercise often, but my bone density tests continued to slowly worsen. Osteoporosis is common in my family and I was told it was genetic, and to basically expect to suffer from this condition as well. I recently had my test re-done and it showed that the bone loss has stopped, and after doing this program for another year I am going to have it re-done again. I am confident that it will show even more improvement."

"When I started this program my blood calcium levels were high and I was very ill. It took Donna many weeks to convince me to *increase* my calcium intake. It scared me, because my doctors told me to do the opposite. But it made sense, and my calcium level was not improving with their advice, so I took the large amount she suggested and sure enough, my next blood calcium test was normal!"

## Watch my Video "Why THIS Program Works for Osteoporosis."
This video, and all of my videos, can be found at *www.UniqueHealing.com* or at *www.YouTube.com/UniqueHealing*.

## Ovarian Cancer
See "Breast/Female Cancers"

## Overweight
See Chapter 4

## Pancreatitis
See "Inflammation" (Chapter Three)

## PANDAS
See "Neurological Disorders"

## Parasite Infections
See "Fungal Infections"

## Parkinson's Disease
See "Neurological Disorders"

## Pneumonia
See "Bacterial Infections"

## Premenstrual Syndrome
See "Female Issues"

# Prostate Disorders
## High PSA Levels, Cancer, Enlarged Prostate, and Other Male Hormone Problems

Prostate problems, largely caused by hormonal imbalances in men, are similar to female hormonal problems, and therefore, the information on breast and other female cancers discussed earlier apply here as well.

## Healing Your Body With This Program Eliminates Prostate Disorders

Un-eliminated acids can aggravate an enlarged prostate, and ultimately, these acids can cause death from prostate cancer, but by in large, this condition, as with breast cancer in women, is largely a hormonal one (which is a "bowel problem").

## Healing Your Bowel With This Program Eliminates Prostate Disorders

Your intestinal bacteria play a key role in regulating the production and balance of male hormones. As with estrogen in women, testosterone is a hormone that helps stimulate the male organs and creates health, but an excess of testosterone can be harmful. Excess levels of testosterone have been implicated in prostate cancer. A healthy bacterial environment in your bowel is necessary to prevent the excessive re-accumulation of testosterone into your body.

Also, your intestinal bacteria fight bacterial infections, and in some cases, prostate enlargement is the result of an infection in your body.

## Why My Crutches Eliminate Prostate Disorders

**Natural Progesterone cream** provides a safe source of natural progesterone, which *balances* hormone levels and eliminates the problems associated with an excess or deficiency of them. Men and women both make progesterone. It helps offset excess testosterone levels, which have been implicated in prostate problems and cancer.

***Unique Healing Colloidal Silver*** has natural anti-bacterial, anti-fungal, anti-parasitic properties, and it eliminates the infections that cause some cases of an enlarged prostrate.

## How much do I take?/Questions about using these

See Chapter 5 for information on using these crutches, including recommendations on the amount to use, as well as a discussion of the misunderstandings about the particular crutch that may, if not understood correctly, cause you to fail to look and feel better while you heal your bowel and body with this program.

## How long will I need to use crutches for my prostate disorder?

The bacterial environment in your bowel affects prostate disorders. To better understand how long you may need crutches for this, refer to Chapter 1 under this subject heading.

# Misunderstandings About Prostate Disorders and Other Information for Your Success

## Acids are more dangerous than excess testosterone

As with breast and female hormonal cancers, it is not the re-absorption of testosterone that is dangerous, rather this condition is a reflection of a very unhealthy bowel, and it is this unhealthy bowel that is dangerous, as it allows for the re-absorption of acids into your body, and accumulated acidity puts you at risk of death from cancer and other diseases. When you are diagnosed with prostate cancer, your primary focus needs to be on eliminating these acids, as this program does.

## Dairy products and prostate cancer

A large study of over 45,000 men found that prostate cancer rose with dairy consumption, which many experts presume was a result of the *hormones* in these products.

A healthy bowel eliminates excess hormones and reduces this risk, but until yours is healthier, it is wise to choose organic dairy foods produced without added hormones.

## Natural progesterone cream is not for women only

You will find this product in the "women's health" aisle of health food stores, but it is not for women only, and it will not "make you a woman," either. Natural progesterone cream will *not* give you female characteristics; on the contrary, it balances your hormones and *increases* your male energy. Likewise, this crutch balances hormones so that you have neither too much nor too little testosterone. In other words, it can reduce the dangerous levels of testosterone in your tissues that trigger prostate caner, but it can increase the levels in your blood that are needed for a healthy sex drive, muscle growth, male characteristics, etc.

## PSA (Prostate Specific Antigen) testing

The medical profession uses blood tests that measure the PSA levels in your blood to help detect prostate cancer. As with all cancers, a biopsy will be done to verify cancer if it is suspected, but this blood test is a clue there may be a problem. Ironically, many of my male clients have never had this test done (which may be in part a reflection of the male population's well-known tendency to avoid doctors more than the female population.) As is true with *all* blood tests, your PSA blood test can be manipulated to look better too (with the use of natural progesterone cream, as recommended earlier).

## Likely much more common than we realize

There is definitely much greater awareness and fear around testing, like mammograms, for female cancer, than there is for male cancers like prostate cancer. While many of my older females clients have had a mammogram done, again, very few of my male clients have had a PSA test.

It seems biased that men are not subjected to a similar fear and push to have PSA tests done. I suspect that if men were subjected to the same fear and mass-testing that women are in this country for breast cancer, a lot more of them would be diagnosed with prostrate cancer/disease.

In fact, it is estimated that 16% of men born today will be diagnosed with prostate cancer during their lifetime (and only 12% of women will be diagnosed with breast cancer). It is ironic, don't you think, that prostate cancer, which affects more men than breast cancer affects women, has not had nearly the amount of coverage (in the media, by fundraising groups, etc.)?

## Have you had, or do you have, prostate cancer?

If so, many of the concepts about female hormonal cancers like breast cancer apply to you as well, so read the section earlier on "Breast and Other Female Cancers."

# Success With Prostate Disorders

Over the last 19 years, the majority of my clients have been women. Additionally, because very few of my male clients have even had a PSA test done, I rarely come across prostate problems. Finally, few of them have willingly volunteered to discuss their male health problems with me, and that is okay.

Nevertheless, male clients who arrive at my door with elevated PSA do see them go down on this program, and more importantly, I have never had a male client get prostrate cancer while healing his bowel and body with my guidance in this program.

### Watch my video,
### "Why THIS Program Eliminates Prostate Disorders"

This video, and all of my videos, can be found at *www.UniqueHealing.com* or at *www.YouTube.com/UniqueHealing*.

## Psoriasis
### See "Skin Conditions"

## Rashes
### See "Skin Conditions"

## Reflux
### Heartburn, Indigestion

Before a drug was invented for this condition, my clients rarely came in with this diagnosis (how interesting!). Once drugs were available, numerous clients, who had always had these symptoms, arrived at my door with a diagnosis of reflux and a prescription drug to treat it. Now, it is one of the more common conditions that I see, and help, clients with.

# Healing Your Body With This Program Eliminates Reflux

When un-eliminated acids are reabsorbed, eventually they find their way to the "middle of your pipe," or esophagus and stomach (review Chapter Three of *Unique Healing* for a description of "the pipe."). Here, they can trigger discomfort and symptoms known as reflux. If these acids continue to accumulate, they can eventually cause dangerous damage and scarring of your esophagus.

Your stomach makes hydrochloric acid, a strong acidic enzyme that is needed for the digestion of protein in your diet. With reflux, this stomach acid "leaks" back up into your esophagus, causing symptoms of heartburn and indigestion. (This occurs if the muscles between the esophagus and stomach do not "close off" the opening between these two areas.) When your blood becomes overly acidic, these muscles may become aggravated, allowing for this stomach acid to leak into your esophagus. Healing your body with this program eliminates the excess acidity that prevents these muscles from functioning properly.

Healing your body with this program eliminates the acids that may be leaked out of your stomach into your esophagus. Antacids that are prescribed for this condition work in a similar way. They buffer these acids; this program eliminates them, which is far superior and permanent.

(Note: When I was first very ill I was prescribed an antacid. This drug caused a remarkable improvement in my symptoms. I went from being very disabled and unable to work, to being able to return to work (still not feeling great but at least functioning). It was unbelievable. Interestingly, I can't remember why I stopped taking it (and once I did, I was back in bed and out of work again), but had I been wise enough to put two and two together (to associate my debilitating symptoms with acids), I may have figured out how to heal myself long ago).

Healing your body with this program heals your stomach and esophagus so that even if there are acids, your body is strong enough to handle them without a reaction (it fixes the holes on your roof so that even if it does rain, your house does not get wet).

# Healing Your Bowel With This
# Program Eliminates Reflux

High levels of the "bad" bacteria H-Pylori have been found in some individuals with this condition. Your healthy bowel bacterial environment is responsible for destroying bad bacteria like H-Pylori.

In addition to its many other important functions, a healthy bacterial environment in your bowel is a necessity for the complete elimination of acids (toxins, heavy metals, pesticides, etc.) from your body. A healthy bowel prevents the re-absorption of acids into your blood that aggravate your esophagus and stomach and allow for stomach acids to leach into your esophagus and trigger discomfort and the symptoms of acid reflux.

## Why My Crutches Eliminate Reflux

***Body Bentonite*** binds to and eliminates acids (toxins, heavy metals, chemicals, etc.) from your body. It helps prevent them from becoming re-absorbed into your bloodstream, where they trigger irritation to your stomach and esophagus.

***Unique Healing Calcium Citrate*** is an alkalinizing mineral that helps neutralize the acids that your bowel does not eliminate. When these acids are buffered, they do not aggravate your stomach or esophagus. (Calcium is included in some over-the counter antacids for its ability to reduce heartburn symptoms).

***Unique Healing Colloidal Silver*** has natural anti-bacterial, anti-fungal, anti-parasitic properties. It eliminates the infections that can aggravate/cause some cases of reflux.

### How much do I take?/Questions about using these

See Chapter 5 for information on using these crutches, including recommendations on the amount to use, as well as a discussion of the misunderstandings about the particular crutch that may, if not understood correctly, cause you to fail to look and feel better while you heal your bowel and body with this program.

### How long will I need to use crutches for my reflux?

Reflux occurs at Level 2 of your pipe. It is the second area of your body to heal (assuming that other areas are unhealthy too). Refer to the diagram "Sequence of Healing" in Appendix A at the end of this book to better understand this concept, as well as to Chapter 1 under this subject heading.

The bacterial environment in your bowel also affects reflux. To better understand how long you may need crutches for this, refer to Chapter 1 under this subject heading.

# Misunderstandings About Reflux and Other Information for Your Success

## Keep your stools well-formed

Because reflux is caused in part by un-eliminated acids, and because well-formed stools prevent the re-absorption of acids into your blood, you will suffer from the least amount of reflux symptoms if you keep your stools well-formed while you are healing your bowel and body.

If you do not have a very good handle on how to define well-formed stools, review Chapter 6 of *Unique Healing* now. (And remember, when your stools are hard and slow you are eliminating more acids, and will therefore feel better, than when your stools are one or more times a day but not all extremely well-formed.)

If your stools are not well-formed, the following changes can help: increase your *Body Bentonite* intake; reduce your carbohydrate intake (pasta, breads, grains, cereals, yogurt, etc.); reduce your sugar intake (including natural healthy sugars such as agave, honey, raw sugar, cane juice, etc.); reduce your alcohol, salt, coffee, and/or soda intake; do not have a massage, chiropractic adjustment, or any other body work; drink a lot of water; rest; and keep your exercise aerobic (see Chapter 4 for more information on how to attain this, and why it is important.)

If these changes do not noticeably help the form of your stools in two days, take them further (i.e. take more *Body Bentonite*, reduce your carbohydrate intake more, etc.)

Out of all of these recommendations, increasing your *Body Bentonite* intake is one of the most productive and helpful. It heals your body, unlike many of the other recommendations. It will do the most to lead you to a place where looking and feeling good is effortless, and some of the other suggestions, such as reducing sugar intake, are simply "too hard to do when your blood is too acidic."

(Note: the exception to this information is when your poorly formed stools are caused by an infection, in which case *Unique Healing Colloidal Silver* is needed to reduce your symptoms. Refer to Chapter 5 for information on when and how to use this crutch.)

## Stopping stomach acid production with drugs is not a wise decision

Unlike antacids, which buffer the acids in your blood and the reflux symptoms associated with them, most of the now-popular drugs for the treatment of reflux work by inhibiting the production of stomach acid. The less acid that is produced in your stomach, the less that can "leak out" into your esophagus. The problem with this approach is that you need stomach acid for the proper digestion of the protein in the foods you eat. Improper protein digestion causes toxic by-products, and it reduces your ability to gain healthy muscle weight. Your body uses amino acids, which are created when proteins are properly digested, for a whole host of functions, like immunity, tissue repair, etc. You reduce the availability of these when you reduce your stomach acid production.

Rather than stop stomach acid production, as these drugs do, it is far more valuable and safer to eliminate the excess acidity that causes your stomach and esophagus muscles to malfunction in the first place, as this program does.

## Drugs for reflux and esophageal damage and scarring

A common argument for the use of drugs to treat reflux is that they can prevent your esophagus from scarring; you may be scared into thinking that if you do not use their drug, you are putting yourself in harms way of this occurring.

Just because you have reflux does not mean that your esophagus will suffer scarring and damage (cellular damage). You must get to the "top of your pipe" before this happens. This program prevents acids from getting to the top of your pipe, and it prevents scarring and damage. The first area of your body that heals with this program, in fact, is the top of your pipe. Drugs do not stop cellular damage form incurring. If anything, they accelerate it.

## Difficulty swallowing pills

In my experience, clients who have inflammation in their esophagus, even in the absence of reflux symptoms, experience difficulty with swallowing pills.

This is a difficult situation, and a bit of a catch-22. Taking pills, like *Bowel Strength* and *Body Bentonite*, helps eliminate the inflammation in your esophagus that causes difficulty swallowing, but how do you accomplish this if you can't swallow pills well?

If you are in this situation, use *Unique Healing Probiotic Powder* and *Body Bentonite* in liquid or powder form until your body is healthier, and you can easily swallow pills.

## Cleansing foods (like tomatoes) increase acids in your blood, and symptoms of reflux

Most of you with reflux have been told to avoid highly acidic foods like coffee and alcohol, but tomatoes are also often on this list too, but not for the reason you are told. Tomatoes are not acidic; they are alkalinizing. But tomatoes *are* cleansing (as many alkalinizing foods are) and they cause acids to dump from your organs into your blood, which trigger symptoms, like reflux, if not completely eliminated from your body and bowel. This applies to *all* cleansing foods. In other words, grains, even gluten-free grains like breads, pastas, crackers, etc., yogurt, and fruit can trigger reflux as well, for the same reason given above. This effect is highly unknown by the majority of you with this condition. You know about it now.

Once again, this program is needed because when you heal your bowel and body with it, you will desire less coffee, alcohol, and other highly acidic beverages, and once you heal your bowel and body, you will be able to tolerate the cleansing effects of healthy foods like tomatoes without discomfort, which will encourage you to eat a healthy diet, as is needed to maintain a long, healthy life.

# Success With Reflux

"I was taking Prilosec but still had a lot of symptoms of reflux. I started this program and very quickly saw an improvement in my symptoms."

"My doctor told me that if I did not take Prilosec I was at a very high risk for damage to my esophagus. I did not take Prilosec and years later, after doing this program, my esophagus is healthy and fine."

"Many foods used to trigger symptoms of reflux for me. Now I can eat anything and still be symptom free."

"I had a very hard time swallowing pills when I came to Donna, which made this process challenging, as she wanted me to take a lot of pills! She told me that as I healed my body that I would one day be able to swallow these easily, and she was right. I can now take handfuls of the capsules with no problems."

"I tried a dairy-free and wheat-free diet for my reflux but still had it frequently. This program worked, and I even eat dairy and wheat now!"

## Watch my Video, "Why THIS Program Eliminates Reflux."

This video, and all of my videos, can be found at *www.UniqueHealing. com* or at *www.YouTube.com/UniqueHealing*.

# Reynaud's
See "Circulatory Problems"

# Sexual Health Problems
## Low or Excessive Sex Drive, Impotence, and Others

Healthy sexual function is helpful in maintaining a healthy relationship, but more importantly, it is a sign of good health.

# A Healthy Body Eliminates Sexual Health Problems

Modern and ancient aphrodisiacs "work" because they enhance one of three functions in your body: One, circulation (think Viagra), which brings more blood flow to your sexual organs and enhances erection and orgasm. Two, hormonal balance (think "bioidentical hormone or other hormone therapy). Your hormonal system largely influences desire as well as proper lubrication of your sexual organs and pleasure. Three, your immune system (think oysters, which are high in zinc, an immune system nutrient). Studies have conclusively found that low levels of zinc lead to infertility, impotence, and improper maturity of your sexual organs.

Healing your body with this program eliminates the acids that cause low oxygen levels and poor circulation (as oxygen is "used up" to buffer and protect you from un-eliminated acids). Healing your body with this program also eliminates the acids that cause low nutrient levels, like low levels of zinc (as nutrients are "used up" to buffer and protect you from un-eliminated acids.)

Your liver, adrenal glands, and bowel regulate hormonal function, and these organs become healthier when you heal your body. Your immune, or lymphatic system, is also part of your "pipe" that heals as a result of this program.

# A Healthy Bowel Eliminates Sexual Health Problems

Your intestinal bacteria play a key role in regulating the production and balance of hormones in both women and men. Un-balanced hormone levels have been implicated in lowered sex drive, difficulty with orgasm in women, and the inability to sustain an erection in men.

In addition to its many other important functions, a healthy bacterial environment in your bowel is a necessity for the complete elimination of acids (toxins, heavy metals, pesticides, etc.) from your body. A healthy bowel prevents the re-absorption of acids into your blood that reduce your circulation, interfere with hormonal regulation, and deplete your immune system of zinc and other nutrients.

# Why My Crutches Eliminate Sexual Health Problems

***Body Bentonite*** binds to and eliminates acids (toxins, heavy metals, chemicals, etc.) from your body. It helps prevent them from becoming re-absorbed into your bloodstream, where they trigger a response by your body to protect you from them. It eliminates the acids that interfere with your circulation, cause stress on your hormonal-regulating organs, and deplete your body of zinc and other immune-system nutrients needed for healthy sexual function.

***Unique Healing Calcium Citrate*** is an alkalinizing mineral that helps neutralize the acids that your bowel does not eliminate. When these acids are neutralized, your circulation improves, and your levels of nutrients, like zinc, increase.

**Natural Progesterone** provides a safe source of natural progesterone, which *balances* hormone levels and eliminates the sexual health problems associated with an excess or deficiency of them.

## How much do I take?/Questions about using these

See Chapter 5 for information on using these crutches, including recommendations on the amount to use, as well as a discussion of the misunderstandings about the particular crutch that may, if not understood correctly, cause you to fail to look and feel better while you heal your bowel and body with this program.

## How long will I need to use crutches for my sexual health problems?

Sexual health problems occur at Levels 2, 3, and 4 of your pipe. They are the second, second to last, and last areas of your body to heal (assuming that other areas are unhealthy too). Refer to the diagram "Sequence of Healing" in Appendix A at the end of this book to better understand this concept, as well as to Chapter 1 under this subject heading.

The bacterial environment in your bowel also affects sexual health problems. To better understand how long you may need crutches for this, refer to Chapter 1 under this subject heading.

# Misunderstandings about Sexual Health Problems and other information for your success

## Keep your stools well-formed

Because sexual health problems are caused in part by un-eliminated acids, and because well-formed stools prevent the re-absorption of acids into your blood, you will suffer from the least amount of sexual health problems if you keep your stools well-formed while you are healing your bowel and body.

If you do not have a very good handle on how to define well-formed stools, review Chapter 6 of *Unique Healing* now. (And remember, when your stools are hard and slow you are eliminating more acids, and will therefore feel better, than when your stools are one or more times a day but not all extremely well-formed.)

If your stools are not well-formed, the following changes can help: increase your *Body Bentoni*te intake; reduce your carbohydrate intake (pasta, breads, grains, cereals, yogurt, etc.); reduce your sugar intake (including natural healthy sugars such as agave, honey, raw sugar, cane juice, etc.); reduce your alcohol, salt, coffee, and/or soda intake; do not have a massage, chiropractic adjustment, or any other body work; drink a lot of water; rest; and keep your exercise aerobic (see Chapter 4 for more information on how to attain this, and why it is important.)

If these changes do not noticeably help the form of your stools in two days, take them further (i.e. take more *Body Bentonite*, reduce your carbohydrate intake more, etc.)

Out of all of these recommendations, increasing your *Body Bentonite* intake is one of the most productive and helpful. It heals your body, unlike many of the other recommendations. It will do the most to lead you to a place where looking and feeling good is effortless, and some of the other suggestions, such as reducing sugar intake, are simply "too hard to do when your blood is too acidic."

(Note: the exception to this information is when your poorly formed stools are caused by an infection, in which case *Unique Healing Colloidal Silver* is needed to reduce your symptoms. Refer to Chapter 5 for information on when and how to use this crutch.)

## Your sex drive should be neither too high nor too low

Just as your blood pressure should neither be too high or too low; your blood sugar should neither be too high or too low; your energy should neither be too high (hyperactive) or too low; your sex drive should also be neither too high nor too low, either.

As a low sex drive indicates poor health, so too does a sex drive that is too high. In this case, you "need" a high amount of sexual activity to feel good physically. Sex creates an elevation of "feel-good" chemicals in your brain; chemicals that your healthy bowel and body should be producing.

If all sex addicts were treated with this type of program, the addiction might end. Unfortunately, our society still views alcoholism, eating disorders, and sex addictions as purely psychological problems. It is for this very reason that people seeking treatments often fail, and will continue to do so, until the physiological imbalances are addressed.

# Success With Sexual Health

Sexual health is often not discussed in my office. I try to respect every client's privacy and comfort level, and so I do not bring it up unless my client has done so first. Likewise, I have not received very many direct testimonials about the improvements in my clients' sexual health problems, but some have shared with me that their sexual health has improved significantly while following this program.

## Watch my Video, "Why THIS Program Eliminates Sexual Health Problems."

This video, and all of my videos, can be found at *www. UniqueHealing. com* or at *www. YouTube.com/UniqueHealing*.

# Seizures
### See "Neurological Conditions"

# Shingles
### See "Viral Infections"

# Sinusitis
### See "Bacterial Infections" and "Viral Infections"

# Skin Conditions
## Acne, Bumpy Skin, Dry Skin, Eczema, Itchy Skin, Psoriasis, Rashes, and Others

Skin issues are a priority with my clients because they are noticeable and affect their looks, and confidence.

Your skin is a reflection of the health of your bowel and body. But good skin does not mean you are healthy, per se. I had great skin when I was horribly ill. More so, skin issues, like all symptoms discussed in this book, is a warning that you are not as healthy as you could be, and that if you do not heal your bowel and body, one day something worse may take its place.

Many skin problems are bacterial, fungal, and/or inflammatory in nature. Hence, common treatments for the symptoms of eczema, psoriasis, and acne include antibiotics like tetracycline (to kill these fungal and bacterial infections), and steroids and other anti-inflammatory medications (to reduce the inflammatory nature of them). Healing your bowel and body with this program eliminates infections and inflammation, naturally, and permanently.

# Healing Your Body With This
# Program Eliminates Skin Conditions

Un-eliminated acids trigger the release of inflammatory chemicals, whish are used to protect you from these acids. Inflammation of your skin can cause acne, eczema, etc.

Rashes can occur when your bowel is overburdened with acids and your body turns to your skin as an alternative means for eliminating them. This can cause irritation to your skin and a rash as a result.

Dry skin is a reflection of dehydration in your body. When your blood is excessively acidic, your body may steal water from your skin to buffer these acids, making your skin dry.

Many over-the-counter treatments for acne, for example, contain a "pH balancing" ingredient. In other words, "they" know that excess acids can trigger this problem. What "they" are not doing, however, is healing your body so that you can *eliminate* these acids and create permanent, complete, effortless results in achieving healthy skin.

Healthy skin does not have issues. Your skin is an organ like any other organ in your body, and like any other organ in your body, it is healed when you heal your body with this program.

# Healing Your Bowel With This
# Program Eliminates Skin Conditions

A healthy bowel bacterial environment fights, and eliminates, bacterial and fungal infections. Many cases of eczema, psoriasis, acne, and others are caused, either in total or in part, by fungal or bacterial infections.

In my experience, itchy skin conditions, as well as bumps on the back of your arms, are almost always fungal/bacterial in nature. A healthy bowel bacterial environment kills fungus and bacterium that cause itchy and bumpy skin conditions.

One study reported less incidence of eczema in children at the age of two who had been given daily probiotics for the first year of their lives versus children who had not received them. No side effects were found. "Probiotics in Prevention of IgE-Associated Eczema: A Double Blind, Randomized, Placebo-Controlled Trial," Journal of Allergy and Clinical Immunology, 2007 March 7; 8/2007. *Thomas.Abrahammson@lio.se.*

In addition to its many other important functions, a healthy bacterial environment in your bowel is a necessity for the complete elimination of acids (toxins, heavy metals, pesticides, etc.) from your body. A healthy bowel prevents the re-absorption of acids into your blood that cause skin irritation, inflammation, and dehydration.

# Why My Crutches Eliminate Skin Conditions

***Body Bentonite*** binds to and eliminates acids (toxins, heavy metals, chemicals, etc.) from your body. It helps to prevent them from becoming re-absorbed into your bloodstream, where they trigger a response by your body to protect you from them. It eliminates the acids that trigger the release of inflammatory chemicals, and cause dehydration.

***Unique Healing Calcium Citrate*** is an alkalinizing mineral that helps neutralize the acids that your bowel does not eliminate. When these acids are neutralized, your body does not need to produce inflammatory chemicals, or rob your tissues of water, to buffer them.

***Unique Healing Colloidal Silver*** has natural anti-bacterial, anti-fungal, anti-parasitic properties. It eliminates the skin conditions that are caused by these infections.

## How much do I take?/Questions about using these

See Chapter 5 for information on using these crutches, including recommendations on the amount to use, as well as a discussion of the misunderstandings about the particular crutch that may, if not understood correctly, cause you to fail to look and feel better while you heal your bowel and body with this program.

## How long will I need to use crutches for my skin condition?

Skin conditions occur at Level 4 of your pipe. It is the last area of your body to heal (assuming that other areas are unhealthy too). Refer to the diagram "Sequence of Healing" in Appendix A at the end of this book to better understand this concept, as well as to Chapter 1 under this subject heading.

The bacterial environment in your bowel also affects skin conditions. To better understand how long you may need crutches for this, refer to Chapter 1 under this subject heading.

# Misunderstandings about Skin Conditions and Other Information For Your Success

## Keep your stools well-formed

Because skin conditions are caused in part by un-eliminated acids, and because well-formed stools prevent the re-absorption of acids into your blood, you will suffer from the least amount of problems with your skin if you keep your stools well-formed while you are healing your bowel and body.

If you do not have a very good handle on how to define well-formed stools, review Chapter 6 of *Unique Healing* now. (And remember, when your stools are hard and slow you are eliminating more acids, and will therefore feel better, than when your stools are one or more times a day but not all extremely well-formed.)

If your stools are not well-formed, the following changes can help: increase your *Body Bentonite* intake; reduce your carbohydrate intake (pasta, breads, grains, cereals, yogurt, etc.); reduce your sugar intake (including natural healthy sugars such as agave, honey, raw sugar, cane juice, etc.); reduce your alcohol, salt, coffee, and/or soda intake; do not have a massage, chiropractic adjustment, or any other body work; drink a lot of water; rest; and keep your exercise aerobic (see Chapter 4 for more information on how to attain this, and why it is important.)

If these changes do not noticeably help the form of your stools in two days, take them further (i.e. take more *Body Bentonite*, reduce your carbohydrate intake more, etc.)

Out of all of these recommendations, increasing your *Body Bentonite* intake is one of the most productive and helpful. It heals your body, unlike many of the other recommendations. It will do the most to lead you to a place where looking and feeling good is effortless, and some of the other suggestions, such as reducing sugar intake, are simply "too hard to do when your blood is too acidic."

(Note: the exception to this information is when your poorly formed stools are caused by an infection, in which case *Unique Healing Colloidal Silver* is needed to reduce your symptoms. Refer to Chapter 5 for information on when and how to use this crutch.)

## Antibiotic skin treatments can cause *greater* skin problems in the future

Antibiotics destroy some of the beneficial bacteria in your bowel, the ones that are supposed to eliminate bacterial infections which cause many cases of acne, in the first place. In other words, your use of these products can produce an immediate improvement in your skin, but a worsening of it once you stop the treatment. Antibiotics are also very acidic, and if your acne is in part or in total the result of an acidic skin condition, this treatment could make your acne worse. When you use *Unique Healing Colloidal Silver* to treat acne, it does not increase the chance that your acne will become worse in the future, and it is not acidic, so it also does not increase acne that is due to excess acidity, as antibiotics can, either.

And as always, when you use an antibiotic to treat a symptom, you avoid the fact that your bowel is unhealthy, which, if not healed, leads to a greater re-absorption of acidity and more symptoms, weight problems, addictions, and disease down the road.

## Milk consumption and teenage acne

In a review of the dietary history of 47,000 women, it was found that milk, more than any other food, was linked to higher rates of teenage acne. The study found that those women who drank more than three glasses a day as teens were 22% more likely to report severe acne those who drank much less. The rate was even higher (44%) for women who had favored skim milk. Researchers aren't sure why this is.

I find this a fascinating study and "puzzle" to solve. Skim milk contains more milk protein than regular-fat milk, and for some of you, it is the protein in milk that is especially difficult to digest. Undigested food creates acids, and as described earlier, excess acids are a contributing factor in acne. Of course, this is just an educated guess.

The irony in this study is the fact that over the years, the advice given to and taken by heart—and weight-conscious people to switch to skim milk, may be causing more problems, not less. (In my house, we always buy regular-fat dairy products, or low-fat when that is the only option.)

## Keep your pores clean, and open

Your skin is an organ of elimination. Your pores excrete waste products/acids/toxins from your body. Un-eliminated acids trigger inflammation and many skin problems. The more you do to keep your pores clean and open, the better these acids will be able to escape, and the less there will be to trigger an inflammatory or dehydrating skin response.

Facials, exfoliating your skin, and using a good moisturizer that does not contain mineral oil or chemicals (which can be found at health food stores, spas, and other stores), are valuable tools for keeping your skin clean, and your pores open.

For more information on how you can help your skin eliminate skin irritating acids, see Chapter 8 of *Unique Healing*.

## Success With Skin Conditions

"For years my son struggled with bad acne. Medications, over the counter products, and even a wheat free diet, as was recommended by my Naturopath, did nothing to improve his skin. He did an aggressive program with Donna and his acne not only cleared up, but stayed clear even once he stopped this program."

"I always had bumps on the back of my arms, and never thought much about it, until I saw it on the questionnaire that I filled out when I went to see Donna. I was told they were caused by a fungal infection, and sure enough, as soon as I started taking the colloidal silver, they went away."

"I struggled with horrible eczema for years. I took massive amounts of vitamins and spent thousands of dollars trying to get rid of it. This program worked, and now even if I am stressed, or I eat something that in the past would send my skin into a major flare-up, like sugar, or alcohol, I remain symptom-free."

"My two year old daughter had eczema and we really didn't want to put steroid cream all over her, as suggested by her doctor. We did this program instead, and her skin looks great now."

### Watch my Video,
### "Why THIS Program Works For Skin Conditions"
This video, and all of my videos, can be found at *www.UniqueHealing. com* or at *www.YouTube.com/UniqueHealing*.

## Schizophrenia
See "Neurological Disorders"

# Sleep Disorders
## Insomnia, Sleep Apnea, Snoring, Difficulty Falling Asleep, Nighttime Urination, Nighttime Waking, Night Sweats, and Others

Sleep disorders affect millions of people (60 million prescriptions for sleep aids were written in 2010 alone), and sleep disorders are a very common complaint of my clients.

Sleep is needed for your body to heal. This is the time that it can focus on repairing your old cells and creating new, healthier ones. A lack of sleep is a big catch 22; you need to be healthy to sleep well, but you also need to sleep well to be healthy. (A healthy body needs eight hours of uninterrupted sleep a night.)

A good night of sleep is a priority when you are healing your bowel and body. It is a condition that needs a crutch soon, preferably a natural crutch, but in some cases, the short-term use of a medical crutch/sleeping aid is advisable. Even though medications are acidic, it can be *more* harmful to not get a good night of sleep. As your body and bowel become healthier, these will no longer be needed.

Additionally, some of these problems, like snoring, affect not only you, but also your partner and relationships, which affect the quality of your life as well.

# A Healthy Body Eliminates Sleep Disorders

**Sleep apnea** The most significant physiological contributor to this disorder is a lack of oxygen, which causes you to "wake up."

**Falling asleep** Difficulty falling asleep is primarily due to "too much on the mind" or to irritation of your nervous system, which prevents your body from calming down.

**Sinus problems and snoring** When your sinuses become clogged with mucus, it causes a loud noise when you breathe in and out heavily, as during sleep.

**Nighttime urination** When your bowel does not eliminate all of the acids that it should have during the day, your kidneys help out by increasing the urination of them out of your body, and this typically results in nighttime urination as well.

Healing your body with this program eliminates the acids that trigger low oxygen levels, irritate your nervous system, cause your body to produce mucus, and cause your kidneys to work overtime trying to eliminate these acids.

## A Healthy Bowel Eliminates Sleep Disorders

**Difficulty staying asleep** If you fall asleep and wake up in the middle of the night for no reason (i.e. a loud wind or noise did not wake you, for example) and you have difficulty falling back asleep, this is most usually due to poor hormonal regulation of your sleep cycle.

A healthy bowel bacterial environment ensures that your sleep cycle is regulated, as one of its jobs is to produce melatonin. Melatonin helps regulate your internal clock, including your sleep cycles.

**Nighttime urination** A bacterial infection in your bladder can also cause nighttime urination. A healthy beneficial bowel bacterial environment keeps harmful bacteria from populating.

**Night sweats** These can be extremely disruptive to a menopausal woman's sleep, and they can be caused by an imbalance of hormones. The bacteria in your bowel play key roles in balancing hormones, and thereby reduce/eliminate sleep disturbances caused by night sweats.

**Prostrate health** Your bowel bacterial environment also needs to be healthy for your prostate to be healthy as well, as it regulates hormonal regulation, and an imbalance in male hormones can trigger prostate disease. An enlarged prostate can cause nighttime urination.

In addition to its many other important functions, a healthy bacterial environment in your bowel is a necessity for the complete elimination of acids (toxins, heavy metals, pesticides, etc.) from your body. A healthy bowel prevents the re-absorption of acids into your blood that cause low oxygen levels (sleep apnea), lymphatic congestion (excess nasal mucus), nighttime urination, and irritation to your nervous system.

## Why My Crutches Work For Sleep Disorders

*Body Bentonite* binds to and eliminates acids (toxins, heavy metals, chemicals, etc.) from your body. It helps prevent them from becoming re-absorbed into your bloodstream, where they trigger a response by your body to protect you from them. It eliminates the acids that reduce oxygen levels, trigger the production of mucus, and trigger the production of more urine to flush these harmful acids out of your body.

*Unique Healing Calcium Citrate* is an alkalinizing mineral that helps neutralize the acids that your bowel does not eliminate. When these acids are neutralized, your body does not need "use" oxygen, create mucus, or create "more urine" to buffer them.

*Unique Healing Colloidal Silver* has natural anti-bacterial, anti-fungal, anti-parasitic properties. It eliminates the infections that can cause nighttime urination.

**Natural Progesterone Cream** provides a safe source of natural progesterone, which *balances* hormone levels and can eliminate the sleep problems associated with an enlarged prostate and nighttime urination, or night sweats.

**Melatonin** regulates your sleep cycles, which can help you sleep through the night, as well as help you fall back to sleep quickly if you do awaken.

## How much do I take?/Questions about using these

See Chapter 5 for information on using these crutches, including recommendations on the amount to use, as well as a discussion of the misunderstandings about the particular crutch that may, if not understood correctly, cause you to fail to look and feel better while you heal your bowel and body with this program.

## How long will I need to use crutches for my sleep disorders?

Sleep disorders occur at Level 3 of your pipe. It is the second to last area of your body to heal (assuming that other areas are unhealthy too). Refer to the diagram "Sequence of Healing" in Appendix A at the end of this book to better understand this concept, as well as to Chapter 1 under this subject heading.

The bacterial environment in your bowel also affects sleep disorders. To better understand how long you may need crutches for this, refer to Chapter 1 under this subject heading.

# Misunderstandings About Sleep Disorders and Other Information for Your Success

## Keep your stools well-formed

Because sleep problems are caused in part by un-eliminated acids, and because well-formed stools prevent the re-absorption of acids into your blood, you will suffer from the least amount of sleep problems if you keep your stools well-formed while you are healing your bowel and body.

If you do not have a very good handle on how to define well-formed stools, review Chapter 6 of *Unique Healing* now. (And remember, when your stools are hard and slow you are eliminating more acids, and will therefore feel better, than when your stools are one or more times a day but they are not all extremely well-formed.)

If your stools are not well-formed, the following changes can help: increase your *Body Bentonite* intake; reduce your carbohydrate intake (pasta, breads, grains, cereals, yogurt, etc.); reduce your sugar intake (including natural healthy sugars such as agave, honey, raw sugar, cane juice, etc.); reduce your alcohol, salt, coffee, and/or soda intake; do not have a massage, chiropractic adjustment, or any other body work; drink a lot of water; rest; and keep your exercise aerobic (see Chapter 4 for more information on how to attain this, and why it is important.)

If these changes do not noticeably help the form of your stools in two days, take them further (i.e. take more *Body Bentonite*, reduce your carbohydrate intake more, etc.)

Out of all of these recommendations, increasing your *Body Bentonite* intake is one of the most productive and helpful. It heals your body, unlike many of the other recommendations. It will do the most to lead you to a place where looking and feeling good is effortless, and some of the other suggestions, such as reducing sugar intake, are simply "too hard to do when your blood is too acidic."

(Note: the exception to this information is when your poorly formed stools are caused by an infection, in which case *Unique Healing Colloidal Silver* is needed to reduce your symptoms. Refer to Chapter 5 for information on when and how to use this crutch.)

## Melatonin is not a narcotic

Melatonin is not only safe, with no side effects, but it works best if it is taken at least several hours before bed (contrary to the advice on many of the labels of this product. As you will learn, the recommendations on supplements are often extremely limiting and ineffective, and are not based on sound scientific research.) Take melatonin a few hours before bed because it takes time for your body to absorb and assimilate this, and this process needs to occur in order for the melatonin to be available to your body when you need it, which is when you are sleeping. *You will not immediately fall asleep after taking it* (unless you are exhausted when you take it and fall asleep early in the evening as a result, but it will not be a result of your taking melatonin.)

Melatonin is not addicting, as many other sleep medications are.

If melatonin sounds like it would be helpful for your particular sleep problem, start with 10 mg/day. If 10 mg does not help after three days, try 20 mg. A dark room is also important for adequate melatonin production, so always turn down your lights, and the television off, at least thirty minutes before bed.

For more information on melatonin usage, see Chapter 5.

## Relax your nerves

*Unique Healing Calcium Citrate*, a hot Epsom bath before bed, valerian root, lavender, GABA, and other supplements and herbs (commonly found in sleep aid products in the health food store), can help sleep problems caused by stress or acidic irritation to your nervous system. As always, if the amount you are taking does not help in a couple days, consider that you are taking the wrong crutch (maybe you need melatonin), or that you are not taking enough of the right crutch (if 2,500 mg of calcium does not help, 4,000 mg might, and it is safe and advisable that you try this before assuming nothing will help.)

## Calcium is not a sleeping pill, either

Like melatonin, *Unique Healing Calcium Citrate* will not cause you to fall asleep right away, so take it during the day and do not use it like a drug (i.e., do not wait to take it until the problem occurs), lying in bed waiting to fall asleep, or in the middle of the night, if you awaken.

## Short-term use of medications

Rarely do clients fail to experience improved sleep with the crutches listed above. However, if they do not work for you, you may want to consider the short-term use of a sleeping pill. See your doctor for advice on this matter.

If you have already tried a drug and it hasn't helped, you may be addressing the wrong problem. For example, the drug may help you fall asleep, but it may not prevent you from waking up in the middle of the night. In this case, the use of melatonin may be more appropriate and helpful. In other words, don't give up!

## The cleansing and eliminating effects of sleep

Much of the cleansing of your organs, the movement of acids from your organs into your blood and bowel, occurs at night. In the morning, your bowel muscles contract in an attempt to eliminate this acidity/waste. Your maid works while you sleep to clean your house, and your trash man arrives in the morning to take away the trash.

In addition to the important cleansing effects of sleep, it is also important for the elimination of acids from your body. When you are at rest, your body is not busy thinking, eating, or doing other things, and it can focus on eliminating acids from your body. If you get poor and inadequate sleep, your bowel and blood will be more acidic as a result. If you feel lousy and your bowels are not good, getting extra hours of sleep can be immensely helpful for improving these.

## Get eight hours a night

You need eight hours of sleep a night, even if you are very healthy. If you are "getting away with less" you are only fooling yourself. The harmful effects of this on your health will catch up with you one day. I used to get by on much less when I was in high school and college, and then suddenly one day, I was diagnosed with chronic fatigue and needed to sleep all the time.

If you don't respect your need for sleep now, you will likely be forced to do so later in life due to a serious illness. This is not a good alternative.

It is especially important that you get more sleep in the winter, just like a bear. The sunlight has a positive effect on our immunity and health, and when there is less, we need more sleep to compensate for this.

Think of sleep as productive. This concept was useful to me, a classic type "A" person. I always felt like I needed to be productive and was constantly running around. I felt guilty if I sat down and did nothing. But sleep and rest are not "nothing." They are very productive because they help make a healthier you. And a healthier you can be much more productive when you are awake! I sleep more than I did for many years, but I am able to accomplish much more than ever before.

## It's a balancing act

If you have not respected your body's need for sleep for many years you may find that as you heal your body, you need more than before. Think of it as your body catching up with what it needed but never got. Like all aspects of the healing process, this is a temporary condition, and one that will eventually be replaced with restful nights and high-energy days.

# Success With Sleep Disorders

"I took melatonin for years but still could not sleep. When I increased it to the amounts Donna suggested, I immediately started to sleep through the night."

"I used to sleep a solid four hours at night at a time, and that was it. The next day I was exhausted. Since healing my bowel and body with this program for the last several years, my sleep problems have completely gone away, and I don't take anything—vitamins or drugs—to help me sleep."

"I was diagnosed with sleep apnea and given a CPAP machine to use. Because of this program, I was able to stop using it."

"Insomnia was destroying my life. I now sleep better than I have in ages."

"The use of colloidal silver completely stopped my nighttime urination."

"I no longer wake up due to night sweats. I used to wake up 8-10 times a night. It was horrible."

## My story

My earliest recollection of sleep difficulties was in middle school. I was always very fearful at night. My nervous system felt on edge, and I had a lot of difficulty falling asleep. When I entered ninth grade I discovered pot and alcohol. I found that ingesting either or both helped me fall asleep, and I enjoyed this. It was a relief and perhaps a contributing factor to my using these substances as often as I did. The pot mellowed me out so I wasn't so stressed, and the alcohol literally knocked me out.

When I became ill and quit these substances, my sleep problems resurfaced with a vengeance. They were worse than ever, due to the fact that as this time I was much less healthy than ever and my "sleep crutches," the pot and alcohol, were gone. For years, I barely slept. I constantly felt like I was going to have a heart attack. At night I was jittery, anxious, and in pain. I was exhausted but completely wired at the same time.

As I became healthier, I was able to fall asleep easily and to sleep restfully without waking up—no drugs or alcohol needed.

## Watch My Video, "Why THIS Program Eliminates Sleep Disorders "

This video, and all of my videos, can be found at *www.UniqueHealing.com* or at *www.YouTube.com/UniqueHealing*.

## Smoking Dependency
See "Addictions"

## Staph Infections
See "Bacterial Infections"

## Strep Infections
See "Bacterial Infections"

## Stress
See "Mental Health"

## Stroke
See "Cholesterol/Heart Disease/Stroke"

## Sugar Addictions
See "Addictions"

## Thyroid Problems
### Hyperthyroid/Hypothyroid/TSH Levels

A diagnosis of thyroid problems, especially high Thyroid Stimulating Hormone (TSH) levels on a blood test, is one that clients very commonly present themselves with when they first come to see me.

A blood test that shows that your TSH levels are too high (or too low) is the *same* as *all* blood tests, in that it does not accurately reflect the health of your thyroid. And while this program can manipulate your tests to look better, as many drugs, diets, and supplements do, more importantly, this program also heals your body so that your thyroid levels are permanently and effortlessly maintained.

# Healing Your Body With This
# Program Eliminates Thyroid Problems

Thyroid problems are usually lymphatic (immune) system problems, not really thyroid problems. While your pituitary gland is largely involved in the release of thyroid hormones into your blood, thyroid problems have been medically described as autoimmune problems, meaning a problem with your immune (or lymphatic) system. It is thought that inflammatory chemicals, released by your immune system when it is under stress (from an excess of acidity), reduce your pituitary gland's ability to regulate this hormone.

Healing your body with this program eliminates the acids that cause inflammation. (For more information on how this program eliminates inflammation, see Chapter 3.)

It is my experience that when you do not have excess un-eliminated acids in your blood, and your lymphatic system is healthy, TSH levels are normal. Healing your body with this program also heals your lymphatic system.

# Healing Your Bowel With this
# Program Eliminates Thyroid Problems

In addition to its many other important functions, a healthy bacterial environment in your bowel is a necessity for the complete elimination of acids (toxins, heavy metals, etc.) from your body. A healthy bowel prevents the re-absorption of acids into your blood that cause blood tests, including thyroid tests, to be out of balance. It eliminates the acids that cause inflammation.

# Why My Crutches Work for Thyroid Problems

*Body Bentonite* binds to and eliminates acids (toxins, heavy metals, chemicals, etc.) from your body. It helps prevent them from becoming re-absorbed into your bloodstream, where they trigger a response by your body to protect you from them. It eliminates the acids that trigger the release of inflammatory chemicals and improper regulation of your TSH levels.

***Unique Healing Calcium Citrate*** is an alkalinizing mineral that helps neutralize the acids that your bowel does not eliminate. When these acids are neutralized, your body does not need to produce inflammatory chemicals to buffer them, resulting in balanced TSH levels.

## How much do I take?/Questions about using these

See Chapter 5 for information on using these crutches, including recommendations on the amount to use, as well as a discussion of the misunderstandings about the particular crutch that may, if not understood correctly, cause you to fail to look and feel better while you heal your bowel and body with this program.

## How long will I need to use crutches for my thyroid problems?

Thyroid problems occur at Level 3 of your pipe. It is the second to last area of your body to heal (assuming that other areas are unhealthy too). Refer to the diagram "Sequence of Healing" in Appendix A at the end of this book to better understand this concept, as well as to Chapter 1 under this subject heading.

The bacterial environment in your bowel also affects thyroid problems. To better understand how long you may need crutches for this, refer to Chapter 1 under this subject heading.

# Misunderstandings About Thyroid Problems and Other Information for Your Success

### Keep your stools well-formed

Because un-eliminated acids cause thyroid problems, and because well-formed stools prevent the re-absorption of acids into your blood, you will suffer from the least amount of thyroid problems, and unbalanced TSH levels, if you keep your stools well-formed while you are healing your bowel and body.

If you do not have a very good handle on how to define well-formed stools, review Chapter 6 of *Unique Healing* now. (And remember, when your stools are hard and slow you are eliminating more acids, and will therefore feel better, than when your stools are one or more times a day but not all extremely well-formed.)

If your stools are not well-formed, the following changes can help: increase your *Body Bentonite* intake; reduce your carbohydrate intake (pasta, breads, grains, cereals, yogurt, etc.); reduce your sugar intake (including natural healthy sugars such as agave, honey, raw sugar, cane juice, etc.); reduce your alcohol, salt, coffee, and/or soda intake; do not have a massage, chiropractic adjustment, or any other body work; drink a lot of water; rest; and keep your exercise aerobic (see Chapter 4 for more information on how to attain this, and why it is important.)

If these changes do not noticeably help the form of your stools in two days, take them further (i.e. take more *Body Bentonite*, reduce your carbohydrate intake more, etc.)

Out of all of these recommendations, increasing your *Body Bentonite* intake is one of the most productive and helpful. It heals your body, unlike many of the other recommendations. It will do the most to lead you to a place where looking and feeling good is effortless, and some of the other suggestions, such as reducing sugar intake, are simply "too hard to do when your blood is too acidic."

(Note: the exception to this information is when your poorly formed stools are caused by an infection, in which case *Unique Healing Colloidal Silver* is needed to reduce your symptoms. Refer to Chapter 5 for information on when and how to use this crutch.)

## A blood test is an inaccurate way to measure the health of your thyroid

Un-eliminated acids in your bowel and blood affect blood tests, like TSH tests. They do *not* accurately reflect the health of your body.

Remember, you can have a lot of holes in your roof, but if it is not raining, your house will be dry. You can have an unhealthy thyroid, but if there is not excess acidity in your blood (maybe because you eat a low carbohydrate diet) you may wrongly be told your thyroid, and you, are healthier than you really are.

On the other hand, you can have a pretty healthy thyroid, and have your blood TSH levels come back bad, if you have a lot of acids in your blood (maybe you ate a lot of fruit before the test, which sent a lot of old acids from your organs into your blood), and be wrongly told that you are less healthy than you really are. You may have only a few holes in your roof, but if it has just rained very hard and your house is very wet, you may be led to believe that you have a lot more holes in your roof than you really do.

If you still do not understand why blood tests are a horrible way to assess your health, review Chapter 2 of "Unique Healing," and watch my video "The Dangers of Blood Tests," available at ***www.UniqueHealing.com*** (it can be found under the link to watch my videos), or at www.YouTube.com/UniqueHealing.

## How to manipulate/improve your blood thyroid/TSH tests

Like all blood tests, your thyroid test, or TSH levels, can be quickly manipulated/improved by improving the form of your stools. You can put a tarp over the holes in your roof so that the doctor "finds a dry house when he walks in;" so your blood tests look better.

To improve your blood TSH levels, make sure that your stools are firm and well-formed a couple days before, and the day of, your blood test (as described earlier).

If you don't like the idea of manipulating your TSH levels with my advice, then if your levels come back too high or too low, do not take Synthroid, as this drug is simply manipulating these results for you too. Meaning, be consistent in your approach.

It is far healthier to use *Body Bentonite* and follow my instructions for manipulating these tests than it is to take a toxic, acidic medication to do this for you. Also, *Body Bentonite* helps heal your body and addresses the cause of these problems in the first place; drugs do not.

When your bowel and body are healthy, as a result of your following this program, you will not need to manipulate your tests. Your blood tests will be in balance regardless of your diet, drugs or supplements you take, or any other means used to manipulate these tests.

## Better blood tests *and* better health with this program

By healing your bowel and body with this program, your immune system, pituitary, thyroid, *and* your TSH levels improve/become healthier.

Other crutches—diets, vitamins, drugs, exercise, etc.—may improve your *blood* thyroid tests, but they do *not* improve the health of your immune system, pituitary, or thyroid glands (which is why you are told you will need to use these "forever"). Also, as is the definition of a crutch, when you stop these other approaches, your TSH levels usually immediately worsen again, as nothing has been done to improve the underlying cause of the problem.

When your bowel and body are healthy, you will not need crutches—diets, supplements, acupuncture, exercise, drugs, etc.—to have healthy thyroid blood tests.

## Hyperthyroidism and hypothyroidism have the same cause, and are eliminated the same way

If your body secretes too much or too little TSH, you will get diagnosed with hypothyroidism or hyperthyroidism, but the truth is, these stem from the same cause (as do conditions like hypoglycemia and hyperglycemia, and hypotension and hypertension.) The difference in all of these is that a condition of "hyper" something indicates more un-eliminated acidity, and often a less healthy body, than a condition of "hypo" something. Likewise, it is worse if you are diagnosed with hyperthyroidism than hypothyroidism.

Hyper—and hypothyroid conditions are *both* triggered by an excess of acidity in your bowel and blood, and *both* of these conditions are eliminated when these acids are eliminated and you heal your bowel and body with this program.

## Thyroid problems are not the cause of your weight gain

For decades now, millions of you have been sold on the idea that there is a simple, magic pill for weight loss—thyroid medication. Yet millions of you who are taking these medications are still overweight. Thyroid medications do not address the cause of your weight gain, which is the retention of excess water and fat in response to un-eliminated acids in your body.

Healing your bowel and body with this program eliminates weight problems; thyroid medications do not. Think about it. If they did deliver on this promise, no one would be overweight, yet the rate of obesity steadily climbs every year.

## Thyroid treatments are not a magic cure-all

Likewise, many clients who come to see me are taking thyroid medications, yet they present themselves with numerous symptoms, illnesses, addictions, and bad blood tests, even though they are diligently taking their drugs, and in most cases, have been taking them for many years.

You will not magically solve your problems with thyroid medications. If it is a crutch that is helping you feel better, that is great. But be careful when you are led to believe it is the answer to all of your problems. It is just a crutch, and crutches do not heal, nor do they prevent the continued worsening of your health, or premature death from diseases like cancer or heart attack.

## An excess of thyroid medications can be problematic

If you are taking Synthroid or any other thyroid medication, be careful. As you become healthier, it will likely become too strong, and this can produce jittery, shaky, and/or heart racing symptoms, and it may be unsafe to continue with this. Your doctor may not expect this result (that your mediation will become too strong), because thyroid medications are crutches, and if you take them and do not heal your bowel and body (which really, no one else is doing), you will likely need them forever (as is true with all crutches).

If you have these symptoms, call your doctor immediately and insist that he re-check your TSH levels and ask for his advice as to whether you should continue with your medication.

# Success with Thyroid Problems

"I took Synthroid for many years, and I was able to stop it when I healed my bowel and body with this program."

"I ended up in the hospital with extremely high levels of TSH. At the time, my stools were very loose. Donna told me my blood had become much too acidic due to an intense exercise program I had just begun and had me stop, and increase my bentonite. Within a couple of days my levels were normal again." (Note: when you exercise to an anaerobic state, which creates excess lactic acid, blood tests can worsen, including TSH or thyroid blood tests.)

"I was diagnosed with Grave's Disease over ten years ago, and thought I would need medications for this forever (that's what the doctor's told me). With this program, I was able to get off them, and I am amazed."

(I have had *numerous* clients who have been able to successfully stop their thyroid medications and maintain balanced TSH blood test levels without it.)

### Watch my Video, "Why THIS Program Works for Thyroid Problems."

This video, and all of my videos, can be found at *www.UniqueHealing.com* or at *www.YouTube.com/UniqueHealing*.

# Tourette's Syndrome
See "Neurological Disorders"

# Tuberculosis
### See "Bacterial Infections"

## Underweight/Difficulty Gaining Weight

While people seeking to lose weight are far more prevalent than those who are seeking to gain it, underweight conditions are a problem, and they are a reflection of a body and bowel that are less healthy than they can be. These conditions can lead to more serious conditions down the road, and if you are underweight, you need to focus on improving your health by healing your bowel and body with this program just as much as the overweight person does.

## Healing Your Body With This Program Eliminates Underweight/Difficulty Gaining Weight

Un-eliminated acids can cause bloating, gas and other stomach/intestinal discomforts that reduce your appetite. Food consumption (i.e. an appetite), especially protein intake, is needed to build healthy weight. These acids can also cause sugar cravings and a greater desire for sugar, coffee, alcohol, and carbohydrates, which do *not* build muscle weight. Muscle weight is the healthy type of weight that you want to gain if you are underweight.

Healing your body with this program eliminates the acids that trigger bloating, gas, and a reduced appetite as a result. Healing your body with this program eliminates the acids that cause low blood sugar and cravings for "non-weight-building" foods.

## Healing Your Bowel With This Program Eliminates Underweight/Difficulty Gaining Weight

A healthy bowel is needed for a healthy appetite, as well as for the efficient conversion of dietary protein into muscle weight. High animal protein foods, like chicken, fish, turkey, and beef, do not build muscle; the protein in these foods needs to be digested and turned into amino acids, as it is the amino acids that are used to build muscle. Difficulty gaining healthy muscle weight is often a result of poor amino acid absorption. In other words, just because you eat foods like chicken and beef does not guarantee that the protein in them will be converted into amino acids and then muscle weight.

A healthy bowel eliminates infections, which can also cause bloating, gas, and discomforts that reduce your appetite and intake of needed "muscle-building" foods.

In addition to its many other important functions, a healthy bacterial environment in your bowel is a necessity for the complete elimination of acids (toxins, heavy metals, pesticides, etc.) from your body. A healthy bowel prevents the creation of gas, bloating, and other stomach discomforts, and the re-absorption of acids into your blood that cause sugar cravings.

# Why My Crutches Eliminate
# Underweight/Difficulty Gaining Weight

*Body Bentonite* binds to and eliminates acids (toxins, heavy metals, chemicals, etc.) from your body. It eliminates the acids that cause bloating, gas, discomforts and a reduced appetite, as well as low blood sugar and sugar cravings.

*Unique Healing Calcium Citrate* is an alkalinizing mineral that helps neutralize the acids that your bowel does not eliminate. When these acids are neutralized, you experience less gas and bloating and more stable blood sugar levels.

*Unique Healing Colloidal Silver* has natural anti-bacterial, anti-fungal, anti-parasitic properties, and it eliminates infections that cause gas, bloating, and a reduced appetite.

## How much do I take?/Questions about using these

See Chapter 5 for information on using these crutches, including recommendations on the amount to use, as well as a discussion of the misunderstandings about the particular crutch that may, if not understood correctly, cause you to fail to look and feel better while you heal your bowel and body with this program.

## How long will I need to use crutches for my underweight/ difficulty gaining weight issues?

Underweight/difficulty gaining weight occurs at Level 4 of your pipe. It is the last area of your body to heal (assuming that other areas are unhealthy too). Refer to the diagram "Sequence of Healing" in Appendix

A at the end of this book to better understand this concept, as well as to Chapter 1 under this subject heading.

The bacterial environment in your bowel also affects underweight/ difficulty gaining weight. To better understand how long you may need crutches for this, refer to Chapter 1 under this subject heading.

# Misunderstandings About Underweight/Difficulty Gaining Weight and Other Information for Your Success

## Keep your stools well-formed

Because underweight conditions/difficulty gaining weight is caused in part by un-eliminated acids, and because well-formed stools prevent the re-absorption of acids into your blood, you will suffer from the least amount of underweight problems if you keep your stools well-formed while you are healing your bowel and body.

If you do not have a very good handle on how to define well-formed stools, review Chapter 6 of *Unique Healing* now. (And remember, when your stools are hard and slow you are eliminating more acids, and will therefore feel better, than when your stools are one or more times a day but not all extremely well-formed.)

If your stools are not well-formed, the following changes can help: increase your *Body Bentonite* intake; reduce your carbohydrate intake (pasta, breads, grains, cereals, yogurt, etc.); reduce your sugar intake (including natural healthy sugars such as agave, honey, raw sugar, cane juice, etc.); reduce your alcohol, salt, coffee, and/or soda intake; do not have a massage, chiropractic adjustment, or any other body work; drink a lot of water; rest; and keep your exercise aerobic (see Chapter 4 for more information on how to attain this, and why it is important.)

If these changes do not noticeably help the form of your stools in two days, take them further (i.e. take more *Body Bentonite*, reduce your carbohydrate intake more, etc.)

Out of all of these recommendations, increasing your *Body Bentonite* intake is one of the most productive and helpful. It heals your body, unlike many of the other recommendations. It will do the most to lead you to a place where looking and feeling good is effortless, and some of the other suggestions, such as reducing sugar intake, are simply "too hard to do when your blood is too acidic."

(Note: the exception to this information is when your poorly formed stools are caused by an infection, in which case *Unique Healing Colloidal Silver* is needed to reduce your symptoms. Refer to Chapter 5 for information on when and how to use this crutch.)

## Simply eating more food isn't the answer

If you are underweight, you have difficulty putting on healthy muscle weight, as your digestive system is too unhealthy to effectively convert the protein you eat into amino acids and muscle. The advice to simply eat more food, as is typically dispensed by the medical community, is wrong and often ineffective. It puts more stress on your already stressed digestive system, and can cause greater difficulties with healthy weight maintenance in the future. It can cause unhealthy fat and water weight gain. It is another of the numerous examples of what happens when you treat a symptom with something that makes the cause of the problem worse in the long run. Quality, not quantity, produces results.

## Eat proteins that are easy to digest

To gain healthy weight while you are healing your bowel and body, focus on eating high quality proteins that are easy-to-digest, such as soft cooked eggs, fish, whey and rice protein powders, nut butters, unsweetened yogurt, and cheese, if a milk allergy does not exist. Digestive enzymes, which can be purchased at the health food store and taken with your meals as directed, can also be helpful.

## Amino acid supplementation

For decades, body builders have used amino acid supplements (along with protein powders) to increase muscle weight gain. These are valuable for you too, if you need to gain weight. You will not turn into a "muscle man" unless you ingest extremely large amounts, coupled with a very intense weight lifting program, so if you have no interest in this type of physique, don't worry, it won't happen to you unless you incorporate these additional practices.

You can purchase amino acid supplements from health food and other nutrition stores. Take these as directed, and like all other crutches, there are zero negative side effects to their use. If your weight gain is slow, consider increasing the amount you consume.

## You cannot eat anything you want, without eventually paying a price for it

It is not safe to eat anything you want if you are underweight. If you need to gain weight, you need to be just as concerned with choosing a healthy diet, and healing your bowel and body, as overweight people do. Being thin does not make you immune to the negative, dangerous, life-threatening side-effects of too much acidity in your diet.

## You may lose weight before you gain it

When you are underweight, you have a low level of muscle weight, but some of your existing weight is toxic/acidic fat and water weight.

When you start this program, you will likely eliminate this toxic weight faster than you heal your bowel and build healthy muscle weight. You may lose weight before you gain it.

> During this program, you may initially lose weight, only to gain healthier muscle weight later. Do not let this initial weight loss concern you. It is temporary.

It is as though you have a bunch of old shoes in your closet and you need to get rid of those before there is space for new shoes. For a little while, your closet will be empty, but only for a short time, as this makes space for your new shoes. For a little while, the toxic weight you lose with this program will make your weight go down, but it will soon be replaced with healthier muscle weight.

If you are concerned, I urge you to use protein powders and/or amino acids, increasing these if you are particularly concerned.

Losing toxic weight with this program is not only safe, but you are safer when this happens.

## . . . but you will not lose healthy muscle weight

While you may initially lose some toxic fat and excess water weight with this program, you *will not* lose healthy muscle weight. This only occurs if you starve yourself, or follow a high protein diet, because ironically, even though you may be consuming a lot of protein, your body becomes starved for glucose (usually obtained from eating carbohydrates), and with low carbohydrate consumption, your body may convert some muscle into glucose (which can also produce toxic and harmful compounds called ketones).

## Your goal should be healthy muscle weight gain, not just weight gain

Your doctor or family may pressure you to gain weight if you are too thin, but be careful. Common advice to consume a lot of calories can lead to toxic fat and water weight, as well as excess acidity that trigger symptoms, illness, and addictions. Do not trade your thin frame for one that is heavier, but less healthy.

Being thin is a symptom of an unhealthy bowel and body. It is rarely a problem in and of itself. It is your unhealthy bowel and body that is not safe, not so much the fact that you are thin. So be patient and as you do this program and feel better, know that you are on the right track, even if your weight is not immediately increased.

In other words, if you start this program and are thin, but have low blood iron levels, and your blood pressure levels are too low, you are healthier, and safer, if you eliminate the acids that trigger low iron and low blood pressure; you are healthier if your iron level and blood pressure normalize with this program, even if you are still too thin.

## Our weight charts are "too heavy"

As your bowel and body become healthier, you will not become too thin. However, you are likely to weigh less than the standard weight charts that are used in this country to access if you are at a "normal" weight. You don't want to be "normal," as "normal" people suffer from numerous diseases, symptoms, and addictions.

If the weight charts that are used in this country were applied to other countries, like China, many of their citizens would be considered dangerously underweight, yet overall, they suffer from much less disease than we do. They are much healthier, even though they are "thinner" than our standard.

## Underweight and overweight problems have the same cause

Just as too low blood pressure and too high blood pressure, too low blood sugar and too high blood sugar, diarrhea and constipation (examples of conditions that seem to be complete opposites) stem from the same cause, so too do the conditions of underweight and overweight.

And just as healing your bowel and body will eliminate blood pressure that is too high or too low, blood sugar that is too high or too low, and stools that are too hard or too loose, so too does this program eliminate weight that is too high or too low.

## You will not gain *too* much weight, and you will only gain weight if you need to

When you follow this program, you will not gain too much weight. Also, weight gain will occur only if you are underweight, so if you are overweight, do not worry!

When you do not heal your bowel and body, and instead follow a traditional and popular approach to weight gain, you can easily gain too much weight, much of which is water and/or fat weight. This is because these programs' objective is simply "weight gain;" no differentiation is made between healthy muscle weight, and toxic fat and water weight.

You will *not* gain toxic fat and water weight on this program because un-eliminated acids cause these problems, and this program is designed to eliminate acids from your body (i.e. eliminate toxic water and fat weight).

## Underweight is not always a sign of an eating disorder

It is easy to judge an overly thin person as someone with emotional issues and an eating disorder. This is not fair, and it is not an assumption that should be made.

I have met many clients who were emotionally distraught over their lack of weight. They didn't want to be overly thin. They were not trying to lose weight; they just didn't know how to gain it, and no one had given them the correct answer to do so.

I have been in these shoes. When I was extremely ill and completely disabled, a nutritionist put me on a very toxic, very low carbohydrate diet, and it caused me to lose a lot of weight. I was *too* thin. I ate a lot of food, as instructed, because my weight concerned me, and I was following my nutritionist's instructions "to a tee" with the absolute determination to get healthy as soon as possible. (I now know that his advice never could have healed me, but that even worse, it was harming me.) But the point is that at the time that I was very thin, I was eating a lot of food, and I was trying to gain weight. It was very hurtful to be judged (and I was) as having an eating disorder. I never tried to lose weight or ever even thought about it when I was sick. The only thing I thought about was getting healthy so that I could live and function again. I ate two or three times more calories than I did prior to becoming ill. Starving myself was my way of controlling my weight previously, so this was a large deviation from that. But never once did I worry that eating more would cause me to gain weight. At the time, I would have given a million dollars to be overweight, but at least healthy and able to live my life again.

Don't judge others until you know their whole story, and if you know someone who is underweight, share my program with them.

(For more information on eating disorders, see "Eating Disorders.")

# Success With Underweight/Difficulty Gaining Weight

"In high school I always had a hard time gaining weight. I came to Donna because of colitis, and all I really cared about was getting rid of that, but in the process of healing my bowel and body, I gained 15 pounds of muscle weight."

"In the beginning of this program I was too thin. Everyone thought I had an eating disorder, but I didn't. I just couldn't gain weight. I had recently lost eight pounds and I was concerned, as were my family members. Donna assured me that this was not a concern and that later on, I would gain healthy muscle weight. Sure enough, I did, and now everyone does not constantly wonder if I have an eating disorder, because I look so much healthier."

## My story

When I was very ill and too thin, as described above, I followed a diet that made me thinner, and sicker. I eventually quit eating this high protein diet and "went to the other extreme." It seemed to make sense that if my high protein diet was causing me to lose weight and feel even worse, maybe I should do the opposite. I was desperate.

So I stopped the high protein diet and for the next seven months, I ate nothing but millet, vegetables, and rice protein powder. Even though I was eating protein powder, my *total* protein intake was *much* lower than when I was on the high animal protein diet. My new diet, which was much less toxic/acidic, and which contained protein that was much easier to digest and absorb, resulted in my gaining significant muscle weight. I looked a lot better, and I felt a lot better too.

## Watch my Video, "Why THIS Program Works for Underweight/Difficulty Gaining Weight"

This video, and all of my videos, can be found at *www.UniqueHealing. com* or at *www.YouTube.com/UniqueHealing*.

# Urinary Problems
## Bedwetting, Cystitis, Frequent Urination, Infrequent Urination, Nighttime Urination, Bladder Pain/Discomfort, and Others

Pee is important too! I spend a lot of time talking about the importance of healthy bowel movements/stools, and you should know how to safely and accurately define healthy stools. (See Chapter 6 of *Unique Healing* if you do not.) But it is just as important that you understand how to correctly define healthy urination.

Healthy urination has the following characteristics: No nighttime urination; not difficult or urgent; no odor; occurs approximately every four to five hours (too infrequent or too frequent is bad). Your urine should be light yellow in color, not clear or dark yellow.

Healthy urination is synonymous with healthy hydration. See Chapter 3 for more information on how this program eliminates dehydration.

# A Healthy Body Eliminates Urinary Problems

Your kidneys are organs of elimination, and they are another "trash can" in your house, or body, that is used for the elimination of acids. When your main trash can, your bowel, does not completely eliminate all of the acids that enter into it, your kidneys/bladder are called upon to help out.

Just as your bowel movements will become "bad" (too soft, loose, or too hard) when an excess of acids are irritating it, your urine becomes "bad" too when an excess of acids irritate your kidneys/bladder. This leads to many urinary problems, including nighttime urination, difficulty holding your urine, and bedwetting. It also contributes to urination that is too frequent or too infrequent.

Urination that is very infrequent (less than four times a day) is a sign of greater ill health than urination that is too frequent (more than once every couple of hours, for example). It is also a sign of greater dehydration, and it results in greater symptoms and weight as well.

Healing your body with this program eliminates the acids that trigger bladder/kidney discomfort and irritation, as well as dehydration. Healing your body with this program heals your kidneys/bladder so that even if there are acids, your body is strong enough to handle them without a reaction (it fixes the holes on your roof so that even if it does rain, your house does not get wet).

## A Healthy Bowel Eliminates Urinary Problems

The beneficial bacteria in your bowel are responsible for fighting bacterial infections. Bacterial infections are the cause of many cases of cystitis, frequent urination, bladder pain, and nighttime urination.

A healthy bowel regulates your hormone levels, eliminating urinary problems associated with an enlarged prostate.

In addition to its many other important functions, a healthy bacterial environment in your bowel is a necessity for the complete elimination of acids (toxins, heavy metals, pesticides, etc). from your body. A healthy bowel prevents the re-absorption of acids into your blood that cause kidney/bladder stress, dehydration, increased or decreased urination, and difficulty holding your urine.

## Why My Crutches Eliminate Urinary Problems

*Body Bentonite* binds to and eliminates acids (toxins, heavy metals, chemicals, etc.) from your body. It helps prevent them from becoming re-absorbed into your bloodstream, where they trigger a response by your kidneys/bladder to protect you from them. It eliminates the acids that trigger nighttime urination, difficulty holding urine, bedwetting, and other urinary discomforts and issues.

*Unique Healing Calcium Citrate* is an alkalinizing mineral that helps neutralize the acids that your bowel does not eliminate. When these acids are neutralized, your kidneys/bladder do not have to react, and become irritated, by them.

*Unique Healing Colloidal Silver* has natural anti-bacterial, anti-fungal, anti-parasitic properties. It fights the bacterial infections that contribute to bladder infections, frequent urination, bladder pain, cystitis, and some cases of nighttime urination.

**Natural Progesterone Cream** provides a safe source of natural progesterone, which *balances* hormone levels and eliminates the urinary problems associated with an excess or deficiency of them.

## How much do I take?/Questions about using these

See Chapter 5 for information on using these crutches, including recommendations on the amount to use, as well as a discussion of the misunderstandings about the particular crutch that may, if not understood correctly, cause you to fail to look and feel better while you heal your bowel and body with this program.

## How long will I need to use crutches for my urinary problems?

This condition occurs at Level 4 of your pipe. It is the last area of your body to heal (assuming that other areas are unhealthy too). Refer to the diagram "Sequence of Healing" in Appendix A at the end of this book to better understand this concept, as well as to Chapter 1 under this subject heading.

The bacterial environment in your bowel also affects urinary problems. To better understand how long you may need crutches for this, refer to Chapter 1 under this subject heading.

# Misunderstandings About Urinary Problems and Other Information for Your Success

### Keep your stools well-formed

Because urinary problems are caused in part by un-eliminated acids, and because well-formed stools prevent the re-absorption of acids into your blood, you will suffer from the least amount of urinary problems if you keep your stools well-formed while you are healing your bowel and body.

If you do not have a very good handle on how to define well-formed stools, review Chapter 6 of *Unique Healing* now. (And remember, when your stools are hard and slow you are eliminating more acids, and will therefore feel better, than when your stools are one or more times a day but not all extremely well-formed.)

If your stools are not well-formed, the following changes can help: increase your *Body Bentoni*te intake; reduce your carbohydrate intake (pasta, breads, grains, cereals, yogurt, etc.); reduce your sugar intake (including natural healthy sugars such as agave, honey, raw sugar, cane juice, etc.); reduce your alcohol, salt, coffee, and/or soda intake; do not have a massage, chiropractic adjustment, or any other body work; drink a lot of water; rest; and keep your exercise aerobic (see Chapter 4 for more information on how to attain this, and why it is important.)

If these changes do not noticeably help the form of your stools in two days, take them further (i.e. take more *Body Bentonite*, reduce your carbohydrate intake more, etc.)

Out of all of these recommendations, increasing your *Body Bentonite* intake is one of the most productive and helpful. It heals your body, unlike many of the other recommendations. It will do the most to lead you to a place where looking and feeling good is effortless, and some of the other suggestions, such as reducing sugar intake, are simply "too hard to do when your blood is too acidic."

(Note: the exception to this information is when your poorly formed stools are caused by an infection, in which case *Unique Healing Colloidal Silver* is needed to reduce your symptoms. Refer to Chapter 5 for information on when and how to use this crutch.)

## Urine should be light yellow, not clear

For many years, it has been promoted that if your urine is yellow, it means you are dehydrated. This information has been most loudly voiced to athletes in various sports publications. The solution given is to drink a lot of water, until your urine becomes clear. Although water consumption is healthy for you, this advice is wrong (and in fact, ingesting too much water can be dangerous).

Healthy urine is light yellow. A healthy bacterial environment in your bowel is responsible for the light yellow color. If you drink a lot of water, your urine should still be light yellow. If your urine is clear, it is an indication of an unhealthy bacterial environment. Many of my clients have commented that their once clear urine turned light yellow during this process.

On the other hand, urine that is dark yellow, or that has a strong odor, is not healthy either, and reflects a high level of dehydration, an infection, or a high level of kidney or bladder stress.

## Vitamin B-2 can turn your urine neon yellow

If you are taking a supplement that has vitamin B-2 in it, it is perfectly normal for your urine to turn neon yellow. If you take supplements like a multivitamin, B-complex, or others that contain vitamin B-2, stop them for a day or two so that you can accurately observe the current and accurate color of your urine.

## Water is a great crutch *and* healing agent for urinary problems

Increasing your water intake is a great crutch for urinary problems that are caused by excess un-eliminated acids. Drinking more water helps your kidneys eliminate these acids, and takes the stress off them as a result. Additionally, there are only four ways to eliminate acids from your body, and urination is one of these. Water helps eliminate acids from your body and is therefore a healing agent as well.

# Success with Urinary Problems

"At age 8, my son continued to have bedwetting accidents at night. They stopped when we started giving him *Body Bentonite*."

"I used to get bladder infections all the time. Since healing my bowel, they have stopped."

"I was diagnosed with interstitial cystitis many years ago. My symptoms are gone and I have my life back."

"I used to wake up three to four times a night to urinate. Then it would sometimes take me hours to fall back asleep. I would be exhausted during the day because of this. Now I wake up only occasionally, I sleep great, and I feel great."

"I used to urinate every hour or two. It was annoying. When that stopped with this program, I also lost weight."

"I was diagnosed with an enlarged prostate, and I was told that was the reason I urinated frequently at night. I haven't been back to the doctor so I am not sure if it is improved, but the nighttime urination has."

"At age 43, I always had to know where a bathroom was, and I occasionally had a problem with a leaky bladder. It was very embarrassing and sometimes I simply didn't want to go out of the house as a result of it. Now I have bladder control and I feel a confidence I have not felt in years."

## My story

Before healing my bowel and body with this program, I had my fair share of problems with frequent nighttime urination. I hated that symptom, as I love a good night of uninterrupted sleep. Now, while I drink a lot of water, as before, I do not wake up to urinate.

Worse, when I was young, I had a very weak bladder. If I laughed too hard I would lose control. Having this happen to me in fourth grade was one of the most embarrassing moments of my life. This problem followed me for a while and made me very nervous and self-conscious. Now, I can laugh my head off and my bladder is as strong as an ox!

### Watch my Video,
### "Why THIS Program Eliminates Urinary Problems"

This video, and all of my videos, can be found at *www.UniqueHealing. com* or at *www.YouTube.com/UniqueHealing*.

## Uterine Cancer
See "Breast/Female Cancers"

## Viral Infections
### Colds, Congestion, Croup, Earaches, Fever, Flu, Hepatitis, Herpes, HIV, Mononucleosis, Warts, and Others

Infections are either viral or bacterial. Viral infections are prevented by your lymphatic, or immune system; the healthy/beneficial bacteria in your bowel prevent bacterial infections. (Bacterial infections were discussed earlier in this chapter.)

Additionally, in many cases where there is an autoimmune disease, viral infections are common. See the section in this chapter on autoimmune diseases for more information on these as well.

## Healing Your Body With This
## Program Eliminates Viral Infections

It is the job of your lymphatic, or immune, system to produce anti-viral compounds that destroy viral infections when you are exposed to them, eliminating any possible discomfort or signs of infection.

Un-eliminated acids deplete your lymphatic/immune system, making it less capable of protecting you against viral infections. Also, viral infections are more prevalent when your blood is overly acidic due to un-eliminated acids. In other words, flies do not come to clean trashcans; rather, they are attracted to dirty ones. Viruses are also attracted to dirty, or acidic, conditions in your body.

A healthy body eliminates the acids that trigger immune responses from your lymphatic system in response to un-eliminated acids, such as mucus production (which entraps acids), fever (as elevated body temperatures can destroy infections), inflammation, inflamed lymph nodes, etc.

Many germs live only in an anaerobic environment, which is lacking in sufficient oxygen. Healing your body with this program eliminates the acids that cause low oxygen levels, and creates an environment that is non-conducive to germ growth. It is not the virus that is the ultimate cause of an infection, rather it is the environment that it is exposed to that determines if it creates symptomatic reactions in your body.

Healing your body with this program heals your lymphatic/immune system so that even if there are acids, your body is strong enough to handle them without a reaction (it fixes the holes on your roof so that even if it does rain, your house does not get wet).

## Healing Your Bowel With This Program Eliminates Viral Infections

In addition to its many other important functions, a healthy bacterial environment in your bowel is a necessity for the complete elimination of acids (toxins, heavy metals, etc.) from your body. A healthy bowel prevents the re-absorption of acids into your blood that cause lymphatic/immune system responses and symptoms.

## Why My Crutches Work for Viral Infections

**Body Bentonite** binds to and eliminates acids (toxins, heavy metals, chemicals, etc.) from your body. It helps prevent them from becoming re-absorbed into your bloodstream, where they trigger a response by your body to protect you from them. It eliminates the acids that trigger the production of mucus, fever (elevated body temperature) and the release of inflammatory chemicals. It eliminates the acids in your blood and lymph that "feed" the virus.

**Unique Healing Calcium Citrate** is an alkalinizing mineral that helps neutralize the acids that your bowel does not eliminate. When these acids are neutralized, your body does not need to produce mucus, raise your temperature (fever), or produce inflammatory chemicals to buffer them.

## How much do I take?/Questions about using these

See Chapter 5 for information on using these crutches, including recommendations on the amount to use, as well as a discussion of the misunderstandings about the particular crutch that may, if not understood correctly, cause you to fail to look and feel better while you heal your bowel and body with this program.

## How long will I need to use crutches for my viral infections?

Viral infections occur at Level 3 of your pipe. It is the second to last area of your body to heal (assuming that other areas are unhealthy too). Refer to the diagram "Sequence of Healing" in Appendix A at the end of this book to better understand this concept, as well as to Chapter 1 under this subject heading.

# Misunderstandings About Viral Infections and other Information for Your Success

## Keep your stools well-formed

Because un-eliminated acids cause viral infections, and because well-formed stools prevent the re-absorption of acids into your blood, you will suffer from the least amount of viral infections if you keep your stools well-formed while you are healing your bowel and body.

If you do not have a very good handle on how to define well-formed stools, review Chapter 6 of *Unique Healing* now. (And remember, when your stools are hard and slow you are eliminating more acids, and will therefore feel better, than when your stools are one or more times a day but not all extremely well-formed.)

If your stools are not well-formed, the following changes can help: increase your *Body Bentonite* intake; reduce your carbohydrate intake (pasta, breads, grains, cereals, yogurt, etc.); reduce your sugar intake (including natural healthy sugars such as agave, honey, raw sugar, cane juice, etc.); reduce your alcohol, salt, coffee, and/or soda intake; do not have a massage, chiropractic adjustment, or any other body work; drink a lot of water; rest; and keep your exercise aerobic (see Chapter 4 for more information on how to attain this, and why it is important.)

If these changes do not noticeably help the form of your stools in two days, take them further (i.e. take more *Body Bentonite*, reduce your carbohydrate intake more, etc.)

Out of all of these recommendations, increasing your *Body Bentonite* intake is one of the most productive and helpful. It heals your body, unlike many of the other recommendations. It will do the most to lead you to a place where looking and feeling good is effortless, and some of the other suggestions, such as reducing sugar intake, are simply "too hard to do when your blood is too acidic."

(Note: the exception to this information is when your poorly formed stools are caused by an infection, in which case *Unique Healing Colloidal Silver* is needed to reduce your symptoms. Refer to Chapter 5 for information on when and how to use this crutch.)

## Anti-viral herbs and supplements are crutches; they do not strengthen your immune system

Anti-viral and immune-enhancing medications, as well as herbs and supplements like Echinacea, zinc, vitamin C, and any supplement generally labeled "immune system support," are often touted as products that strengthen your immune system. This is untrue. They are crutches that can help you feel better and fight viral infections, but just because you feel better does not mean that you have made your immune system healthier in the process.

If you use these medications, herbs, or supplements and feel better, that is all that they have done for you. They have not healed your immune system and they have not, and cannot, help protect you from further viral infections.

Healing your bowel and body with this program *does* heal and strengthen your immune system.

## Viral crutches can cause "addictions" because they are just crutches

You may read or hear that you must take immune-supporting supplements and herbs with caution, as there is a risk of becoming "addicted" to them; they may cause your immune system to become less healthy over time, causing you to need more of them.

This is utterly untrue. The reason for this fear and misunderstanding is that these herbs and supplements are simply crutches, but they are sold under the very wrong idea that they heal your immune system. They do not heal your immune system.

Therefore, if you use these, and do not concurrently heal your immune system, as you do with this program, you will likely find that down the road, your immune system has become less healthy. But it is not the use of herbs or supplement and herb crutches that causes this to happen; it happens because these crutches never did, or could, heal your immune system in the first place.

You took a crutch and felt better and were wrongly led to believe this meant you were healthier. You were not. These crutches do nothing to prevent acids from accumulating and making your immune system less healthy over time. Using these crutches hurt you when you are led to think they are making you healthier, and therefore, you don't do anything along with these crutches to really make you healthier, like healing your bowel and body with this program.

*Body Bentonite* and *Bowel Strength* cannot make you "addicted" to it. They cannot weaken your immune system. On the contrary, these products are very healing for your immune system.

## "Immune suppressant" drugs suppress the *reactions* of your immune system, not your immune system itself

Drugs that are called "immune suppressants" are very misleading. Almost always, a client who is given these is led to believe that these drugs are stopping their "bad" immune system from working, and that anything or any supplement that makes their immune system healthier will interfere with the action of these drugs. This is crazy!

Immune suppressant drugs suppress the *reactions* of your immune system to un-eliminated acids; they do *not* suppress the health of this system itself. They stop your body from secreting inflammatory chemicals to protect you from un-eliminated acids, for example. As a result, you feel better. But *you* are not better, and your immune system is not better (or healthier) from having done this, either.

Finally, when you suppress the reactions of your immune system to these un-eliminated acids, you have done *nothing* to eliminate these acids in the first place. You have stopped one of your body's ways of protecting you against these acids, and as a result, another system in your body will have to work harder to protect you. For example, you may have less inflammation or your blood test may show more stable immune markers, like your viral load or white blood cell count, but another system will be stressed, and this is often called a "side effect" of the drug.

For example, now that you have taken a drug that has forced your body to stop producing immune reactants to this acidity, your kidneys may have to step up to the plate and work harder to protect you from these acids. This can result in extra water weight gain as your body retains water to now buffer these un-protected acids. This is a common reaction to steroids, for example. These drugs have simply "shoved the trash from your bedroom into your kitchen." One room looks better, but another looks worse.

When you heal your bowel and body with this program, this does not happen, One room does not get better at the expense of another. One symptom is not replaced with another. Acids are eliminated that trigger *all* of these symptoms.

*Body Bentonite* will not interfere with "immune-suppressant" drugs if you are taking them; it can only help *reduce* your need for these drugs, which is a very good and positive reaction.

## Advice about other immune crutches

If you have a viral infection and extra *Body Bentonite* does not help you feel better in a couple of days (and increasing this should be your first reaction to this infection), and you are taking at least 2,500 mg of *Unique Healing Calcium Citrate* as well, consider taking an additional 200 mg of chelated zinc as an additional crutch.

Additionally, you will recuperate faster if you help create an environment where germs cannot survive. Think of immune supplements as insecticides that kill flies. Cleaning up the trash that *attracted the flies in the first place* will also help eliminate them.

In addition to *Body Bentonite*, you can help your body eliminate the acids that viruses feed upon by drinking a lot of water. Take Epsom salt baths or go in the sauna. Eat very little until you feel better, as the less you eat, the more energy that is available for your body to fight these germs. And most of all, rest, rest, rest, rest, rest.

## Use caution with vitamin C

Vitamin C intake can make your stools loose. If you want to add extra vitamin C, stop it immediately if your bowels get looser on it, because otherwise you may feel worse from the dehydration caused by loose stools. Equally dangerous is the possibility that you will wrongly blame *Bowel*

*Strength* or *Body Bentonite*, the products you need to heal your immune system, for causing your looser stools.

If your stools are already loose, don't use this crutch. In general, I recommended against extra vitamin C. There are other products that can help just as much, like *Unique Healing Calcium Citrate*, that have no chance of complicating the matter.

Sometimes clients think I have something against vitamin C, but I don't. I simply understand the complexities and limitations of using it. When I was very ill, I had 10 grams, or 10,000 mg, of it dripped into my veins during weekly I.V. treatments, and I also took this same amount orally on a daily basis. While my stools never became looser on these high amounts, I also never felt better, either. It simply is not the "magic cure-all" that it has been promoted to be.

## When you are sick, use the right crutch

Taking extra *Body Bentonite* or *Unique Healing Calcium Citrate* (or Echinacea, zinc, or vitamin C, which are common crutches recommended for viral infections) will not help you feel better if your infection is a bacterial one. Likewise, taking natural "antibiotics" like *Unique Healing Colloidal Silver* will not help you feel better if your infection is a viral one.

Because an immune system support product can contain crutches for both viral and bacterial infections (the company selling it will make no attempt to teach you the difference), if you buy these products, you may end up taking some herbs and nutrients you don't need, and not enough of the ones you do. You will feel better much faster if you use the right crutch.

If you are uncertain as to whether your infection is a viral or bacterial one, use crutches for both. It will not hurt you to take one that you don't need. More commonly, however, I see clients who are taking a crutch for a viral infection when they have a bacterial infection, and not getting better because of it.

## The pros and cons of the flu vaccine

**Pros:** It *might* prevent you from getting the flu, and therefore you might avoid some days of discomfort. It may help ease your anxiety and fears of getting sick, or of dying from the flu, and the elimination of fear is the number one ingredient needed for success with this program.

**Cons**: Vaccines give you the false sense of security that your immune system is healthier than it really is. They are a crutch and like all crutches, they do not heal you or make you healthier. There are dangers to vaccines as there are to all drugs, as they are all toxic and acidic (but the dangers of vaccines are also over-rated. Damage from mercury, etc., can only occur if you are already very vulnerable/unhealthy to begin with.) Finally, if you get the vaccine, you may still get the flu.

My kids and myself have never, and never will, get a flu vaccine. But if you do, it will not prevent you from healing your bowel and body with this program.

## Put your coat on when it's cold outside

A reality that has puzzled researchers is why, despite the fact that people congregate at work, the mall, and daycare in the spring and summer months, are influenza "A" outbreaks much more rare in the warmer months?

Not long ago a study was done involving college students who were placed out in the cold without warm clothes, and another group who were placed out in the cold dressed appropriately. The underdressed kids had significantly higher incidences of catching colds, lasting up to three days after the exposure of the cold.

*The cold virus does not cause colds. It is only a trigger.* If it caused colds, then everyone who was exposed to it would get one, which means that all of us would have colds almost all of the time. Because only some people get sick when exposed to the cold virus, it is obvious that some variables differ among people that affect their susceptibility to getting sick.

When you go out into the cold without a coat on, your body becomes very cold. In this state it needs to expend a lot of energy to warm itself up, because a cold body is not conducive to the proper functioning of your body. The energy expended to warm itself up is diverted from other, more important jobs, like eliminating acids and killing off germs; eliminating trash and killing off flies. This makes you more likely to become sick. It does not guarantee that you will; it simply increases the likelihood.

## The microbe is nothing, the terrain is everything

It is claimed that before the death of Louis Pasteur, the father of our modern germ theory, he stated, "The microbe is nothing, the terrain is everything."

My analogy has always been, "Flies will not be attracted to a clean trash can, but only to one that is full of waste." If your body is unhealthy and there are many un-eliminated acids floating around your bloodstream, you are likely to catch everything that is going around. When you heal your body and your bowel with this program, you will not. Not only will you rarely get sick, but it is also much less stressful to live without the constant worry of contamination. Luckily, we have a lot more control over our terrain than we have over the presence of microbes. This is a very empowering concept.

## Getting sick does not mean you are very unhealthy

It is extremely common for a client to present themselves to me with a very unhealthy body—with cancer, lupus, fibromyalgia, autism, etc.—and comment that they rarely "get sick," which usually means that they rarely get colds or the flu.

It is only once they become healthier that colds and the flu may manifest, temporarily. Compared to the previous, more disabling condition they presented themselves with, these are a blessing. They are only a curse when they *wrongly* invoke a fear that colds and flu are signs of a less healthy body.

This concept was covered in Chapter 2 of *Unique Healing*. If you are sick and this is discouraging to you, go back to this chapter and read the section titled "The problems with using symptoms to assess your health" again.

You are in the process of healing your body with this program, and it is only once you have significantly healed your immune system that illness will become an infrequent event. Twelve months into this program, many of my clients find that they get sick much less often than they used to.

Keep your focus on healing your body and do not let an illness get you down or discouraged. Keep your mind focused on the future and what it holds for you. And last but not least, remember that colds and flu do not happen unless your body is "strong" enough to react this way. When I was disabled with an autoimmune disease I never had a cold or flu. I never had a cold or flu in college either, the time right before my illness when my body was extremely unhealthy. When I healed my body and my health dramatically improved, I experienced a handful of colds and flu that were one thousand times more tolerable than the ill health and symptoms I had before.

> If you have been healing your bowel and body with this program and you get sick, it does not mean that you are not getting better.

When you are ill, be patient. Illness often occurs because you have been doing too much, or eating too many highly acidic foods, like sugar and alcohol at the holiday time. Illness often comes as a reminder from your body that you are not respecting its needs and you should be thankful for this reminder. When you listen, it helps prevent a more serious disease from developing later on. While you are ill, reflect on what you can do to get some of the craziness out of your life. Be careful that you do not view healing your body as an opportunity to continue with a crazy life. If you do, you will find that it takes much longer to heal.

## Do not use *Bowel Strength* or probiotics, like *Unique Healing Probiotics,* as a crutch

They are not ones, contrary to some much-heeded advice. These products are not crutches and *cannot* help you get better right away. *Bowel Strength* and probiotics like *Unique Healing Probiotics* heal your bowel and *eventually* prevent viral infections from occurring. They are not crutches that can immediately fight off an infection once it has occured.

# Success With Viral Infections

"I had herpes for eight years and broke out often. I've now gone a record ten months without a breakout, even though I have been completely stressed, which always made things worse in the past."

"My daughter kept getting ear infections and Donna had me give her *Body Bentonite*. Since then she has not had a single one."

"I had a cold and took *Body Bentonite* and it went away in one day. I don't understand why this helped, but I don't care. I just care that it helped."

"I was diagnosed with HIV and my viral load was consistently extremely high. As soon as I started this program it began to fall, and now it is non-detectable."

"I was diagnosed with hepatitis and liver damage. I took large amounts of milk thistle and did a lot of acupuncture, but my blood tests kept coming back showing these were problems. I am now told my liver is completely healthy, and my blood tests show that the hepatitis is gone, too."

## My story

When I first became ill, I was diagnosed with mononucleosis. Soon thereafter, as I never recovered from this, I was diagnosed with an autoimmune disease. While I was *extremely* ill and completely disabled, I never got colds or other viral infections. This is not because I was healthy; it was because I was too *unhealthy* to react to these germs with the symptoms most notable with these.

It was only once I healed my body that my disabling symptoms went away, replaced temporarily with an increase in viral infections, like colds and earaches. This was a very positive experience, because these "new" and more familiar symptoms were tolerable; my autoimmune symptoms were not. My "new" symptoms were familiar and not scary; my old symptoms were frightening.

Now my immune system is very healthy. I no longer have an autoimmune disease. However, it "screams" at me if I over-extend myself for too long (when my stress levels are out of control for months on end), and I am grateful for the reminder and warning that I need to change my lifestyle and reduce my stress.

## Watch my Video,
## "Why THIS Program Eliminates Viral Infections"

This video, and all of my videos, can be found at *www.UniqueHealing. com* or at *www.YouTube.com/UniqueHealing*.

# Weight Problems
## See Chapter 4

# Chapter 3

## D.O.I.C.N.
## (Dehydration, Oxygenation, Inflammation, Circulation, Nutrient Levels)

Healing your bowel and body with this program reduces dehydration, improves oxygenation, reduces inflammation, increases circulation, and increases the nutrient levels in your body.

The improvements in the above conditions are at the foundation of the majority of the symptoms, weight problems, illness, and addictions listed in Chapter 2. These conditions are at the core of numerous other symptoms and diseases that I did not include in this chapter, as well.

It is my hope that by addressing these conditions in a separate chapter, I might further help you understand the wide impact, and amazing potential, that this program has for eliminating disease, symptoms, addictions, and weight problems.

## Dehydration

Nothing is more important for good health than proper hydration of your body, and nothing accomplishes this better than healing your bowel and body with this program.

The average person could live forty days without food, but only three to five days without water. Approximately two-thirds of your body weight is water. Blood is 82% water, and your brain and muscles are 75% water. The major ingredient of all fluids in your body is water, including saliva, gastric juices, bile, pancreatic juices, and intestinal secretions. In other words, proper digestion and elimination depend on water, and your health and weight depend on healthy digestion and elimination. Water also helps carry essential nutrients to your cells and aids in circulation.

Hydration is healing, and addressing the cause of poor hydration, or dehydration, is one answer to excellent health.

Dehydration is very common. The vast majority of you are in this state. Some of the most obvious symptoms of dehydration are dry skin and hair, swollen ankles, rings that get too tight on your fingers, and infrequent or too frequent urination. Yet almost every health symptom, including headaches, acne, asthma, sugar cravings, joint pain, poor memory, fatigue, irritability, depression, high cholesterol, high blood pressure, and many others, occur concurrently with a state of dehydration.

Dehydration is also a leading factor in weight gain, because as you become dehydrated, your body retains extra water to protect you, and extra water retention equals extra weight.

## Healing Your Body With This Program Eliminates Dehydration

Dehydration occurs when there are excess un-eliminated acids in your blood. To protect you from the dangers of these, your body may draw water from your tissues/organs into your blood to dilute these acids, making the acids less harmful, and you dehydrated.

When your stools are mushy, skinny, or loose, you are eliminating the *least* amount of acids. The poorer the form of your stools, the more dehydrated you will be.

Healing your body with this program eliminates the acids that cause dehydration.

## Healing Your Bowel With This Program Eliminates Dehydration

When your bowel bacterial environment is healthy, you are not vulnerable to bacterial/fungal/parasitic infections and the diarrhea that these can trigger. Diarrhea is a leading cause of dehydration.

In addition to its many other important functions, a healthy bacterial environment in your bowel is a necessity for the complete elimination of acids (toxins, heavy metals, pesticides, etc.) from your body. A healthy bowel prevents the re-absorption of acids into your blood that trigger the removal of water from your tissues to buffer them, and dehydration.

# Why My Crutches Eliminate Dehydration

*Body Bentonite* binds to and eliminates acids (toxins, heavy metals, chemicals, etc.) from your body. It helps to prevent them from becoming re-absorbed into your bloodstream, where they trigger a response by your body to protect you from them. It eliminates the acids that cause water to be drawn out of your tissues, and the resultant dehydration.

**Unique Healing Calcium Citrate** is an alkalinizing mineral that helps neutralize the acids that your bowel does not eliminate. When these acids are neutralized, your body does not need to rob your tissues of water to dilute them.

*Unique Healing Colloidal Silver* has natural anti-bacterial, anti-fungal, anti-parasitic properties. It fights the infections that cause dehydration from diarrhea.

## How much do I take?/Questions about using these

See Chapter 5 for information on using these crutches, including recommendations on the amount to use, as well as a discussion of the misunderstandings about the particular crutch that may, if not understood correctly, cause you to fail to look and feel better while you heal your bowel and body with this program.

(Note: Dehydration, low oxygenation, inflammation, poor circulation, and low nutrient levels are pervasive and can occur for some time while you are healing your bowel and body with this program, which means that you may need to use these crutches for these conditions throughout the length of this program.)

# Misunderstandings About Dehydration and Other Information for Your Success

## Keep your stools well-formed

Because dehydration is caused in part by un-eliminated acids, and because well-formed stools prevent the re-absorption of acids into your blood, you will suffer from the least amount of dehydration if you keep your stools well-formed while you are healing your bowel and body.

If you do not have a very good handle on how to define well-formed stools, review Chapter 6 of *Unique Healing* now. (And remember, when your stools are hard and slow you are eliminating more acids, and will

therefore feel better, than when your stools are one or more times a day but not all extremely well-formed.)

If your stools are not well-formed, the following changes can help: increase your *Body Bentoni*te intake; reduce your carbohydrate intake (pasta, breads, grains, cereals, yogurt, etc.); reduce your sugar intake (including natural healthy sugars such as agave, honey, raw sugar, cane juice, etc.); reduce your alcohol, salt, coffee, and/or soda intake; do not have a massage, chiropractic adjustment, or any other body work; drink a lot of water; rest; and keep your exercise aerobic (see Chapter 4 for more information on how to attain this, and why it is important.)

If these changes do not noticeably help the form of your stools in two days, take them further (i.e. take more *Body Bentonite*, reduce your carbohydrate intake more, etc.)

Out of all of these recommendations, increasing your *Body Bentonite* intake is one of the most productive and helpful. It heals your body, unlike many of the other recommendations. It will do the most to lead you to a place where looking and feeling good is effortless, and some of the other suggestions, such as reducing sugar intake, are simply "too hard to do when your blood is too acidic."

(Note: the exception to this information is when your poorly formed stools are caused by an infection, in which case *Unique Healing Colloidal Silver* is needed to reduce your symptoms. Refer to Chapter 5 for information on when and how to use this crutch.)

## Body Bentonite reduces dehydration

A common concern of clients is that *Body Bentonite* can increase dehydration. I have found three primary reasons why some of you have *wrongly and dangerously* been led to believe that using *Body Bentonite* increases dehydration. They are as follows.

1.  **Constipation is not caused by dehydration**. Some of you will experience constipation as you heal your body with this product, and most of you have been wrongly led to believe that constipation is caused by dehydration. On the contrary, if you have daily but not perfectly firm and formed stools (as fitting the description in Chapter 6 of *Unique Healing*) you are the most dehydrated. In this state you have a large number of un-eliminated acids in your bowel, leading to a greater susceptibility to dehydration (and symptoms and weight gain.)

If you start this program and have daily but not perfectly formed stools (as is true of at least 85% of the clients I see), as you take *Body Bentonite*, you will likely go through a state of constipation. In this state, there are *fewer* un-eliminated acids than when you had daily, but not perfectly formed, stools. In this state, you are *less* dehydrated than you were before.

While constipation is not the ideal elimination, it is an improvement for most of you. To better understand the health benefits of constipation over daily but not perfectly well formed stools, review Chapter 6 of "Unique Healing" and watch my video, "Stop Freaking Out About Constipation," available at www.YouTube.com/UniqueHealing.

2. **Craving or desiring more water is a sign of *better* hydration. It is not a sign of dehydration.** Our body is amazing, but it has some flaws. One of them is the fact that when you are dehydrated, you crave less of what you need (i.e. water), than when you are well hydrated.

   Excess acids in your blood can make you feel full and bloated, and drinking liquids of any kind, water included, is often unappealing when this is occurring. Excess acids also reduce your blood sugar levels, and this can cause you to want to drink a beverage, like coffee, soda, alcohol, and sweetened drinks, to raise your blood sugar so you feel better. Water does not increase your blood sugar levels. So if you are very acidic and dehydrated, you are not likely to desire water.

   If you are doing this program and find, like many of my clients, that your desire to drink water increases, hooray! This is a sign that you are in better health. It is also very positive because drinking water is a valuable way to help your body eliminate the acids that lead to symptoms, weight gain, addictions, disease, and premature death.

3. **The wrong thing is blamed.** This has happened thousands of times, and will surely continue to happen thousands more. Practitioners of all kinds, such as conventional doctors, acupuncturists, chiropractors, herbalists, naturopaths, as well as health food store workers, blame the wrong thing for your symptoms and weight all the time. Unfortunately, they are allowed

to write about, and discuss with you, their wrong conclusions and state these as though they are fact.

While you are taking *Body Bentonite* you can become dehydrated, but this is *not* caused by bentonite use. It can happen because you can very easily be taking *too little* bentonite; just because you are taking bentonite does not mean that you are eliminating all of the acids in your bowel and blood that cause dehydration. *More*, not less, *Body Bentonite* is needed if you become dehydrates while using it.

In other words, when a practitioner recommends the use of this product (whish is rare, and when it is done, it is at a dosage that is extraordinarily too low to help), and you get dehydrated during its use, this practitioner may blame (and has wrongly blamed) the bentonite for this symptom. If this happens, it is because this practitioner does not understand the physiology of how excess acidity in your blood causes dehydration and how your diet and other variables affect this. If you eat a bowl of cleansing fruit, which moves acids into your blood from your organs, for example, at the same time you take a pathetically small amount of bentonite, this bentonite will not be strong enough to offset the acids dumped into your blood from eating this fruit. The bentonite may get blamed, when in truth, the real blame lies in the fruit consumption. Unfortunately, some of these practitioners have gone on to spread the word "that bentonite caused dehydration" (verbally to other clients, through internet articles, articles in magazines, etc). Then you read this, and how do you know that they blamed the wrong thing? You don't.

There are zero studies that show that bentonite causes dehydration. A study consists of taking a variable and testing to see if there is a relevant cause and effect relationship. In other words, no studies have every been done where "X" amount of people were given bentonite and then compared to a control group who were not, to see the effects of this on hydration levels (or health, weight, addictions, or symptoms). I know of zero practitioners, including alternative ones, who have recommended extremely large amounts bentonite over a long period of time, and therefore, I know of zero practitioners who have the knowledge and experience to comment on the effects of using this product.

I have over a decade of experience using bentonite with clients, in amounts much larger than is routinely recommended, and I have never seen this cause dehydration.

## Dehydration co-exists with many other conditions

Un-eliminated acids cause dehydration, and they cause many symptoms, too. Your body reacts to un-eliminated acids with the production of inflammatory chemicals to buffer these acids, for example. Hence, when you have a headache, you often have dehydration as well. Your body may use *both* the removal of water from your tissues, and the production of inflammatory chemicals, to buffer these acids.

These two conditions often co-exist, but that does not mean that dehydration is the *cause* of headaches, or other symptoms, as is often stated. Un-eliminated acids are the cause of the symptoms that are associated with dehydration.

## Water intake and dehydration

Drinking five glasses of water daily is said to decrease the risk of colon cancer by 45%, breast cancer by 79%, and bladder cancer by 50%. Why? Water eliminates acids that cause cellular destruction and cancer. Water eliminates acids that reduce the production of neurotransmitters to your brain. Water eliminates acids that trigger the release of buffering, inflammatory chemicals, for example.

Improper bowel elimination increases dehydration, and all of the efforts to combat this by drinking more water are aimed at the *symptom* of dehydration, not the *cause*. While I strongly promote increased water consumption, and drink quite a bit daily myself, it is nevertheless important that you not rely solely on water, but on a healthy bowel, to keep you properly hydrated. In this program, you heal your bowel and body and ultimately, this leads to a permanent solution for your dehydration, and a much greater outcome in your health and weight.

## Should you still drink water?

If your bowel elimination is not good, drinking more water *will* help offset some of the symptoms of water retention and dehydration, but you are treating the symptoms of the problem, not the cause. It is not a lack of eight glasses a day that causes dehydration. If your bowel is eliminating acids properly, drinking water will be an added boost to your system, and this should not be overlooked. When your bowel and body are healthy, you will not be dehydrated, but you still need to drink water.

## You will desire more water as you become healthier

Often I see clients who don't want, or crave, water. The recommendation to drink more is very difficult for them to follow. The more acidic and dehydrated you are, the *less* you will desire water. I had to force myself to drink it when I was ill; I did not drink it out of desire.

Ironically, the more hydrated you become, the more water you will desire, yet this comes at a time when you "need" it the least.

## Too much water can cause problems

Excessive quantities of water, especially when consumed within a very short period of time, can cause electrolyte imbalances that can lead to death. Drinks with electrolytes are safer to drink in larger amounts, but more importantly, if you need a lot of water to feel better, then you may be overlooking a more significant problem, which is an unhealthy bowel and poor elimination.

# Success with Dehydration

"I lost five pounds of water weight in the first two weeks of starting this program and using *Body Bentonite*."

"I never used to want to drink water, even thought I knew it was good for me. Now I love it. I don't want most of the other sugary drinks that I used to love."

"My hair stylist told me that my hair looks the healthiest that she has ever seen!"

"My electrolytes were low on my blood test and after I started taking *Body Bentonite*, they became normal."

"I used to get dehydration headaches constantly. They are now rare and when they do happen, I take more *Body Bentonite* and they go away!"

## My story

When I was ill I consistently drank approximately twelve glasses of water a day. I felt a little better when I drank a lot, so I used this crutch heavily. As my bowel and body health improved, I felt and looked better drinking much less water. My healthy bowel and body improved my hydration much more than water consumption ever did.

### Watch my Video, *"Body Bentonite* REDUCES Dehydration"

This video, and all of my videos, can be found at *www.UniqueHealing. com* or at *www.YouTube.com/UniqueHealing*.

# Oxygenation

Low levels of oxygen in your blood are associated with many symptoms and diseases as well. Low oxygen levels in your blood translate into low brain function, as your brain needs large amounts of oxygen to function correctly. Low brain function can be experienced as fatigue, mental fogginess, slow response times, irritability, depression, and even neurological conditions such as Alzheimer's, brain tumors, and autism. In one study, 86% of children with autism were found to have low levels of oxygen flowing to their brain.

Low oxygen levels are also implicated in slow healing times, and lung problems, like asthma. It occurs with sleep apnea and anemia. Low oxygen levels in your blood can cause your red blood cells to clump together, which can cause a blood clot and a subsequent heart attack or stroke. Low levels of oxygen in your blood also create an environment in which harmful bacteria and Candida can flourish. These immune invaders are anaerobic; they thrive in a non-oxygenated environment. If enough oxygen is present they cannot survive. And scientists have found that cancer cannot survive in a highly oxygenated environment, which is why many alternative cancer clinics employ means of oxygenating the blood in their treatment programs. Additionally, your muscles need oxygen to perform. Low levels of oxygen lead to muscle fatigue, pain, and cramping.

The majority of your symptoms, disease, addictions, and weight problems co-exist with low levels of oxygen in your body.

## Healing Your Body With This Program Increases Oxygenation

When there are excess un-eliminated acids in your blood it is dangerous, and your body responds to protect you from them. Excess acids are represented by positive hydrogen ions, or H+. Your body can attach these

H+ ions to O2, or oxygen, in an attempt to buffer these acids, and protect you from them. This buffering action, however, results in lowered oxygen levels in your blood. Healing your body with this program eliminates the acids that lower your blood oxygen levels.

Your lungs oxygenate your blood, and eliminating acids from your body also heals your lungs so they can perform this job effectively.

## Healing Your Bowel With This Program Increases Oxygenation

In addition to its many other important functions, a healthy bacterial environment in your bowel is a necessity for the complete elimination of acids (toxins, heavy metals, pesticides, etc.) from your body. A healthy bowel prevents the re-absorption of acids into your blood that cause low oxygen levels in your body.

## Why My Crutches Increase Oxygenation

**Body Bentonite** binds to and eliminates acids (toxins, heavy metals, chemicals, etc.) from your body. It helps to prevent them from becoming re-absorbed into your bloodstream, where they trigger a response by your body to protect you from them. It eliminates the acids that reduce your oxygen levels.

*Unique Healing Calcium Citrate* is an alkalinizing mineral that helps neutralize the acids that your bowel does not eliminate. When these acids are neutralized, your body does not need to rob it of oxygen to buffer these acids.

### How much do I take?/Questions about using these

See Chapter 5 for information on using these crutches, including recommendations on the amount to use, as well as a discussion of the misunderstandings about the particular crutch that may, if not understood correctly, cause you to fail to look and feel better while you heal your bowel and body with this program.

# Misunderstandings About Oxygenation and Other Information for Your Success

## Keep your stools well-formed

Because un-eliminated acids cause poor oxygenation, and because well-formed stools prevent the re-absorption of acids into your blood, you will suffer from the least amount of the problems associated with low oxygen levels if you keep your stools well-formed while you are healing your bowel and body.

If you do not have a very good handle on how to define well-formed stools, review Chapter 6 of *Unique Healing* now. (And remember, when your stools are hard and slow you are eliminating more acids, and will therefore feel better, than when your stools are one or more times a day but not all extremely well-formed.)

If your stools are not well-formed, the following changes can help: increase your *Body Bentonite* intake; reduce your carbohydrate intake (pasta, breads, grains, cereals, yogurt, etc.); reduce your sugar intake (including natural healthy sugars such as agave, honey, raw sugar, cane juice, etc.); reduce your alcohol, salt, coffee, and/or soda intake; do not have a massage, chiropractic adjustment, or any other body work; drink a lot of water; rest; and keep your exercise aerobic (see Chapter 4 for more information on how to attain this, and why it is important.)

If these changes do not noticeably help the form of your stools in two days, take them further (i.e. take more *Body Bentonite*, reduce your carbohydrate intake more, etc.)

Out of all of these recommendations, increasing your *Body Bentonite* intake is one of the most productive and helpful. It heals your body, unlike many of the other recommendations. It will do the most to lead you to a place where looking and feeling good is effortless, and some of the other suggestions, such as reducing sugar intake, are simply "too hard to do when your blood is too acidic."

(Note: the exception to this information is when your poorly formed stools are caused by an infection, in which case *Unique Healing Colloidal Silver* is needed to reduce your symptoms. Refer to Chapter 5 for information on when and how to use this crutch.)

## Oxygen therapy

Ironically, most of you have been manipulated to view oxygen therapy as strange and barbaric (think of the public's general negative perception of Michael Jackson's use of the oxygen chamber that he had in his home.) You may have also heard about oxygen therapy, and more fear and criticism of it, if you are a tennis fan (as I am). In September 2011, the number one ranked men's player in the world, Novak Djokovic, disclosed that he had been sitting in a "pressurized egg," which, among other things, increases oxygen levels. This drew more ridicule and criticism from others, but it shouldn't. (Perhaps his win at the 2011 U.S. Open, during which his use of this egg was publicized, quieted some of the naysayers?) Increasing oxygen levels to improve athletic performance is not entirely rare, and according to *The Wall Street Journal*, 8/29/11, others think this is a good idea too, including ultra cyclist George Vargas and rock star Axl Rose. Others don't. Referring to Djokovic, one former tennis player commented that he does not share his "daredevil mentality." Wow. Really, what is "dare devilish" about increasing your oxygen levels?

I'm not sure why people find this bizarre, but they don't find it strange when an ill patient is given oxygen in the hospital/emergency room? In fact, the medical profession *uses oxygen therapy all the time.* Likely you have seen someone tooling around with an oxygen tank. This is a common prescription given by doctors for people with lung inflictions like emphysema. Have you ever heard of sleep apnea treatments? Well guess what, these force more air, i.e. more oxygen, into your body. During a stroke, your brain is robbed of oxygen. HBOT, or hyperbaric oxygen therapy, has been found to be healing to these patients and remarkable improvements in their symptoms have been seen.

I don't have an oxygen chamber, but if someone I loved were very ill or disabled, I would certainly support and encourage them to consider using one.

## Altitude sickness

Some of you find that when you go to a higher altitude, like the mountains, you feel fatigued, short of breath, or get headaches. At higher altitudes, there is less oxygen, and an aggravation of your symptoms can easily occur when you go to a higher altitude where there is less oxygen to buffer the un-eliminated acids in your blood. And this list is not limited to only those symptoms we have commonly associated with "altitude sickness," like fatigue or headaches. For example, because un-eliminated acids affect your weight, inflammation, and even thyroid levels, and these too can become aggravated at higher altitudes.

If you start your trek to the mountains with an acidic bloodstream, you will be the most susceptible to these reactions, because you will already be starting off with lower than ideal levels of oxygen in your blood. The additional lowering of these levels when you hit the higher altitudes can be enough to put you over the edge into a state of symptomatic reactions.

My clients consistently remark about how much better they feel at sea level. (Having recently lived in Boulder for 18 years, at over 5,000 feet, this experience is one that many of my local clients observed.)

If you travel to an area with a higher altitude, consider taking more *Body Bentonite*. Also, if you do not feel well during this trip, blame the altitude, and not any of the healing products you are taking, for causing this.

## Iron supplementation

Anemia is commonly treated with iron because iron oxygenates your blood. A better way to treat this is to heal your bowel and body with this program, which eliminates the acids that cause low oxygen levels, and subsequently a reduction in your iron levels, in the first place. My clients have eliminated anemia without the use of iron supplements.

## Antioxidant therapy

Coenzyme Q10, Vitamin E, and other anti-oxidants improve the oxygenation of your blood. In other words, they "work" in part because of the resultant increase in oxygenation of your blood. (But they also "don't work" because they do nothing to eliminate the acids that *cause* low oxygen levels in the first place.)

## Aspirin and oxygen

Aspirin is commonly prescribed to prevent heart attacks because it has the ability to thin your blood, thereby reducing the clumping of red blood cells (also called "stickiness") that can lead to a heart attack. Ultimately, oxygenating your blood by eliminating acids, and reducing blood stickiness, is much safer than relying on aspirin to do this for you.

## Aerobic exercise oxygenates

Aerobic means "oxygen." Aerobic exercise helps oxygenate your blood, and this is one reason why it is beneficial to your body. Yet it is even more beneficial to have a constant supply of oxygen going to your organs, as occurs when you heal your bowel and body with this program, and which does not happen when you exercise, as in this case, the increased oxygenation of your blood is limited to a very short period of time (during the exercise and for a short period of time afterwards).

Likewise, during anaerobic exercise, you exercise beyond your body's ability to eliminate the creation of lactic acid that develops during exercise, which therefore *reduces* your oxygen levels. Exercising to this point is harmful to your health, yet many people do, with the mentality that "more is always better."

You will feel better and lose weight faster if you keep your exercise aerobic. To ensure that yours is, check the Internet for "target heart rate" (aimed to keep you in an aerobic state), and find out what yours should be while you exercise, and/or buy a heart rate monitor, a device that can be worn during exercise that constantly monitors this for you electronically.

## Oxygen bars, etc.

In Boulder, there is a "bar" that sells herb drinks and other concoctions, along with the ability to sit down and inhale oxygen for a small fee. I never visited this bar, but I like this idea. You can also buy oxygenated water called "Penta" water and oxygen drops from the health food store, all of which goes to show you that the awareness of the value of increasing oxygen levels is perhaps more popular than you realize.

## The magic of David Blaine

In 2006, infamous magician and entertainer David Blaine performed a stunt whereby he was immersed in water for seven days, and then attempted to break an 8 minute 58 second record for holding his breath. During the week that he was in water he was not given any food, only an intravenous fluid of glucose and electrolytes, and possibly some other nutrients. For many, this week of "starvation" made his attempt to break this breathing record at the end even more unbelievable. Most of you think that a week of no food should and would kill you, or at the very least, make it impossible to perform a difficult feat such as holding your breath a long time.

On the contrary, his spectacle of immersing himself in this bubble of water, where he was on display outside for all to see in New York City, made it *easier*, not harder, for him to hold his breath. I am sure he knows this, and am impressed at his brilliance and ability to manipulate millions into thinking otherwise. As I was watching this, I thought it was an excellent opportunity to help you apply the principles in my books.

When Blaine ate no food for one week and was administered high levels of electrolytes, his blood was being cleared of acidic toxins. "Fasting," or eating no food, gives your body time to eliminate acids, much more time than it has when it is busy digesting food. See Chapter 9 of *Unique Healing* for a complete explanation of digestion. The I.V. of electrolytes provided him with alkaline buffers to reduce these acid levels further. *Excess acids in your blood reduce oxygen levels.*

By reducing the acids in his blood, he reduced the oxygen consumption of his body, and increased the oxygen saturation of his blood. *This made it easier for him to hold his breath for a long time.* The less oxygen that is used up to buffer acids, the more that is available to feed your brain and muscles. Holding your breath and reducing the oxygen coming into your body is easier to do when your body's need for oxygen is reduced, as was accomplished during this week of fasting and electrolyte administration.

I am not saying that I was not impressed with this feat, and there are many others he has done that I can't figure out. I am just saying that this one was easier than it appeared. He applied the principles of pH chemistry that I am teaching you. Who knows what all of you may do with this one day!

## Success With Oxygenation

"I went to a nutritionist who did a live blood cell analysis and was told that my blood cells were clumping and that I showed signs of low oxygen levels. I tried all of the supplements he gave me, hundreds of dollars of them, and sometimes this got better, but it quickly got worse as soon as I stopped the supplements. Most of the time I was exhausted, couldn't sleep, was depressed, and felt horrible. After following this program for just a couple of months, all of these conditions have improved tremendously."

"I always found that when I went up to Vail to ski, my headaches got worse. Donna explained how the altitude has less oxygen, and how this program would oxygenate my blood. Since I have been on this program I have been skiing many times, and my headaches have not returned."

"My wife and kids and I went to the mountains with some friends, and their 12-year-old daughter experienced altitude sickness, which was eliminated in 24 hours after convincing the family to give her large amounts of bentonite."

## My story

At one point when I was very ill, I had oxygen and megavitamins pumped into my veins through an I.V. I was incredibly acidic and toxic at the time and one symptom I had was severe brain fog and irritation. This lifted for a few hours after the treatment, but because nothing was done to improve my body's ability to eliminate the acids that cause oxygen depletion, the symptoms always returned shortly after the treatment was over.

### Watch My Video, "Why THIS Program Improves Oxygenation"

This video, and all of my videos, can be found at *www. UniqueHealing. com* or at *www. YouTube.com/UniqueHealing*.

# Inflammation

Inflammation is at the core of many symptoms and diseases. Any condition or disease that ends in "itis," which means "inflammation," is an example of an inflammatory condition. Consider the following examples of these: arthritis, bursitis, colitis, cystitis, dermatitis, diverticulitis, hepatitis, laryngitis, mastitis, meningitis, nephritis, neuritis, pancreatitis, prostatitis, sinusitis, tonsillitis, and vaginitis.

Inflammation is also at the core of many other conditions as well, like asthma, autism, headaches, aches and pains, gout, lupus, fibromyalgia, and TMJ, for example.

## Healing Your Body With This Program Eliminates Inflammation

The inflammatory process is a reaction from your lymphatic system to the presence of acids that have not been eliminated from your body. Inflammatory chemicals are released to buffer un-eliminated acids. Therefore, when you heal your body with this program and these acids are eliminated, the release of these chemicals no longer occurs.

Healing your body with this program also heals your lymphatic system so that even if there are acids, your body is strong enough to handle them without a reaction (it fixes the holes on your roof so that even if it does rain, your house does not get wet).

# Healing Your Bowel With This Program Eliminates Inflammation

The healthy bacteria in your bowel are responsible for fighting bacterial, fungal, and parasitic infections. Because these infections can trigger inflammation, healing your bowel with this program reduces inflammation caused by these infections. Your healthy bowel bacteria are also responsible for digesting gluten and lactose. When these are not digested completely, they create toxic by-products that can also trigger inflammation.

In addition to its many other important functions, a healthy bacterial environment in your bowel is a necessity for the complete elimination of acids (toxins, heavy metals, pesticides, etc.) from your body. A healthy bowel prevents the re-absorption of acids into your blood that cause an unhealthy body, and triggers the release of inflammatory chemicals into your blood.

# Why my Crutches Eliminate Inflammation

*Body Bentonite* binds to and eliminates acids (toxins, heavy metals, chemicals, etc.) from your body. It helps to prevent them from becoming re-absorbed into your bloodstream, where they trigger a response by your body to protect you from them. It eliminates the acids that trigger the release of inflammatory chemicals.

*Unique Healing Calcium Citrate* is an alkalinizing mineral that helps neutralize the acids that your bowel does not eliminate. When these acids are neutralized, your body does not need to produce inflammatory chemicals to buffer them.

*Unique Healing Colloidal Silver* has natural anti-bacterial, anti-fungal, anti-parasitic properties. It is valuable for eliminating inflammation that can occur due to an infection.

## How much do I take?/Questions about using these

See Chapter 5 for information on using these crutches, including recommendations on the amount to use, as well as a discussion of the misunderstandings about the particular crutch that may, if not understood correctly, cause you to fail to look and feel better while you heal your bowel and body with this program.

# Misunderstandings About Inflammation and Other Information for Your Success

## Keep your stools well-formed

Because inflammation is caused in part by un-eliminated acids, and because well-formed stools prevent the re-absorption of acids into your blood, you will suffer from the least amount of inflammation if you keep your stools well-formed while you are healing your bowel and body.

If you do not have a very good handle on how to define well-formed stools, review Chapter 6 of *Unique Healing* now. (And remember, when your stools are hard and slow you are eliminating more acids, and will therefore feel better, than when your stools are one or more times a day but not all extremely well-formed.)

If your stools are not well-formed, the following changes can help: increase your *Body Bentonite* intake; reduce your carbohydrate intake (pasta, breads, grains, cereals, yogurt, etc.); reduce your sugar intake (including natural healthy sugars such as agave, honey, raw sugar, cane juice, etc.); reduce your alcohol, salt, coffee, and/or soda intake; do not have a massage, chiropractic adjustment, or any other body work; drink a lot of water; rest; and keep your exercise aerobic (see Chapter 4 for more information on how to attain this, and why it is important.)

If these changes do not noticeably help the form of your stools in two days, take them further (i.e. take more *Body Bentonite*, reduce your carbohydrate intake more, etc.)

Out of all of these recommendations, increasing your *Body Bentonite* intake is one of the most productive and helpful. It heals your body, unlike many of the other recommendations. It will do the most to lead you to a place where looking and feeling good is effortless, and some of the other suggestions, such as reducing sugar intake, are simply "too hard to do when your blood is too acidic."

(Note: the exception to this information is when your poorly formed stools are caused by an infection, in which case *Unique Healing Colloidal Silver* is needed to reduce your symptoms. Refer to Chapter 5 for information on when and how to use this crutch.)

## Injuries and inflammation

Technically, when you are injured, your blood vessels dilate, as this brings more blood to the injured site. Your blood contains the oxygen and nutrients needed to help with healing. Phagocytes, like white blood cells, are also released, which "eat up" the waste products, and harmful bacteria that may be present at the site. Chemicals are released that include histamine, kinins, and prostaglandins (pg's). Pg's magnify pain, and kinins affect nerve endings and create pain, too. Neutrophils clear toxic debris. Increased circulation at the injury causes heat, redness, and swelling.

When your bowel and body are healthy, as created in this program, your ability to heal and recover from injuries is much improved. A healthy body has adequate amounts of oxygen and nutrients available for this healing to occur. It eliminates the "waste products," or acids, that are created when there is an injury. And a healthy body has a healthy lymphatic system, which is involved in the production of many of these healing agents, like white blood cells and histamines, etc. A healthy bowel prevents the infections that can occur with an injury.

## Essential fatty acids and inflammation

Essential fatty acids have anti-inflammatory effects, but I am not a fan of these for two reasons. One, I have found that it takes very large amounts (much larger than the majority of you take and/or are advised to take), to provide anti-inflammatory relief. You would be better off taking large amounts of *Body Bentonite* instead, because it eliminates the acids that cause inflammation, and it has a cumulative healing effect, unlike essential fatty acids. Two, many supplements are concentrated and difficult to get in through your diet alone. For example, you could not come remotely close to consuming 30,000 mcg/day of vitamin B-12 in your diet. But essential fatty acids are simply oil in capsules, and this is extremely easy to replicate in your diet (and should be a part of your daily diet anyway). It would be more valuable to eat olive oil, avocadoes, nuts, and seeds than to take these oils in capsule form (and less expensive, too).

# Success With Inflammation

"I was diagnosed with Crohn's disease (inflammatory bowel disease). I stopped eating wheat and gluten, sugar, and dairy, but I continued to have symptoms often. Living like a hermit and eating a very limited diet was a struggle and even that only helped a little. I was miserable and completely lost. I tried everything to help this prior to doing this program. Now I can eat anything and not have my symptoms come back. I am completely cured."

"I had knee surgery and my doctors were completely amazed by how fast I healed and how little pain and inflammation I had afterwards."

## My story

Inflammatory conditions were the ones that plagued me, and disabled me, the most prior to healing my bowel and body with this program. I remember having joint pain as young as a teen, and experiencing knee pain if I walked a long distance. When I first became very ill. I experienced excruciating neck pain, as well as severe chest pain (which sent me to the hospital at least once, thinking that I was dying of a heart attack). This pain eventually subsided, but the neck pain persisted for a number of years. I tried thousands of supplements, had hundreds of chiropractic adjustments, many massages, and many more treatments to eliminate this pain. These crutches gave me minimal relief, and of course, it was always short-lived. When I began healing my bowel and body with this program, the neck pain subsided substantially, and for a period of time, it was replaced with headaches (which I surprisingly never had when I was younger and unhealthy). The headaches were uncomfortable, but compared to the neck pain they were immensely more bearable. It was progress. As I continued with this program the headaches disappeared as well. Now, the only experiences with inflammation that I have are due to injury (a few broken bones, a herniated groin, etc.). I was criticized for not seeking medical care for any of these injuries, but they healed without this intervention.

## Watch My Video, "Why THIS Program Eliminates Inflammation"

This video, and all of my videos, can be found at *www.UniqueHealing. com* or at *www.YouTube.com/UniqueHealing*.

More information on inflammation can be found in Chapter 2 under "Aches and Pains."

# Circulation

Healthy circulation, or blood flow, is a necessity for life. Your heart, lungs, arteries, capillaries, and veins are the main components of your circulatory system. Blood delivers needed oxygen and nutrients to the cells and organs of your body. Without these your cells, and you, would die. Poor circulation also impedes healing, results in cold hands and feet, and increases aches and pains. Reynaud's is a condition of extremely poor circulation, and even more extreme circulatory problems can occur with other conditions, like diabetes.

As is true with dehydration, oxygenation, inflammation, and nutrient levels, poor circulation coexists with the majority of symptoms, diseases, addictions, and weight problems that you have.

## Healing Your Body With This Program Increases Circulation

Excess acidity weakens your circulatory organs and reduces blood flow. Healing your body with this program eliminates acids from your body, which improves your circulation.

## Healing Your Bowel With this Program Increases Circulation

In addition to its many other important functions, a healthy bacterial environment in your bowel is a necessity for the complete elimination of acids (toxins, heavy metals, pesticides, etc.) from your body. A healthy bowel prevents the re-absorption of acids into your blood that cause poor circulation.

## Why My Crutches Increase Circulation

*Body Bentonite* binds to and eliminates acids (toxins, heavy metals, chemicals, etc.) from your body. It eliminates the acids that reduce blood flow/circulation.

***Unique Healing Calcium Citrate*** is an alkalinizing mineral that helps neutralize the acids that your bowel does not eliminate. When these acids are neutralized, your blood flows (i.e. circulates) more effectively.

## How much do I take?/Questions about using these

See Chapter 5 for information on using these crutches, including recommendations on the amount to use, as well as a discussion of the misunderstandings about the particular crutch that may, if not understood correctly, cause you to fail to look and feel better while you heal your bowel and body with this program.

# Misunderstandings About Circulation and Other Information for Your Success

## Keep your stools well-formed

Because poor circulation is caused in part by un-eliminated acids, and because well-formed stools prevent the re-absorption of acids into your blood, you will suffer from the least amount of circulatory problems if you keep your stools well-formed while you are healing your bowel and body.

If you do not have a very good handle on how to define well-formed stools, review Chapter 6 of *Unique Healing* now. (And remember, when your stools are hard and slow you are eliminating more acids, and will therefore feel better, than when your stools are one or more times a day but not all extremely well-formed.)

If your stools are not well-formed, the following changes can help: increase your *Body Bentonite* intake; reduce your carbohydrate intake (pasta, breads, grains, cereals, yogurt, etc.); reduce your sugar intake (including natural healthy sugars such as agave, honey, raw sugar, cane juice, etc.); reduce your alcohol, salt, coffee, and/or soda intake; do not have a massage, chiropractic adjustment, or any other body work; drink a lot of water; rest; and keep your exercise aerobic (see Chapter 4 for more information on how to attain this, and why it is important.)

If these changes do not noticeably help the form of your stools in two days, take them further (i.e. take more *Body Bentonite*, reduce your carbohydrate intake more, etc.)

Out of all of these recommendations, increasing your *Body Bentonite* intake is one of the most productive and helpful. It heals your body, unlike many of the other recommendations. It will do the most to lead you to a place where looking and feeling good is effortless, and some of the other suggestions, such as reducing sugar intake, are simply "too hard to do when your blood is too acidic."

(Note: the exception to this information is when your poorly formed stools are caused by an infection, in which case *Unique Healing Colloidal Silver* is needed to reduce your symptoms. Refer to Chapter 5 for information on when and how to use this crutch.)

## Many treatments are aimed at increasing circulation

Many alternative treatments improve circulation in your body, including but not limited to: acupuncture, physical therapy, chiropractic, massage, and "energy" work. In most cases, "energy" and "circulation" are synonymous.

Applying "Vicks" to your chest when you are sick increases the circulation to your lungs; using "Ben-Gay" on sore muscles does the same thing. Jacuzzis are helpful for sore muscles for the same reason. Exercise improves circulation, and some herbs, like cayenne, do as well. Gently brushing your gums with your toothbrush, a practice many dentists recommend, improves circulation to your teeth and gums.

As with many other conditions, it is immensely more valuable to have your healthy bowel and body regulate your circulation 24 hours-a-day then it is to have to rely on an external treatment/method to do this for you (as this delivers much less than a 24 hours-a-day improvement in your circulation, becomes costly and time-consuming, and does not heal your body and prevent premature death and disease as a healthy body does, either.)

## Microcurrent Electrical Stimulation (MENS)

Microcurrent electrical stimulation, or MENS is another therapy that increases circulation. It is explained that the electric current stimulates cellular activity, or energy/circulation. This energy, along with an improvement in protein synthesis and nutrient absorption that accompanies it, creates an ideal environment for better healing.

A number of famous athletes have used this device to treat their aches and pains. It has also found a market in the skin care industry, and mini face-lifts are achieved with its use, as the improved circulation helps to reduce inflammation and tone your skin.

This is just but one of many age old methods for improving circulation. Like all of these methods, however, it is safe, but it has limited value, as it does nothing to heal your bowel and body, which creates a natural, complete, and permanent improvement in your circulatory system.

I went to a physical therapist many years ago who used this same therapy to treat my excruciating neck pain. Unfortunately, in my case, I never experienced any improvements in my neck pain as a result.

## Compression garments

Compression shorts are garments marketed to athletes to promote increased athletic performance due to a reduction in muscle soreness and increase in recovery rates. These shorts "squeeze" your muscles, improving the blood (circulation), oxygen, and nutrients that reach them, which reduces lactic acid and increases your recovery time. And a device (which will set you back a whopping $4,850) that provides two-second pulses of compression along your leg in a programmed sequence has been tested on Olympic athletes and has been found to reduce muscle soreness. (A less expensive version of this machine is apparently available for use in a center in my old hometown of Boulder.)

The point is, many entrepreneurs "get" that circulation, oxygen, and higher nutrient levels enhance performance. This program does it even better.

For $4,850 you can create a healthy bowel and body with this program, and as a result, have natural, 24-hour-a-day, increased levels of circulation, oxygen, and nutrients (along with an elimination of all of your symptoms, disease, addictions, and weight problems).

## Heat, not cold, is healing

When I was very ill with excruciating neck pain, a chiropractor told me to ice it. I remember one time when it was particularly bad and I sat with ice on my neck, and the pain got worse, not better. I thought it didn't make sense, but of course I wasn't the expert, and this was a time when I still listened to everyone else. Years later, as I continued to battle the pain, I found great relief in a warm cloth or heating pad on my neck.

Applying ice to an injury does not heal it; it slows down the healing process. In the immediate term, it can make things feel better. But feeling better does not mean you are healthier, or that the method you used to feel better is beneficial to your body.

It is like a drug; you feel better, but you are interfering with the healing process, so that in the long run, you are worse off for having taken it.

The common advice to ice everything that is injured is a product of our "treat the symptoms" mentality. A lot of things that we do to make things feel and look immediately better, like high protein diets, are harmful in the long run. Yet millions follow this type of advice daily.

Ice stops blood from going to your injury, and it therefore stops the delivery of healing oxygen and nutrients to it that are needed for this area to heal. But this blood also causes swelling and pain, and this is what many are trying to avoid when injured. This swelling and pain are your body's attempt to heal itself, and encouraging this with heat would be best. These symptoms are also your body's wonderful way to try to get you to stop what you were doing that caused the injury in the first place. Drugging yourself so you are out of pain, so you can run around on this injury, is not wise. This often eventually leads to greater, more serious problems in the long run, like a torn meniscus in your knee, or a ruptured disc in your back, for example.

Researchers in Australia studied 200 individuals with tennis elbow. They were split into three treatment groups: one group received a corticosteroid injection; one group received eight sessions of physiotherapy; and one group were on the "wait and see" plan of doing neither. In the short run, the steroid and physiotherapy group experienced improvements over the wait and see group. But in the long term (at 52 weeks) *the steroid group experienced much higher rates of recurrence and poorer outcomes than the physiotherapy group. In the long run, the physiotherapy group experienced no difference in outcome versus the group who did nothing.*

This study shows that taking a drug to treat a problem, and getting short-term benefits from it, can result in a worse outcome in the long term.

I believe that the only time you should ice an injury is if you need to immediately and unavoidably perform. For example, if you are making $10 million dollars a year as a basketball player and you are injured in the first half of a playoff game, ice, and other "drugs" like Tylenol, are good choices! Or if you have a big presentation at work and you need to show up. In other words, any time you need an immediate reduction in pain, ice is a great crutch, just keep in mind that this is hampering the healing of your injury, and it should be stopped as soon as possible.

In simple terms, heat promotes healing, and cold prevents it.

## Ice cube baths and fevers

I heard differing reports regarding the day that Anna Nicole Smith died. In one, her nurse put her in a bathtub full of ice on the morning of her death. In another, this happened one or two days before her death. Either way, this was wrong and it most certainly hurt, not helped her. Smith had a very high fever (over 104 degrees) prior to her death. When an adult has a fever above 102 degrees, they should be admitted to the hospital. An I.V. to hydrate the body is in order, and would be very helpful in helping relieve the body of the stress of fighting off whatever is causing this high fever.

A fever is your body's way of protecting itself. A fever raises your internal body temperature, *because high temperatures destroy deadly germs.* Cooking chicken well does the same thing to help prevent salmonella poisoning.

Putting someone in an ice cold bath reduces this germ killing mechanism, and that is very dangerous. If anything, when one is ill with a fever, this heat producing affect should be encouraged with a warm bath or by lying under heavy blankets. When one adopts a simplistic mentality that cold will cure a fever and illness, they are ignorant of, and abusing, the way the body heals. An I.V. would have helped because the electrolytes in it buffer acids in the body, and *germs live in an acidic environment.* If you have a high fever, you have an overload of acids in your blood, and often, an overload of germs.

Anna Nicole Smith was not a healthy woman. Her diet program was unhealthy, and the drugs she used were harmful as well. Ultimately, the cause of her death was attributed to an overdose of drugs. Nevertheless, it is possible that she would still be here today if her nurse had insisted that she be hospitalized. The ice bath may have been the icing on the cake.

Regardless, I share this story to give you another opportunity to learn how to create and maintain health, and if any of you, or your children, is ill with a fever, you will know what to do.

Electrolyte beverages, warmth, and rest are the best medicine when you are ill with a fever. Drugs like Tylenol, which reduce fever, can be harmful; fever is healing, but we like these drugs because we fear a high fever. Ideally, refrain from these if you have one, and if your child has a fever above 104, call your doctor. If an adult has one above 102, call your doctor too.

## How much is the therapy helping?

When I was ill, I worked for a very successful chiropractic office in Newport Beach, California. I saw thousands of patients enter the office. After an injury, many got better, but for many others, who came as a result of a chronic condition, the improvements were hard to see, and the visits were endless. I wondered about this.

Back pain after an injury is not the same as back pain due to chronic ill health.

If these people with back pain due to an injury had just slowed down and not been adjusted, would they have healed anyway? I thought the answer was yes. And did these people who did get adjusted think that the adjustments healed them? And did they then go around telling everyone how well these adjustments worked? I began to think so. So when someone with a chronic problem entered the office and felt better for a very short time but did not get better, did they blame themselves? Did they think something was wrong with them that they weren't improving? Did they ever think to blame the approach instead? I was adjusted three to four times a week for five years, and while it brought temporary relief of my pain, my neck pain persisted. When I started to heal my bowel and body, it not only got better, but it stayed better. This elimination of my neck pain has maintained itself for over fifteen years now.

## Success With Circulation

"Before the start of this program I was experiencing horrible back pain. After lifting something very heavy, my back went into spasms, and this was not the first time. My back was very weak, and I had flare-ups pretty often. I had to take a week off of work, went to physical therapy, but continued to be in pain. Three weeks later, still in pain, I contacted Donna. The first thing she had me do was stop icing it and use a heating pad all day, as well as use Ben-Gay on my back all day long. I must admit, this felt a lot better than the ice! She also recommended a huge amount of bentonite. I was willing to try anything. My back did not get better right away, but pretty soon after I started all of this, it did. It has now been ages since my back has been a problem. I think she probably saved me from a back surgery!"

## My story

I spent my teenage years in New York, and I was in agony during the winter months. My hands and feet froze easily and I never could get warm. I hated the cold. I went to college in Virginia, because it was the furthest south (i.e. warmer) that my parents would let me travel. After college I moved to Southern California (i.e. even warmer). I became ill while living there, and I also became healthier while living there. As I became healthier, I began to "crave" the cold weather. It was amazing and shocking to me. Who was this woman? I moved to Boulder, Colorado, in part, as a result of my strong desire to live in a colder climate (and then recently moved to Connecticut). Sure I get cold at times, but I do not get the freezing hands and feet I used to when I was younger, and I do not mind the cold temperatures, as I did back then too. My circulation is much healthier than it used to be.

### Watch My Video,
### "Why THIS Program Improves Your Circulation"

This video, and all of my videos, can be found at *www.UniqueHealing. com* or at *www.YouTube.com/UniqueHealing*.

# Nutrient Levels

Thousands of studies have been conducted, and continue to be done, that show the benefits of nutrients for your health and well-being. In the past fifteen years, the sale of vitamin supplements has skyrocketed into billions of dollars as a result. Very few people will deny that nutrient levels in your body are important.

Numerous explanations are given for why nutrients help the health of your body and I won't repeat them all here. Likely you've heard them all already. What you probably haven't heard is that *the greatest cause of nutrient depletion in your body is un-eliminated acids.*

# Healing Your Body With This Program Improves Nutrient Levels

When your blood is overly acidic, due to the inefficient elimination of these acids by your bowel, your body "soaks up" nutrients to buffer and protect you from these acids. This causes your nutrient levels to decrease.

For example, antioxidants reduce the damage of the free radicals caused by excess acidity. Excess acidity reduces the assimilation of fat-soluble vitamins (A, D, E, and K), which need a correct pH in your bile and pancreatic juices to be assimilated by your body.

As you eliminate acids from your body with this program, your *entire* vitamin/nutrient needs plummet (calcium, B-vitamins, vitamin D, vitamin E, you name it.)

> A body that is not overly acidic is a nutrient-rich body. Focus on "acids out" rather than "nutrients in" and you will be much healthier and much more successful in eliminating your symptoms, weight problems, addictions, and illnesses.

## Healing Your Bowel With This Program Improves Nutrient Levels

A healthy bowel bacterial environment plays a key role in the utilization of vitamin B-12, absorption of calcium, and the manufacture of vitamin K and some of the B vitamins as well.

Good bacteria break down impacted material on your intestinal walls, which in turn increases your absorption of all nutrients.

Candida, yeast that multiplies in your bowel when the beneficial bacterial levels are low, produces an enzyme called thiaminase that destroys Vitamin B-1 in your bowel. When your bowel is healthy, you will have healthy levels of Vitamin B1.

In addition to its many other important functions, a healthy bacterial environment in your bowel is a necessity for the complete elimination of acids (toxins, heavy metals, pesticides, etc.) from your body. A healthy bowel prevents the re-absorption of acids into your blood that cause your nutrient levels to decreases.

## Why My Crutches Improves Nutrient Levels

*Body Bentonite* binds to and eliminates acids (toxins, heavy metals, chemicals, etc.) from your body. It helps to prevent them from becoming re-absorbed into your bloodstream, where they trigger a response by your body to protect you from them. It eliminates the acids that otherwise cause a depletion of your nutrient levels.

*Unique Healing Calcium Citrate* is an alkalinizing mineral that helps neutralize the acids that your bowel does not eliminate. When these acids are neutralized, your body does not need to "use up" nutrients to buffer them.

**Methyl Vitamin B-12** provides your body with this needed nutrient, which will be available in adequate amounts only once the health of your bowel bacterial environment has improved.

### How much do I take?/Questions about using these

See Chapter 5 for information on using these crutches, including recommendations on the amount to use, as well as a discussion of the misunderstandings about the particular crutch that may, if not understood correctly, cause you to fail to look and feel better while you heal your bowel and body with this program.

## Misunderstandings About Nutrient Levels and Other Information for Your Success

### Keep your stools well-formed

Because low nutrient levels are caused in part by un-eliminated acids, and because well-formed stools prevent the re-absorption of acids into your blood, you will have the healthiest nutrient levels if you keep your stools well-formed while you are healing your bowel and body.

If you do not have a very good handle on how to define well-formed stools, review Chapter 6 of *Unique Healing* now. (And remember, when your stools are hard and slow you are eliminating more acids, and will therefore feel better, than when your stools are one or more times a day but not all extremely well-formed.)

If your stools are not well-formed, the following changes can help: increase your *Body Bentonite* intake; reduce your carbohydrate intake (pasta, breads, grains, cereals, yogurt, etc.); reduce your sugar intake (including natural healthy sugars such as agave, honey, raw sugar, cane juice, etc.); reduce your alcohol, salt, coffee, and/or soda intake; do not have a massage, chiropractic adjustment, or any other body work; drink a lot of water; rest; and keep your exercise aerobic (see Chapter 4 for more information on how to attain this, and why it is important.)

If these changes do not noticeably help the form of your stools in two days, take them further (i.e. take more *Body Bentonite*, reduce your carbohydrate intake more, etc.)

Out of all of these recommendations, increasing your *Body Bentonite* intake is one of the most productive and helpful. It heals your body, unlike many of the other recommendations. It will do the most to lead you to a place where looking and feeling good is effortless, and some of the other suggestions, such as reducing sugar intake, are simply "too hard to do when your blood is too acidic."

(Note: the exception to this information is when your poorly formed stools are caused by an infection, in which case *Unique Healing Colloidal Silver* is needed to reduce your symptoms. Refer to Chapter 5 for information on when and how to use this crutch.)

## The trend towards higher nutrient intakes

Over the years, the recommended dosage of supplements has steadily increased. For example, when I was ill, a standard recommended dosage of acidophilus was about 10 million organisms a day; today, twenty years later, it has increased to about 3 billion a day. This is an enormous increase. And while I took massive supplementation when I was ill, it was considered extremely revolutionary and uncommon. Today it is much more widespread.

> The reason you have seen a greater response and benefit from massive nutrient supplementation is because your bodies are becoming increasingly less healthy and more acidic. The less healthy your bowel is, and the more acids you accumulate, the more vitamins/nutrients you need to look and feel better.

The problem is that most of you who take supplements don't know that they are crutches and that you will need to take them long-term, and eventually at even higher doses, as often occurs with medications, to maintain a reduction in your symptoms.

If you don't eliminate acids from your body, more will eventually accumulate, and you'll eventually need a higher dose of a nutrient crutch to buffer these acids and get the same relief. As more trash accumulates in your house, you will need a larger bottle of perfume to eliminate the odor.

This is very profitable for the supplement companies and others who sell them. It is not very profitable for you.

At some point, the larger amounts needed to achieve the same results is very hard to maintain on a daily basis, and it is then that you may seek an new answer to your problems. Many of you are reading this book, and many of you have landed in my office.

When I was very ill, I took thousands of dollars worth of supplements, yet I saw no improvements in my symptoms or health. At one point I was sold on the miracles of mega-nutrient supplement through an I.V. Once again, I was led to believe that this was the answer. I spent many hours in an office hooked up to an I.V. while mega-nutrients were dripped into my veins. I noticed minor improvements in my symptoms with this approach, but they were minor, and very temporary. A few years ago, I saw that this protocol had made its way to Boulder. There are many of you who will be wrongly sold on the idea that this is the answer to your problems.

I believe that until you start addressing the cause of your health and weight problems, as this program does, this trend to higher nutrient intakes will continue, but to a limit. Who wants to rely on an I.V. every week, or every day, to feel better? Worse, because you are only treating the symptoms of your problems, eventually even these won't help, as was my experience. Then you will find that all of that time and money was a waste. Also, many of you become concerned once supplement usage enters into the mega-zone, anyway.

## It's not about taking more vitamins

The average American woman is advised to consume 1,200 mg of calcium of day through diet and supplements, and yet osteoporosis, the disease thought to be helped by this advice, is prevalent in this country. On the other hand, for centuries, Asian women have only been consuming about 400 mg of calcium a day, through diet alone, and their rate of osteoporosis is much lower than ours.

We take in much higher levels of calcium to achieve the same or worse results, because the overall composition of our diet is much more acidic than theirs. I suspect their bowels are much healthier than ours, too.

*Simply ingesting more nutrients is not the answer to better health.*

## Do you need to take vitamins?

When I first see a client, one of the most frequently asked questions is about supplement use. There is a concern that I am not recommending multivitamins and other popular-selling ones. They are suspicious that I don't. To appease them, I tell them they can take all of these things if they want to. After some explanation, most of them decide on their own not to take them. Interestingly, when these same clients reach the end of this program, they *never* ask me "Do I need to take vitamins?" Maybe you, too, will only really get this concept when you get there too; when you heal your bowel and body and find that you look and feel better, and feel safer, than you ever did when you were on a popular supplement usage regimen.

At the end of this program clients do not take extra vitamins and they look and feel much better than they did when their bowel and body were unhealthy and they were ingesting numerous ones.

## You'll easily meet your nutrient needs when your bowel and body are healthy

The more acidic you are, and the less healthy your bowel is, the greater amount of every nutrient that is needed to feel good.

When your bowel and body are healthy, as is created with this program, you won't need extra supplementation to feel good.

A healthy body needs nutrients to function, but a healthy body needs very few of these. Once you have healed your bowel and body with this program, you will desire a nutrient-rich diet of grains, vegetables, cheese, yogurt, beans, eggs, etc. When you are healthy, these foods will provide adequate amounts of nutrition for your body.

When you are healthy, you will no longer desire nutrient-empty foods, like coffee, sugar, soda, and alcohol. Currently, these comprise a large percentage of the American diet and are a leading cause of nutritional deficiencies, not only because they contain little to no nutrients, but also because they are all highly acidic, and again, an increase in acids increases your nutritional needs.

## Nutrients won't save your life; eliminating acids can

Nutrients are present in foods that are low in acidity and easy-to-digest; two qualities of a food that make it healthy for you, that reduce the accumulation of acidity in your body, and that help extend your life.

Unfortunately, it is the nutritional content of these foods, and not the low acidity, easy-to-digest nature of them that has gotten all the credit!

A very large, long-term study recently found that people who ingest handfuls of supplements die at the same age of people who do not.

To extend you life, you need to eliminate acids from your body. When you simply ingest a handful of vitamins and other supplements, you do not get this result. Nutrients do not eliminate acids from your body.

## Success With Improved Nutrient Levels

"When I came to Donna I was taking 32 different supplements, but I still suffered from extreme fatigue, joint pain, insomnia, poor concentration, and gas and bloating. I stopped these supplements about six months into the program and noticed that I felt no worse for doing so. In fact by this time, my symptoms had improved dramatically and I felt 100 times better than I did when I took all of the supplements. I also saved a tremendous amount of money."

"I was diagnosed with low iron levels, and these improved by doing this program, even though I never took an iron supplement."

"I was getting B-12 shots once a month for energy. Donna taught me how this is a crutch that would only help if I did this daily, so I stopped, and now I have an enormous amount of energy."

"My naturopath told me I had numerous nutrient deficiencies and I bought a bagful of supplements from her to treat this. I spent over $400/month on these for almost nine months. I was told my health had improved; but as soon as I stopped taking everything, my symptoms came back. Now I take none of these supplements, and I feel better than ever before."

"I now take no vitamins, I eat a healthy diet, as that is what I crave, and I look and feel great."

### Watch My Video,
### "Why THIS Program Improves Your Nutrient Levels"
This video, and all of my videos, can be found at *www.UniqueHealing. com* or at *www.YouTube.com/UniqueHealing*.

Review Chapter 4 of *Unique Healing* for a better understanding of the shortcomings of vitamin/mineral supplementation, and why it is not safe for you to depend on these to eliminate your symptoms, addictions, weight problems, and prevent disease and extend your life.

By helping your body eliminate acids, a healthy bowel and body reduces dehydration, increases oxygenation, reduces inflammation, increases circulation, and increases the nutrient levels in your body.

# Chapter 4
## Why THIS Program
## Eliminates Your Weight Problems

Weight problems have increased tremendously in the last decade, even though you have spent billions of dollars trying to lose weight; even though you have become "smarter" and have purchased enormous numbers of gym memberships and increased your exercise, and have been on diets (many of them, in fact) of less carbohydrates, less fat, and less calories.

Roughly two-thirds of Americans are either overweight or obese (thirty pounds or more over a healthy weight). The number of Americans who are morbidly obese, or 100 pounds over a healthy weight, has risen dramatically since 2000. Three percent of the population, or 6.8 million adults, are morbidly obese, versus only 2%, or 4.2 million people, in 2000. This is an increase of 2.6 million more people. Researchers are calling this "catastrophic" and a "serious emergency."

A recent article in the *American Psychologist* reviewed 31 diet studies and found that on average, 41% of participants gained back more weight than they had lost. Authors think these estimates are conservative and that people may be too embarrassed to accurately report the amount of weight gained back. The lead author says, "eating in moderation is a must and getting regular exercise may be the key to sustained weight loss." You have heard that message millions of times, so why isn't it working?

Because diet and exercise help people lose weight, a "wrong diet" and a lack of exercise have erroneously been labeled as the cause of weight problems. This assumption is wrong.

Every client I have ever seen with weight struggles has had an unhealthy bowel and body. Put another way, weight gain is not caused by excess calories, carbohydrates, fats, or insufficient exercise. An unhealthy bowel and body cause it. And diets and exercise do not heal your bowel and body. This program does.

Weight loss programs rely on crutches, like reduced carbohydrate or calorie diets, exercise, etc., and weight loss crutches, like *all* crutches, fail in the long-term. The only way to achieve a healthy and thin body in the long-term without effort or failure is to heal your bowel and body and *rely on them*, not the diet, exercise or other weight loss crutch, to keep you thin.

A healthy bowel and body, as created with this program, will keep you thin *without* the need for crutches like diet or exercise. Now *this* is a revolutionary approach to weight loss!

Additionally, this program creates permanent weight loss. Sure, others have promised you this too, but when you rely on a crutch for weight loss—*and they all do*—this promise, cannot, and should not, be made.

Most of you blame yourself when you fail with these programs because you believe that if the diet helped you lose weight initially, it can't be the diet that caused you to fail later on. This is not true.

When you follow a diet or other weight loss program and lose weight, only to gain it back later, do not blame yourself. The real blame lies in the program itself. The approach you took failed, not you. Weight loss programs are failing *you!*

*The information you are given is wrong. You are doing your best.*

The success of a diet, or health program, needs to encompass long-term results. Billions of dollars are taken every year by the weight loss industry because you keep blaming yourself and not their advice. This has to stop.

More importantly, this program will help you lose weight and gain health so that as you age, you can look and feel great. Too many programs deliver weight loss with health loss. What is the value of being thin and looking great, if you are 55 and dying of cancer? I want to be thin and die at a very old age. If you do too, you need to heal your bowel and body.

If you think there is no hope because you have tried every diet without long-term success, you are wrong. Until you have healed your bowel and body with this program, you haven't tried everything yet to lose weight.

# Healing Your Body With This Program Eliminates Weight Problems

Your have a number of organs and glands that, when healthy, help keep you thin. Your *thyroid gland* regulates your metabolism, or how fast you burn food/calories; your *liver* breaks down fat; your *adrenal glands* help regulate your blood sugar, which reduces your cravings for sugar, alcohol, coffee, and other "fattening" foods; your *kidneys* maintain water balance and keep water weight off; and your *bowel* eliminates the acids that cause you to gain fat and water weight (read more on this below).

Healing your body with this program heals your thyroid, liver, adrenal glands, kidneys, and bowel. Healing your body means that you have eliminated acids from it; acids that otherwise reduce the oxygen and nutrients needed for healthy organs and glands. When your organs are healthy, their weight-regulating functions occur effortlessly, and naturally.

## Excess un-eliminated acids cause excess fat production

When your bowel is unhealthy and acids are not completely eliminated from your body, your body comes to the rescue to protect itself against this excess acidity. One way your body protects you is by creating more fat cells, an action that is primarily a response by your liver to this excess acidity.

Think of fat cells as safe homes for un-eliminated acids.

When you eliminate acids from your body with this program, your body no longer needs to store fat, and you lose fat in the process.

A healthy body has a healthy liver, and a healthy liver does not make extra fat, even if there are un-eliminated acids in your blood. (When there are no holes over your kitchen, your kitchen does not get wet, even if it does rain.)

## Excess un-eliminated acids also cause water weight gain

Another way your body protects you from un-eliminated acids is by retaining water, an action that is primarily a response by your kidneys to this excess acidity.

Water weight can cause a significant amount of total body weight. If you are overweight, five to fifty or more pounds of this can be attributable to excess water weight. When your weight fluctuates three or five pounds in one day or one week, this is due to changes in water weight. Many of you carry extra weight as water.

Excess water weight is most noticeable and recognizable as swelling, puffiness, bloating, cellulite, and a lack of muscle definition (which is why bodybuilders are notorious for using dangerous methods to eliminate excess water before a competition). But extra water weight looks a lot like extra fat weight, and many of you wrongly think that your water weight is fat.

Drinking a lot of water helps you lose extra water weight because the water you drink helps flush out the acids that *cause* you to retain water inside your body. Movie stars are frequently captured in photos with a bottle of water in their hands, and Weight Watchers and other diet programs put a heavy emphasis on water consumption, for the same reason.

Many years ago diuretics were very popular for weight loss. They are harmful and can even cause death, and they should never be taken unless directed by a physician. Once it was discovered how dangerous these were, the contribution that excess water weight made to one's overall overweight condition was soon forgotten. This happens often when a quick-fix drug is not available to treat the problem. Rather than acknowledge the problem and search for a safe way to eliminate it, it is simply ignored.

Eliminating acids with this program results in a reduction in water weight—safely, healthfully, and permanently.

A healthy body has healthy kidneys, and healthy kidneys do not cause you to retain water, even if there are un-eliminated acids in your blood. (When there are no holes over your living room, your living room does not get wet, even if it does rain.)

Excess weight exists as excess fat, excess water, or both. Healing your body with this program eliminates excess fat *and* excess water weight.

Watch my Video, "Why THIS Program Eliminates
Fat *and* Water Weight."

This video, and all of my videos, can be found at *www.UniqueHealing.com* or at *www.YouTube.com/UniqueHealing.*

# Healing Your Bowel With This Program Eliminates Weight Problems

A healthy bacterial environment in your bowel is needed for you to attain a healthy weight naturally and permanently, too. The good bacteria in your bowel help produce neurotransmitters that affect sugar, food, alcohol, coffee, and other cravings. The more of these acidic foods and beverages you consume, the more you struggle with weight, as once again, excess weight is the product of un-eliminated acids. When your bowel is healthy your desire for these go down, and the less of these you consume, the lower your weight will be.

Numerous studies have found that individuals lose weight, and gain health, on a high-fiber diet. In one, researchers at Children's Hospital in Boston found that men and women who ate a diet high in fiber gained the least weight over a ten-year period, regardless of how much fat they consumed. The people who gained the most had diets low in both fiber and fat. (Notice that this was a long-term study, which is the most credible type.) Unfortunately, when your bowel bacterial environment is unhealthy, this diet advice can be hard to follow. When your bowel is unhealthy, a high fiber diet can produce excessive amounts of gas and bloating. These discomforts are often enough to, understandably, cause many of you to stop eating this healthy, weight-loss producing, high fiber diet.

## Studies on bowel bacteria and weight

Not surprisingly, there is a limited amount of research that is funded on the link between weight problems and your bowel bacterial health, yet I found some relevant studies/articles, as discussed below.

According to one recent article, titled "Intestinal Bacteria May Explain Obesity," researchers at Washington University found that certain bacteria in your intestines appear to do better than others at helping their hosts turn food into energy. Researcher Buck Samuel inoculated identical mice with different microbes (i.e. bacteria) and found that mice that were inoculated with certain microbes stored more fat than other mice. While this is a very limited study and interpretation of the role of the bowel bacteria, it is a step in the right direction. After reading the article I entered a chat room to see the comments of people in response to it. Every one of them said that only exercise and less calories or more protein could cause weight loss, not intestinal bacteria. This is a belief that you have come to accept as absolute truth. I have a hard task trying to re-educate you about how your body works and why a healthy intestinal environment is, with undeniable certainty, a contributor to healthy weight, but I'll never stop trying!

In the PBS video, "Fat: What No One is Telling You," the work of Dr. Lee Kaplan, a medical doctor affiliated with Mass General and the Harvard Medical School, is highlighted. (The secrets of the bowel are this doctor's passion.) He has found that gastric bypass surgery works, because with this, your stomach is attached to your bowel and some nerves are cut in your gut/bowel, and these alter signals to your brain, signals that tell you to eat. He believes that in the next five to ten years we will learn many more things about how important the gut is. (With the *Unique Healing* books, you can learn about them *now*.)

Dr. Michael Gershan, from Colombia University, also says that your gut affects your brain, and your cravings for food. He says this was discovered long ago but forgotten. Is this because no drug was found that could alter the bowel bacterial environment? It is hard not to think so. (The pharmaceutical giant GlaxoSmithKline largely funded the above video.)

Gershan says that the gut plays a role in deciding when and what we eat, and that the "brain" in the gut disturbs the one in the head. (Furthermore, he found that stimulating nerves in the gut relieves depression, increases memory, and reduces epileptic seizures.)

Finally, as reported in the *Wall Street Journal* (2/7/11), researchers found that 7% of breast-fed babies were considered obese at age three compared with 13% of formula fed children. (Also, obesity levels rose the earlier babies were given solids; if fed solids before age 4 months, there was a six-fold increase in obesity than if solids were not introduced until 4-5 months). No explanation was given for these findings, but I suggest that it is the beneficial bacteria in breast milk, that are not present in formula, that account for these less overweight children.

In addition to its many other important functions, a healthy bacterial environment in your bowel is a necessity for the complete elimination of acids (toxins, heavy metals, pesticides, etc.) from your body. A healthy bowel prevents the re-absorption of acids into your blood that cause fat and water weight production.

# Why My Crutches Eliminate Weight Problems

*Body Bentonite* binds to and eliminates acids (toxins, heavy metals, chemicals, etc.) from your body. It helps prevent them from becoming re-absorbed into your bloodstream, where they trigger a response by your body to protect you from them. It eliminates the acids that trigger the production of fat and the retention of water. It is the most valuable and effective crutch for weight loss.

*Unique Healing Calcium Citrate* is an alkalinizing mineral that helps neutralize the acids that your bowel does not eliminate. When these acids are neutralized, your body does not need to retain water or create fat cells to buffer them.

*Unique Healing Methyl Vitamin B-12 12* provides your body with easy to assimilate levels of this nutrient, which reduces your cravings for "weight-producing" substances like alcohol, coffee, and sugar, for example.

**Note:** The above-mentioned crutches can quickly help you lose water weight. Un-eliminated acids in your blood cause water weight, and there are "only so many of these." Fat weight, on the other hand, is caused by many years of accumulated acidity, and you cannot quickly eliminate this. You will be eliminating it with this program, but to eliminate fat quickly, you need to either reduce calories, or increase your exercise levels. If you are patient, you can simply wait for your healthier body to eliminate the acids that are causing you to hold onto fat weight.

## How much do I take?/Questions about using these

See Chapter 5 for information on using these crutches, including recommendations on the amount to use, as well as a discussion of the misunderstandings about the particular crutch that may, if not understood correctly, cause you to fail to lose weight while you heal your bowel and body with this program.

## Why My Diet Crutches Eliminate Weight Problems

The information provided in Chapter 9 of *Unique Healing* on diet pertains to weight loss as well. Review this chapter now.

To quickly summarize, the low acid, alkalinizing diet recommended in my book reduces the intake of new acidity that causes fat and water weight gain, and helps your body buffer the existing acidity in your blood, reducing water weight gain. My book strives to teach you how to reduce the old acids in your organs from moving into your blood faster than you can eliminate them, and this also reduces water weight as well.

Remember, these dietary recommendations are advisable while you are healing your bowel and body with this program. They are not meant for the long-term. A long-term healthy diet contains a much larger amount of carbohydrates and much less protein than this "transition crutch diet."

## Eat easy-to-digest foods

An easy-to-digest diet yields more energy for acid (and therefore fat and water weight) elimination. When your body is not busy digesting food, it has more time to eliminate acids. Some of the easy-to-digest foods that I especially recommend are vegetables, avocado, cheese, and nut butters.

Eating proteins that are easy-to-digest helps you build muscle faster, and muscle helps your body burn fat. Replace as many of the hard-to-digest proteins that you eat, like chicken, beef, and turkey, with proteins that are easier to digest, like fish, soft-cooked eggs, and protein powders, especially whey and rice protein powders.

## Replace acidic foods with similar, alkaline ones

Replace wine and distilled vinegars with apple cider and balsamic vinegars; replace coffee with unsweetened tea; replace salt with sea salt. Replacing these acidic foods with similar alkalinizing ones reduces the new acids entering your body that cause fat and water production. These foods are also alkalinizing and can buffer the acids in your blood that cause water weight gain.

Several years ago, a client travelled to Jordon with her parents, and while there, she ate three big meals a day and was not exercising. She drank eight bottles of bottled water every day, which was special water from the nearby Dead Sea that contained a high amount of natural sodium. During this vacation, in which diet and exercise were not followed, she lost eight pounds. This was a result of the high amount of alkalinity she was drinking every day from the natural salt water. Alkaline foods buffer the acids that cause water weight.

## And most importantly, do not eat a more cleansing diet, yet

Fruit, carbohydrates such as breads, pastas, cereals and grains (even if they are wheat or gluten-free), sugar (even natural sugar such as agave and honey), and other high carbohydrate foods (foods with more than 15 grams of carbohydrates/serving), such as yogurt, "move" stored acids from your organs into your blood and bowel to be eliminated. This can trigger fat and water weight gain if these acids move into your blood and bowel faster than you can eliminate them.

If your stools are not daily and very well formed, you have excess acids in your blood and bowel, and you will likely have extra weight as a result.

High protein foods like chicken, fish, turkey, beef, eggs, etc. are non-cleansing. While they are not healthy to eat in large amounts in the long-term, eating them can help you lose weight in the short-term, while you are healing your bowel and body with this program.

Note: Even though fruit and natural sugar such as honey and agave are alkalinizing, they are even more cleansing than they are alkalinizing, and eating them, while healthy for you, can easily cause you to gain weight when your bowel and body are not healthy. However, if you have to make a choice between an acidic, cleansing food such as sugar, and an alkaline, cleansing food such as honey or fruit, pick the alkaline one. You can find more information on the acidity or alkalinity of foods in Chapter 9 of *Unique Healing*.

## Vegetables are not cleansing

Vegetables contain carbohydrates, but the amount is minimal. Coupled with the fact that they also contain a large amount of alkalinizing minerals, vegetables are "non-cleansing," and eating them "keeps" the acids in your blood to a minimum, which means they help keep your weight down. This is why they are allowed in abundance on every diet plan imaginable. It is also why "green drinks" are popular weight loss beverages.

The exception to this rule, however, is that very sweet vegetables, such as yams and sweet potatoes, *are* cleansing and may cause you to retain weight if eaten. Regular potatoes have a higher carbohydrate content than green vegetables, and these too may be too cleansing for you; eating too many of them may not allow you to lose weight as quickly as you might like.

On the other hand, sweet potatoes and regular potatoes contain a lot of alkalinizing minerals, so if given a choice, choose these over high carbohydrate foods like breads, pastas, cereals, etc. if you are trying to lose weight.

## Eat more healthy fat

Eating more high quality fats will also help you lose water weight faster. They give you energy and help reduce your cravings for sugars, which trigger water weight. Some fats, such as olive oil and avocadoes, are alkalinizing and "non-cleansing." Also, nuts and seeds, cheese, sour cream, and butter are very low in acidity (and you do need to consume some acidic foods for health), and they too do not cleanse your body.

Be careful however if you are currently eating a very low calorie diet, and you are relying on this to "burn fat." If you increase your intake of calories by eating more fat, you may temporarily gain more weight.

## Avoid allergic foods

As is true in all cases where I make dietary suggestions, if you are allergic to a food, do not consume it until your bowel is healed, and you can consume it without harm or symptoms. In the case of asthma, this is especially important, given the seriousness of this condition and potential danger of it.

I do not conduct food allergy tests because the majority of the clients I see (and you) do not have them. (Re-read the section on "Food Allergies" in this chapter for a better understanding of this concept, including an explanation of why many of your "food allergies" are not true allergies at all.) The majority of the clients I work with who do have them have already had these tested and determined; and because the most common allergens like dairy, wheat, shellfish, nuts, and eggs can be tested on your own by avoiding these and/or observing your reaction to them, I find no need to conduct these tests. If desired, you can likely find a local allergist or practitioner who will do extensive food allergy testing for you.

## An example of a diet you might follow

For breakfast you might choose two eggs with spinach, 1 ounce of cheese and a cup of green tea. For lunch, a large salad with 1/8 cup of sliced almonds, a slice of avocado, vegetables, 2 ounces of feta cheese, and 6 ounces of grilled salmon or chicken, and balsamic vinaigrette salad dressing. As a snack, you might choose cottage cheese with eight to ten whole grain crackers. For dinner, you might choose 6 ounces of fish with cooked vegetables and a baked potato with one tablespoon of butter and sea salt.

Drink large quantities of water, unsweetened tea (green, black, and/or herbal), or tea sweetened with stevia.

## A healthy diet can cause weight gain

Cleansing foods, like fruit, carbohydrates, and yogurt, are healthy for you, but cleansing foods can trigger water weight gain. Here is the great irony and difficulty that many of you face. If you try to eat healthier, you can gain weight, and if you eat a less healthy diet, you may lose weight. Because this less healthy, "quick weight-loss diet" makes your organs less healthy—the ones that are supposed to keep you thin naturally and effortlessly—down the road however, you often find that it is more difficult to lose weight. It can be an ugly, frustrating, vicious cycle. This program will break this cycle for you.

A healthy diet also incorporates a good amount of healthy fats such as nuts, olive oil, avocadoes, and cheese. These foods are also calorie-dense, however, and when your liver is unhealthy, your consumption of them can cause you to create more fat. This will not happen once you have healed your liver with this program.

## This program offsets the damage of an unhealthy diet

Programs that rely solely on a low cleansing (i.e. high protein) diet are dangerous, and they set you up for the vicious cycle of failure described above. This program is different. It is not dangerous (on the contrary, it reverses dangerous health conditions), and it will help you break this vicious cycle.

While I am suggesting you *temporarily* consume more protein than is ideally healthy for you, you will also be healing your bowel and body, and the recommendations for doing this are strong enough to more than offset the harm of this diet. You will be eliminating more acidity than you will be "putting back into you with a higher protein diet." This is not true when you simply follow one of these diets and do not concurrently heal your bowel and body (as is almost always the case otherwise.)

## Can't follow a strict diet?

A low calorie, non-cleansing (i.e. low carb), alkalinizing diet will help keep your weight down while you are healing your bowel and body with this program; while you are waiting for your body to become healthy enough to eat a cleansing (i.e. higher carb) and higher calorie diet without it causing weight gain.

But this is a difficult diet to follow day in and day out, and if you find it too hard to follow, that's okay. This diet is recommended as a crutch to help you lose weight faster. But it is not a necessity for you to lose weight. If you can't follow it, you can simply follow this program and wait for your healthier bowel and body to cause weight loss. What other program can offer you this?

For some of you, this will require a great deal of patience, so it is up to you to decide which is harder: a strict diet, or patience? There are no easy answers. It is only once you heal your bowel and body that maintaining your weight will be extremely easy. If you do not heal your bowel and body, you will likely have a lifetime of difficulty dealing with your weight. Now this takes patience! So ultimately, following this program is much easier than other weight loss programs.

## How long will I need to use crutches for my weight problems?

Weight gain occurs at Levels 2, 3, and 4 of your pipe. It is the second, third, and fourth areas of your body to heal (assuming that other areas are unhealthy too). Refer to the diagram "Sequence of Healing" in Appendix A at the end of this book to better understand this concept, as well as to Chapter 1 under this subject heading.

## You might need to "wait" for fat loss

Excess weight consists of some combination of water and/or fat weight. Water weight goes down when you keep your blood pH from becoming too acidic/when you take *Body Bentonite* and eliminate the acids from your blood that otherwise can trigger water retention, and use *Unique Healing Calcium Citrate* to buffer them. Water weight can be eliminated relatively quickly.

Fat weight, on the other hand, is the result of accumulated fat in response to many years or large amounts of accumulated acids. *Body Bentonite* can quickly eliminate *future* fat weight from occurring, but for fat weight that exists prior to starting this program, my crutches cannot quickly eliminate this. Large accumulations of acidity take time to eliminate, even with an extremely aggressive healing program, like this one. You must invest some time into this program to get this result. (Or use a low calorie and/or exercise crutch to burn this fat.)

Your body holds onto acids in your organs and in your fat cells. If you have a lot of acidity in your organs, this is more dangerous, and when you begin eliminating acids with this program, it is this acidity that is eliminated first. You cannot control the area of your body that heals first, and while this may be frustrating, appreciate the great wisdom of your body, as it heals the most "dangerous stuff" first.

If you have been following this program for more than two months and your stools have been better formed during this time, and you have not changed a crutch (i.e. have not reduced your exercise or increased your calories), but you have not lost more than five pounds, then consider that you had a large amount of dangerous acidity affecting your organs (and longevity). In this case, you *really* needed this program, and in this case, you will need to wait until the dangerous acidity is gone before your body eliminates the acids in your fat cells, and the extra fat surrounding it.

## Why High Protein/Low Carbohydrate/Low Glucose/Low Glycemic Diet Crutches Are Failing You

Glucose is a vital nutrient necessary for life. Your body consistently needs a certain amount to feed your muscles and brain. Your body gets glucose from dietary carbohydrates (i.e. breads, pastas, bagels, cereals, grains, etc.) and sugar-containing foods (i.e. desserts, yogurt, honey, fruit, etc.). Dietary protein (i.e. chicken, turkey, beef, fish, eggs, etc.) does not provide glucose.

Therefore, when you eat a lot of protein, and very few carbohydrates or sugar, your body does not receive the glucose it needs. In response to this, your body converts some stored fat into fatty acids, which are then converted into this needed glucose by your liver. The accepted physiology of weight loss programs is that if you starve your body of glucose by eating a high protein, low sugar, low carbohydrate diet, stored fat will be converted into glucose and you will lose weight. (The terms high protein, low carbohydrate, low glucose, and low glycemic are synonymous and will herein simply be referred to as "high protein.")

Others explain this phenomenon by stating that high blood glucose levels increase the secretion of insulin, and insulin turns sugars into bad fatty acids, which are then turned into fats. I say that excess acidity in your blood triggers the production of fat to protect you from it (and excess acidity in your blood occurs alongside diets high in glucose, as glucose cleanses your organs and causes acids to exit them into your blood).

High protein diets are helpful for quickly losing weight because they contribute to significant loses of water weight as well, which lends to their incredible popularity (exercise and low calorie and low fat diet crutches, on the other hand, do not necessarily help with water weight reduction.)

High protein diets "work" because they stop your body from cleansing, resulting in fewer acids in your blood, which leads to less water and fat production, as described earlier. (Of course, this also results in more acids in your organs, which leads to more disease and death alongside your weight loss results.). Numerous studies have found this to be true. Re-read Chapter 5 of *Unique Healing* for more information on the dangers of these diets.

You may lose weight when you cut down carbohydrates, but that does not mean that eating them caused your problem. You may lose weight when you smoke two packs of cigarettes a day, as nicotine acts as an appetite suppressant, but that does not mean that "not smoking" was the cause of your weight gain, either.

Low carbohydrate, high protein diets do not heal your bowel or body, as this program does. They are crutches that you must depend on and commit to religiously and permanently in order to keep your weight down.

## Nowadays they are *all* high protein diets

High protein, low carbohydrate diets work in the short-term, and fail in the long-term, regardless of how these diets are marketed, named, or described. Some of the other names used for these diets are "South Beach Diet," "The Zone," "Atkins Diet," "The Psoriasis Cure," "Maker's Diet," "Weight Watchers," and "NutriSystem." Every month or so, a new weight loss book hits the shelves, and the majority of them are high protein diets. A recent article on weight loss in *People* highlighted individuals who lost 100 pounds. While they all ate different foods, all of their diets were low calories and high in protein. For one day I counted the percentage of calories from protein and it was approximately 50%. Because you only need 10% of your calories from protein, eating five times more than this is not only considered very high in protein, it is very dangerous as well.

High protein diets are even recommended for people who have undergone gastric bypass surgery, which contributes to the weight loss (and danger and short-term results) seen with many who have undergone these procedures.

## The great appeal of high protein diets

High protein diets are more popular than ever, and I believe this stems from several reasons, including the fact that they are easy. You can find high protein foods at almost any restaurant, and with all the eating out many of you do these days, this makes this type of diet convenient. Most of you also have a lot of experience cooking high protein foods like chicken and steak. Learning to eat the foods on these diets is therefore not much of a stretch for most of you. Finally, high protein diets can result in both the reduction of body fat *and* water weight. Other weight loss crutches, including low calorie diets and exercise, do little to nothing to alter the water weight on your body, which can contribute many pounds to the scale.

## The dangers and long-term effects of high protein diets

High protein diets are dangerous. They recommend an excess of protein consumption; much more than government and dietary agencies recommend. Excess protein is acidic, and excess acidity damages those organs in your body that, ironically, are responsible for keeping fat production and water retention down, naturally and effortlessly, in the first place.

Thousands of studies have found a link between higher protein consumption and higher rates of early death from every disease imaginable. And the medical profession even recognizes the damage that these inflict on your kidneys, as they advise a very low protein diet to patients with kidney disease.

When you stop following a high-protein diet, you are left with a body that is less healthy than it was before. These diets make the cause of your weight problems—an unhealthy bowel and body—worse. As a result, when you stop the diet, you often find yourself gaining back all or more of the weight you lost. This is a documented fact. You fail with these diets because your body always "wins:" eventually it craves some much-needed carbohydrates. Your body's need for glucose eventually becomes stronger than your will power.

When you follow these diets and your bowel and body become less healthy, it becomes harder to lose weight in the future and a vicious cycle ensues in which desperation sets in, creating greater appeal for programs that deliver a quick fix, regardless of their safety. You fall even harder for the dangerous quick fix.

Seven to ten days before Dr. Atkins, the "high-protein diet doctor," died, he went into a coma. The medical autopsy revealed that *during those seven to ten days* he gained *sixty* pounds of water weight! Journalists and scientists attributed this to his horrific high-protein diet, which damages all of your organs, but is especially damaging to your kidneys (which, when healthy, prevent the retention of water in the first place).

Additionally, when un-eliminated acids are "forced out of your blood and into your cells" with high protein diets, your body is more likely to create internal fat that is damaging to your organs, but that does not appear as fat on your body.

A recent article titled *"Thin People May Be Fat Inside,"* by Maria Cheng, demonstrates this concern. It also shows that others are seeing the need for a new definition of health and weight, and that there are some serious dangers in our current interpretations. The article states that internal fat surrounding vital organs could be more dangerous than the external fat that bulges underneath the skin. Dr. Jimmy Bell and his team scanned nearly 800 people with MRI machines to see where it is that people store fat. According to their data, people who maintained their weight through diet rather than exercise were likely to have major deposits of internal fat, even if they were otherwise slim. As many as 45% of the women tested and 60% of the men tested who had normal body mass index (BMI) scores were found to have excessive levels of internal fat. "The whole concept of being fat needs to be redefined," said Bell. Dieting methods were not discussed, but if the average, low calorie, low carbohydrate diet has been followed (and really, this is the only possible scenario), then yes, fat will accumulate internally. *Concern was expressed over the fact that when one is skinny they can dangerously assume they are healthier than they really are.*

Hundreds of books and alternative and medical practitioners recommend these diets, yet few studies have been done that have looked at the link between these diets and long-term weight loss results. The Atkins craze stimulated research into this area and results should be forthcoming. I can tell you right now what this will show. They will show that, again, the majority of people who followed these diets have, in the long-term, gained back all or more of the weight that they had before starting the diet. When we finally look at the *long-term* effects of these high-protein recommendations, the results will be shocking. Hopefully it will be enough to end, once and for all, the high-protein craze. (Note: I originally wrote this section to this book two years ago, yet the results of this research, which should have long been published and discussed by the media by now, never materialized. You and I have not heard about the results. Why?).

Long-term studies show that people who eat a low protein diet are thinner than meat eaters. A 1997 study by the American Cancer Society tracked the dietary and lifestyle habits of 79, 236 healthy adults and found that the more vegetables and less meat subjects ate, the less likely they were to become overweight. And among 80,000 Americans surveyed in 1982, and again 10 years later, people who were most likely to gain weight were those who ate meat frequently. Low protein diets are healthier for you, and over the long-term, they help keep your organs that regulate your weight healthier, too. (You, however, are likely looking for "short-term" results, so again, for now, follow my recommendations for a temporarily higher-than-ideal protein diet, and be grateful that as a result of this program, one day you will be able to eat a lower protein, healthier diet and keep your weight down.)

You need to do this program for many reasons, but especially so that these dangerous diets are no longer appealing to you.

> Too many carbohydrates do not cause overweight conditions. An unhealthy bowel and body cause weight gain.

## Why Low Calorie/Low Fat Diet Crutches Are Failing You

As described previously with regard to high protein diets, restricting calories "works" because when you eat less, there is less glucose available and your body may burn fat into this much needed glucose for you. They "don't work" because you must constantly eat a low calorie diet to maintain this fat-burning mechanism. They are a crutch and once you stop, as is true with *all* weight loss crutches, your excess weight returns. (Because fat is high in calories, a low fat diet turns into a low calorie diet, and the same concepts apply.)

Have you noticed that these diets are returning? Here we go again! The cycle keeps turning and turning. In years past, when these diets were popular, they failed to deliver long-term weight loss or optimum health, and they will do so again.

Eating less calories and starving yourself is not a step towards health. People who are dying lose their appetite. You need to stop viewing having an appetite with weight gain, and in negative connotations. An article in a Naturopathic publication (which treats symptoms), states that "a biological evolutionary design protects us from starvation, but such a mechanism is not as critical or innately fine tuned for the restraint of food intake; thus predisposition toward obesity." In other words, they generally too believe that extra food causes weight gain. They also recognize that strict low calorie diets are close to impossible to follow in the long-term, hence their very common recommendations for dangerous high protein diet crutches for weight loss, as well.

According to the *Wall Street Journal* (4/2/11), the Obama Administration approved the initial spending of $315 million, and then $44 million/year thereafter, to have foods in restaurants and by vendors labeled with calorie content, *even though the posting of calories has not been proven to curtail obesity* (this already has been done in twenty cities and there is no evidence that it helps).

Low calorie, low fat diets do not heal your bowel or body, and they are crutches that you must depend on and commit to religiously and permanently in order to keep your weight down, but at least they can be much healthier and safer than high protein diets.

Too many calories or fat do not cause overweight conditions. An unhealthy bowel and body cause weight gain.

## Why Food Allergy/Gluten-free Diet Crutches Are Failing You

These diets also do not heal your bowel or body (the cause of your weight gain), either, and many of you fail to lose weight on these diets, as they can be high in calories (thereby failing as a low-calorie weight loss crutch) and high in carbohydrates (thereby failing as a low-protein weight loss crutch as well).

Gluten-free does not mean low calorie, or low carbohydrate, in other words. In a recent article titled "Giving Up Gluten To Lose Weight? Not So Fast: Diet is Effective in Treating Celiac Disease, Wheat Allergies, But Not for Shedding Pounds" (Wall Street Journal, 8/24/10), the following statement was made: "The notion that a gluten-free diet can help people lose weight or avoid carbohydrates is a myth." And as stated by Shelley Case, registered dietician, "Many packaged gluten-free products are even higher in carbs, sugar, fat and calories than their regular counterparts . . . . In fact, a serving of regular pasta has 41 grams of carbohydrate while a serving of gluten-free pasta has 46 grams."

These diets "work" only when they also become low calorie, low carbohydrate diets. But then again, they also fail in the long run, and are dangerous in the long run, for all the reasons that all low carbohydrate/high protein diets are, as discussed earlier.

Food allergies do not cause overweight conditions. An unhealthy bowel and body cause weight gain.

# Why Alkalinizing and Detoxifying Diet Crutches Are Failing You

These diets help with weight loss because they reduce the acidity in your blood by buffering it with alkalinizing minerals contained in foods and supplements. Remember, however, that this buffers these acids, yet it does nothing to permanently eliminate them from your body, as this program does, and therefore these diets do not lead to permanent, effortless weight loss, as this program does.

When the acids in your blood (that are not being eliminated because of an unhealthy bowel) are neutralized with alkaline minerals, your body no longer needs to retain water to buffer them, and you lose water weight. Neutralizing these acids also reduces blood glucose levels, which in turn reduces appetite and the secretion of insulin and the resultant production of body fat.

Incidentally, alkalinizing and detoxifying diets are almost always low in calories as well, and they "work" but also "fail you" for the same reasons given for low calorie diets crutches earlier.

*Skinny Bitch,* a recent diet book that relies largely on alkalinizing and low calorie diet crutches for weight loss, is a healthy diet, but it is unfortunately bound to fail. It will fail because it relies on crutches, and because most of you will find this diet too difficult to follow for a long period of time. Also, it is very high in fiber and the frequent bowel movements, gas, bloating, and stomach discomfort that this can cause when you follow this diet and have an unhealthy bowel is likely to make you stop the diet altogether.

Another alkalinizing diet that has been around for decades, that regains surges in popularity from time to time, is the "Master Cleanse." On this diet you consume only drinks made from lemon juice, maple syrup, and cayenne for three to ten days. This is a low calorie diet crutch as well which "works" and "fails you" for the same reason that all alkalinizing and low-calorie diet crutches do. It can also be very cleansing (due to the maple syrup) and this can cause you to look and feel worse, not better. Like all alkalinizing and detoxifying diets, it is very misleading and falsely misrepresents toxin elimination from your body.

Grapefruit is alkalinizing, and grapefruit diets have also been used for years as well. In one twelve-week study participants who ate ½ a grapefruit three times a day lost an average of 3.6 pounds. In another, dieters who ate half a grapefruit, or drank grapefruit juice with every meal, lost seven times more weight than those who didn't. (Be careful before you start eating a lot of grapefruit, however, because grapefruit is cleansing. If you replace white sugar in your diet with grapefruit, your blood will be less acidic and you will likely lose some weight quickly; if you continue eating sugar and add a lot of grapefruit juice to this diet, you are unlikely to lose weight quickly, and may even gain it.)

In a 2005 study published in the *Journal of the American Dietetic Association*, participants who consumed about one tablespoon of (alkalinizing) apple cider vinegar, along with a bagel and fruit juice reduced the post-meal rise in glucose in half compared to those eating the same meal without the additional cider vinegar. The cider drinkers also ended up eating 200-275 fewer calories a day as a result of this vinegar addition to their diet.

In another study, people who drank tea at least once a week had 20 percent less body fat than non-tea-drinkers. And a 2005 study in Japan found that of subjects drinking green tea (4-5 cups a day) lost an average of 5.3 pounds compared to a control group that lost only 2.9 pounds. *Both were on the same low calorie diet.* The researchers comment that green tea appears to rev up the rate at which the liver breaks down fat, decreases fat absorption from the gut, and boosts levels of the neurotransmitter norepinephrine, which plays a role in how the body burns calories. More simply, green tea is highly alkalinizing, and alkalinizing diets are weight loss crutches that work, and eventually fail you, all the time.

The medical profession often criticizes alkalinizing and detoxifying diets. In January 2009, a local medical doctor gave his recommendations on weight-loss programs on the local news. He said, "It is a waste of money to detoxify to lose weight because your liver, kidneys, and skin will detoxify for you." Let me correct this statement for you. All of you who need to lose weight have too many toxins in your body, and if your body automatically detoxified them for you, none of you would be overweight! Every overweight person I see has noticeable ill health in at least two, if not three, of the organs he mentioned. When you are finished healing your body, then, and only then, will you have the natural ability to detoxify without further help. Finally, notice he made no mention of your bowel, which is hands-down, the most important detoxifier (or eliminator) in your body.

Having said that, he is correct in criticizing these diets, as they are just temporary weight loss crutches. More so, *my* criticism is that they do *not* cause the elimination of toxins (acids) from your body that you are led to believe that they do! You can only eliminate toxins through your stool, urine, breath, or sweat. These diets do nothing to increase these, although you are often led to believe that you are eliminating toxins because one, when you feel better, you are told that you have eliminated toxins (not true), and two, if you experience more frequent elimination on these diets (which is common due to the higher fiber and magnesium content of them, and these two substances tend to increase the frequency of your bowel movements), you are told that you have eliminated more toxins through your stool (not true either). If you do not understand why frequent elimination does not mean that you are eliminating more toxins from your body, review Chapter 6 of *Unique Healing* until you do.

Finally, be careful with these diets, as many alkaline-containing foods, like fruit, are very cleansing, and their cleansing attributes usually overshadow their alkalinizing attributes, meaning that you can follow a high-alkalinizing diet and still retain weight due to the increase in un-eliminated acids in your blood that cleansing diets create.

Alkalinizing and detoxifying diets are mostly very safe and healthy, but they are difficult to follow in the long-term, and like *all* diet crutches, the only way to maintain your weight with these diets is to follow them religiously and permanently. Few of you will succeed with these programs. (This was Oprah's latest craze when I originally wrote this section of this book. I wrote this a couple years ago and not surprisingly, I see she is still struggling to lose weight.)

A lack of alkalinizing minerals does not cause overweight conditions. An unhealthy bowel and body cause weight gain.

## Why Exercise Crutches Are Failing You

Exercise is a crutch and most of it is performed in an *effort to lose weight.* In a 1998 national study of 36,598 overweight people, the Centers for Disease Control and Prevention found that 66% of men and 62% of women were trying to lose weight by participating in physical activity. ("Exercise Frequency in the United States," Nutrition Week, May 5, 2000;

30(18): 7.) I do not have recent statistics on this, but my observation and experience is that this number has *increased* over the years.

As described earlier, your blood consistently needs a certain amount of glucose to feed your muscles and brain. If your glucose level gets too low, your body can convert stored fat into fatty acids, which are then turned into glucose by your liver. During any strenuous exercise, such as running, aerobics, and biking, your muscles require a greater supply of energy (glucose) to perform. After a given period of time this can result in a breakdown of stored fat (i.e. weight loss), as this stored fat is converted into fatty acids and then glucose. The primary benefits of exercise, it is said, are an increased *metabolism,* which is really just a term to describe the breaking down of fats into fatty acids.

When you exercise to lose weight, your body breaks down excess fat so that is available as an energy source, but this does *nothing* to eliminate the acids that *caused* the excess fat to be produced and stored in the first place. This means that when you stop it, your weight will increase again. It means that you may look better as a result of this exercise, but you have done nothing to extend your life and prevent death from disease.

In fact, forcing your body to break down fat with exercise can be harmful and dangerous. Without fat to buffer your un-eliminated acids, your body has to buffer them another way. For example, it may turn to your cells' supply of alkalinizing sodium and potassium to buffer these acids, resulting in cellular death, cancer, and your death. This is a possible explanation for why we are seeing more and more thin people die prematurely of cancer and heart disease.

Exercise does not permanently heal your body or bowel, as this program does. It is a crutch that you must depend on and commit to religiously and permanently in order to keep your (fat) weight off.

## And exercise can only cause fat loss, not water weight loss

Exercise can burn fat weight, but it cannot eliminate extra water weight. Many of you have gotten "stuck" with your weight loss programs because of this; you have been led to believe that all of your extra weight is fat and that exercise will get rid of all of it for you. This is not true.

When you watch weight-loss programs on television, or read about celebrities who have lost a lot of weight, the exercise portion of their weight loss is highly emphasized, and this is misleading. They are not just exercising to lose weight; they are also following strict low carbohydrate diets, which cause water weight loss as well.

The *Unique Healing* program eliminates fat weight *and* water weight.

## Keep your exercise aerobic

In many areas of life we have been led to believe that more is always better. This same mentality applies to exercise as well. There *are* some wonderful benefits of exercise, like increased circulation, endorphin production/mental health improvement, and the movement of your lymphatic fluids, but it has many limitations, too. While it is a crutch that can help you lose weight, if done wrong, it can be stressful and trigger health problems, even death. This can occur if you exercise beyond the capacity of your body to eliminate the lactic acid that is generated during it. A recent client had a heart attack while exercising, which was attributed to his exercise, and a Kennedy just died while working out (which may or may not have triggered the death), but still, it is a story that is not uncommon.

During aerobic exercise your body maintains a positive oxygen balance; you increase your blood oxygen levels and this is very healthy for you. During anaerobic exercise, you reduce oxygen levels and this is unhealthy for you. During exercise your muscles produce lactic acid, an acid like all acids that needs to be eliminated. When more lactic acid is produced than your body can eliminate, such as occurs during anaerobic exercise, you harm your body and organs, as they become stressed, buffering this acidity.

If you over-exert yourself and fall into the "more is better" mentality, you can easily move into an anaerobic state. This dangerous possibility is why you are told to consult with your doctor prior to embarking on an exercise program. That alone should tell you something.

There are a few ways to ensure that your exercise is aerobic and healthy. One, you should be able to breathe easily and talk while exercising. You should not be extremely sore the next day. And your heart rate should be maintained within safe limits. This is taught at aerobics classes, and information on this can be found online and in many exercise books. Many athletes depend on a heart rate monitor or are told how to monitor their heart rate so that it stays within safe limits. I highly recommend these. If you exercise to the point where it is difficult for you to catch your breath, you are overdoing it and need to slow down.

Walking, Pilates, and yoga are excellent forms of exercise that keep your body in an aerobic state. During many of these, a focus in placed on deep breathing so that acids are eliminated. You may not burn calories and lose weight as quickly with these as with other forms of exercise, but they can be much healthier for you than other forms of exercise, and ultimately, a healthier body will help you stay thin.

## Other dangers of exercise as a weight loss crutch

One of the greatest dangers of using exercise to lose weight occurs when you believe that your thinner body is a healthier one, and that you are automatically immune to disease, and premature death, as a result.

Fit does not necessarily mean healthy. Being "fit" means that you look good. It does not necessarily mean that your body and organs are healthy.

I was thin and working out four times a week when I became ill with a devastating autoimmune disease. Millions of people who are fit and thin die from cancer and heart disease, and suffer from an endless list of health and mental symptoms, because they are not healthy.

If you are overweight and lose weight, your joints might feel better, for example, because less weight is being placed on them. This is great, but it does not mean that your immune system is healthier (which is the system that should be preventing joint pain/inflammation in the first place). You have simply reduced the rain hitting the roof without fixing the holes. You are often led to assume that these holes are fixed, and this can be dangerous if you think you are invincible and healthier than you really are. This can reduce your need to find the real cause of your joint pain or other symptoms. When you strengthen your immune system with this program, you not only reduce your joint pain, but your chance of getting cancer too, for example.

I lived in Boulder, Colorado for eighteen years. It is a very athletic, active town. Numerous professional athletes train and live there, and on any given warm weekend you can find hundreds of runners, cyclists, hikers, and mountain climbers outside. Yet I have worked with many locals who have unhealthy bowels and bodies and significant health problems, even though they are fit and thin. I have seen the gamut of health problems, including cancer and heart disease, in these fit clients.

A PBS video on weight loss documented the case of an overweight woman with no history of cancer; and her sister who is thin who has had cancer three times. We need to wake up and realize that this is not an uncommon story! Dr. Louis Teichholz, chief of cardiology at Hackensack Hospital in New Jersey, commented that "just because someone is lean doesn't make them immune to diabetes or other risk factors for heart disease." Amen to that, too.

Also, in the February 2008 issue of "Shape" magazine Dr. Kathy Magliato, cardiothoracic surgeon, commented, "Being thin and fit isn't a heart health guarantee." This comment was in part a response to a recent survey from the Society for Women's Health Research that found that almost 36 percent of women didn't know that even if you eat right and exercise, you can still have dangerously unhealthy cholesterol levels."

## You can't "exercise off" the harmful effects of diet

When you are thin and working out, it is easy to adopt the mentality that you don't need to worry about what you eat because you will be burning off the calories.

It is not safe, and you are putting yourself at risk of future weight problems, if you adopt this mentality. Working out does not eliminate the harmful effects that eating poorly has on your health. It can eliminate the chance that these calories become fat, but it does not eliminate the chance that these foods will harm you and cause disease.

If you eat sugar all day and work off the calories from it, you may be thin, but the exercise has not eliminated the damage to your health by this sugar; it has not reduced your susceptibility to early heart disease and cancer, for example. And this sugar also makes your organs less healthy; the ones that are supposed to keep you naturally thin in the first place, so that later on, it is even harder to maintain your weight.

Overweight conditions are not caused by a lack of exercise. An unhealthy bowel and body cause weight gain.

# Why Weight Loss Supplement
# Crutches Are Failing You

As found in many health and drug stores, as well as heavily marketed in infomercials, most weight loss supplements contain herbs and other ingredients that act as stimulants, reducing your desire for food (so you eat a low calorie diet, which works, but fails you, for all of the reasons given earlier in the section on low calorie diet crutches). Some contain natural diuretics that reduce water weight, and while they are safe crutches, they do nothing to heal your kidneys, which should keep extra water weight off of you in the first place. They do not heal your bowel and body and you would need to take these daily to maintain your weight, something few of you want to do, will do, or can afford to do. Likewise, since they do not heal your bowel and body, you can, and most likely will, become less healthy as you continue with these supplements, and eventually find that you need to take larger amounts to maintain the same amount of weight loss as earlier. This increases the likelihood of your not continuing with these crutches on a daily basis, and a return of your weight problems once you stop them, as happens with all weight loss crutches.

Some of these weight loss supplements contain stimulants that can be harmful if your heart is unhealthy, and I do not personally recommend them.

## Why Medical/Drug Crutches Are Failing You

Doctors are taught to treat your symptoms and diseases with crutches, so it should come as no surprise that they take a similar approach to weight loss.

I saw an episode of Dr. Phil in which he promised "a weight loss program that delivers long-term results, where you never have to struggle again." A few people were given a personal trainer for three months and a big prize, like a trip to Hawaii, at the end of the program, if they met their weight goals. No long-term follow-ups were done on these people, even though that's what the show promised—long-term weight loss without the struggle! Are these people going to hire a personal trainer, and have to find someone who will buy them a trip to Hawaii every three months to help motivate them to keep up with a strict exercise program to keep their weight off? Is this the idea behind long-term struggle-free weight loss that he tempted viewers with? I thought the show was very deceptive to make a promise and then not fulfill it.

A while back I also saw Dr. Oz on Oprah promoting his new weight-loss book, which focuses on reducing calories. He wants people to aim for eating 100 fewer calories per day. What is new and revolutionary about the promotion of a low-calorie diet to lose weight? Haven't we heard this same story a trillion times already? Haven't we seen this approach fail to work in the long-term long enough to conclude that we need another approach?

## You could lose weight by snorting cocaine, too

Dr. Oz also says that the goal is not to lose weight but to eat foods with nutrients. For example, he says no diet sodas are allowed. He said he could get someone to lose weight if they took chemotherapy drugs. I think this is a very valuable comment, and I am always saying something similar:

"You could lose weight snorting cocaine because it acts as an appetite suppressant, but that does not mean it (your extra weight) was caused by a cocaine deficiency!" It also does not mean that it is a safe way to lose weight. It certainly is not. Likewise, you can lose weight eating a low carbohydrate diet, but that does not mean that your extra weight was caused by a protein deficiency, or that it is safe.

Drugs are crutches, and drugs that are used for weight loss are as well. Like high protein diets, they are acidic and damage your organs that should be keeping you thin naturally and effortless, and therefore, they have the potential to create greater weight struggles in the future.

There will never be a drug that helps you to lose weight safely, and/ or permanently.

## The connection between smoking/nicotine and weight loss

Nicotine is a drug, and it is one that has been used for weight loss for decades.

According to a study in *Science*, researchers at Yale found that low doses of nicotine reduced body fat in mice by 15% to 20% and food intake by up to 50%. Research showed that nicotine acted on a brain pathway involved in the regulation of appetite. In other words, when you use it to lose weight, you are using a "low calorie" crutch.

Reducing your appetite with a toxic, acidic drug like nicotine is a dangerous and temporary approach to losing weight. You may be thinner, but you are risking a lower quality and shorter life, in return. When you heal your bowel and body with this program, you can be thin, and have a long, high quality life as well.

## Gastric bypass, liposuction, and other weight loss surgeries

These are crutches for losing weight that can be very dangerous and deadly. Upon writing this, Kanye West's mother made the news due to her death following breast surgery and liposuction.

There is always a risk with surgery. I think that the use of these crutches for weight loss should only be used as a last resort. Having said that, I understand how people must become frustrated and desperate enough to use them. I understand the people who are critical of these methods as they are usually people who have made great sacrifices with diet and exercise to lose weight. These people say you must "suffer" to lose weight and do it the "hard way." They want to believe this is true. I do not agree that people who use these procedures are taking the easy way out, as they are often accused of. They have simply been led down the wrong road.

If you are overweight and others don't have compassion for you, it is because they are jealous, fearful, or incapable of admitting that they don't have the answer for you. You deserve better than that.

# Why Mental/Emotional Weight Loss Crutches Are Failing You

When you use weight loss crutches and they fail, your mental/emotional health are inevitably blamed for this failure. It is a weakness in your character, we accuse.

When I was sick, and twenty-five doctors didn't know how to help me, they blamed my symptoms on stress and emotional issues. In truth, they simply didn't know how to help me, so they "blamed me" instead of their lack of knowledge. It is not to say that I, or many of you, did not have room to grow and improve emotionally and mentally, but these problems are separate issues, and they do not cause your health or weight problems.

If you followed a weight loss program and have regained weight, blame the program you followed, not yourself.

I have compassion for anyone and everyone who is struggling, or has struggled, to lose weight. It does not have to be this way, but as long as you keep using weight loss crutches to lose weight, and do not heal your bowel and body, it will always be a struggle.

Today, my ability to effortlessly maintain a healthy weight has nothing to do with my mental or emotional health. In fact, healing my body allowed me to become much healthier in these two regards, not the other way around.

> My ability to effortlessly maintain my weight has nothing to do with me being a better person than you. It has to do with the fact that I am much healthier than you are.

## It's not a lack of discipline or willpower

Even though I have never been overweight, prior to my illness, my weight was on my mind daily, and obsessively. I relied on starvation and frequent exercise to maintain my weight. I had the discipline to do this, but not because I, or anyone else, is better than those of you who do not. In my case, I had a very strong motivating factor to stay thin. I got that my looks opened doors for me. Movie stars do too, and it makes it easier for them to maintain their weight, too. If you were paid $15 million to star in a movie and needed to be thin, you could probably do it too.

Watching a television star lose a lot of weight on a program like NutriSystem and thinking you will get the same results is extremely misleading. If they fail, they will be publicly humiliated in front of millions of people on television who are watching their results as a company spokesperson, for example. You are not in the same boat. You likely do not have the same motivation.

The same is true for people who feel as though they will only be loved if they look good. They may have more motivation, and greater consequences, for maintaining their weight. (But you probably don't want to be in their shoes.)

A PBS documentary reported that your subconscious brain always wins and beats out willpower. For example, if you are running and you try to breathe slowly, you won't be able to do this. You will always end up breathing fast because your body needs the extra oxygen. The same thing happens when you starve your body of calories or glucose on a low carbohydrate diet. Uncontrollable hunger and your body's need for glucose for survival ruins your willpower. Thank goodness this happens.

Unfortunately, rather than recognizing and respecting this, too many of you view this as personal failure, and as your self-esteem goes down, so does your desire for a quick fix. And the vicious cycle ensues—quick fix, short-term results, long-term failure, and desperation for another quick fix.

Your ability to lose weight and keep it off is a product of your ill health, not your will power. Your inability to eat well is also a product of your ill health and not of your willpower, either. I am able to pass on sugary treats and alcohol because I am healthy, not because I have more willpower than you or anyone else who finds it difficult to say no.

*It's not okay to judge people who are overweight.* If you know someone who is, have compassion for them, and give them a copy of my books.

## Food addictions, overeating, and cravings for unhealthy, "fattening" foods like alcohol and sugar

Addictions for food, overeating, and cravings for unhealthy food, are not psychological problems, but physiological ones.

Many foods can make you feel good, but you should feel good, physically and mentally, without it. When you heal your bowel and body with this program, you will not crave unhealthy food, and you will not overeat, either. As you go through this program you will desire less animal protein, less sugar, less coffee, less alcohol, and/or less salt. You will need much less food than you used to in order to maintain your mental and physical energy levels.

Cravings, addictions, and overeating may trigger your weight problems, but they are not the cause. Your unhealthy bowel and body are.

## Stop blaming everyone else

Watching television does not cause weight problems, nor is it caused by Hollywood, restaurants serving big portion sizes, lack of P.E., or the social circles you walk in.

Not long ago, an article in the *Boulder Daily Camera* (7/26/07) had the following headline; "Obesity can spread in social circles," making it sound like an infectious disease that spreads.

A study found that you are much more likely to become obese if your friends and family put on weight. Researchers believe that when your friends and family are obese, you may change your perception of what is an acceptable weight. The value of this research, it is stated, is that it might be helpful to treat obese people in groups instead of just the individual. This is ridiculous.

Get off the blame road and on this healing road. The blame road will not lead you towards a long, healthy life free of weight struggles.

## Weight problems are not caused by stress or sadness

When you are stressed, you have a tendency to take shallow breaths, which increases blood acidity. Sadness can cause a reduction in your happy brain chemicals, and this can cause you to reach for more sugar, for example, to stimulate these chemicals. Excess acidity, and extra sugar, makes an unhealthy body gain more weight.

In health, your bowel eliminates the acids caused by stress, and it eliminates the fat and water associated with un-eliminated acids. In health, your body is able to regulate the production of your brain chemicals so that even if you are sad, you are less vulnerable to the physiological effects of this.

*Stop blaming yourself, and start blaming the approach for your weight-loss failures.*

### Watch My Video,
### "Why Weight Loss Crutches Are Failing You."

This video, and all of my videos, can be found at *www.UniqueHealing. com* or at *www.YouTube.com/UniqueHealing*.

# Misunderstandings About Weight Loss and Other Information for Your Success

## Keep your stools well-formed

Because un-eliminated acids cause weight gain, and because well-formed stools prevent the re-absorption of acids into your blood, you will lose weight the quickest if you keep your stools well-formed while you are healing your bowel and body.

If you do not have a very good handle on how to define well-formed stools, review Chapter 6 of *Unique Healing* now. (And remember, when your stools are hard and slow you are eliminating more acids, and will therefore feel better, than when your stools are one or more times a day and they are not all extremely well-formed.)

If your stools are not well-formed, the following changes can help: increase your *Body Bentonite* intake; reduce your carbohydrate intake (pasta, breads, grains, cereals, yogurt, etc.); reduce your sugar intake (including natural healthy sugars like agave, honey, raw sugar, cane juice, etc.); reduce your alcohol, salt, coffee, and/or soda intake; do not have a massage, chiropractic adjustment, or any other body work; drink a lot of water; rest; and keep your exercise aerobic, as discussed earlier.

If these changes do not noticeably help the form of your stools in two days, take them further (i.e. take more *Body Bentonite*, reduce your carbohydrate intake more, etc.)

Out of all of these recommendations, increasing your *Body Bentonite* intake is one of the most productive and helpful. It heals your body, unlike many of the other recommendations. It will do the most to lead you to a place where looking good is effortless, and some of the other suggestions, like reducing sugar intake, are simply "too hard to do when your blood is too acidic."

(Note: the exception to this information is when your poorly formed stools are caused by an infection, in which case *Unique Healing Colloidal Silver* is needed to reduce your symptoms. Refer to Chapter 5 for information on when and how to use this crutch.)

## Weight loss programs rely on crutches,
## and that is why they are failing you

The majority of weight loss programs do not address the cause—i.e. un-eliminated acids—of your weight problems. They are crutches. They are the tarp that is placed over your roof that has holes in it that does nothing to fix these holes in the first place. Some of them contribute to the further destruction of your roof. Some of these contribute to greater struggles with losing weight in the future.

These programs/crutches do nothing to eliminate the acids that cause your weight problems in the first place. Therefore, once your exercise program slows down and/or you start eating more food or carbohydrates again, your body is still incapable of eliminating the acids that caused your weight problems, and you end up storing excess fat and water again. When you stop spraying perfume on your pile of trash, it's still there, and it starts to stink again!

## The most, and the least, dangerous weight loss crutches

The most dangerous weight loss crutches to use while you are healing your bowel and body with this program, as well as those that cause harm so that it is harder, not easier, to lose and maintain your weight in the future, are: drugs, surgery, and high protein diets.

The safest weight loss crutches to use while you are healing your bowel and body are: the crutches I recommended earlier, aerobic exercise, low calorie diets, alkalinizing and detoxifying diets, and modalities that help with the elimination of acidity, like saunas, deep breathing, and increased water consumption. These crutches can help you break the vicious cycle of losing weight and having more difficulty doing the same in the future. They do not reduce your health, and therefore they do not increase your risk of illness or premature death.

## Health and weight are the same

To succeed in attaining effortless, long-term weight loss, and to live long enough to enjoy it, you have to stop making losing weight your priority. You have to focus on making your body healthier. When you are healthy, you will be thin.

In 2005 Governor of Arkansas Mike Huckabee stated "we have to focus on our health, not losing weight. That's why we fail." I agree. Unfortunately, the wisdom of this man has been lost, and no strides have been made in the collective conscious towards this direction since then.

Weight loss programs are failing you because they focus on weight loss and not on health gain.

## More wrong cause-and-effect conclusions/an "F" in science

I may write a book about these one-day. I could write a very long one. I cannot begin to count the number of statements and conclusions that are made by the medical, and alternative, professions that are based on the hypothesis that because two variables co-exist, one must cause the other. How do they get away with this? This is "anti-science." When my kids were in elementary school they had to do science fair projects. They had to come up with a hypothesis and then test it ten times to see if it held true. Had they come up with the hypothesis but then never tested it, they would have gotten an "F" on their project, as they would not have been following the scientific method. But the science world/medical and other professionals fail to follow this method all the time! They come up with statements/hypotheses, but then never test them to see if they are true (in the meantime, massive harm has been inflicted because the statements are made as though they *have* been proven.)

You may read and/or hear about hundreds of these unproven cause-and-effect assumptions that may counteract the information in my books, so be careful. Make sure that the information you read and trust and follow is based on an actual proven study, or experience, not just an assumed correlation.

One example of these cause-and-effect hypotheses that has never been proven is the statement that diabetes and other health conditions are caused by excess weight; the weight is named the cause of these problems, but this is not true (nor has it been proven). Excess weight is caused by an unhealthy bowel and body, *as are* diabetes and other health conditions. Excess weight does not cause them. (By the way, if it did, then thin people would never have diabetes or other health conditions, but millions of thin people *do* have health problems.)

Another example is a PBS documentary that showed a couple that was having a hard time getting pregnant. This was blamed on their weight, as they were overweight, but again, this is wrong. An unhealthy bowel and body cause you to be overweight, and an unhealthy bowel and body makes it difficult to conceive. I know plenty of thin, "fit" women who have struggled to get pregnant. You can be thin and unhealthy.

Excess weight is a symptom of less than ideal health. I challenge you to find me an overweight person who does not take medications and/or does not have headaches, PMS, gas, allergies, high cholesterol, insomnia, fatigue, osteopenia, or any other symptom of poor health. When you regain your health with this program, you will lose both your extra weight *and* your symptoms.

Likewise, just because you lose weight does not mean that you are healthier, and will live a long, disease-free life.

## You can be in control

Similarly, a recent article about current research on weight loss, stated, "In a study of 100 overweight, *otherwise healthy* women . . ." You have heard this dangerous message millions of times; that overweight people are healthy. *This is absolutely not true.*

More often, you are told that you need to lose weight to improve your health. This is wrong and misleading too. If you lose weight you can feel better, but feeling better does not mean you are healthier.

You need to start thinking, "If I get healthy, I will lose weight."

As long as you continue to be led to ignore your health as the cause of your weight problems, your weight problems will continue. You can lose weight and become less healthy in the process. Millions of people have done this already. Because of this, you keep joining health clubs, buying diet pills, and blaming your lack of willpower or old age or bad genes. This has got to stop. Your health and weight are under your control.

## Diets focus on weight loss and not health gain, hence their failure

Dietary advice is largely geared towards weight loss rather than health gain. But the only way to lose weight and keep it off permanently and effortlessly is to regain your health.

You can eat foods that "quickly" help you lose weight, but there are no foods that can "quickly" help you gain your health.

Your desire for the quick fix has led you astray. Your focus on eating food that helps you lose weight, rather than eating food that is healthy for you, is one of the main reasons you continue to struggle with your weight.

There are many weight loss diets which consist of many highly acidic, health-destroying foods like steak, ham, beef, pork rinds, diet sodas, and sugar-free foods made with artificial sweeteners. While you may lose weight eating this way, you will also lose some of your health. Not only is this dangerous, but once you regain your weight, and you will, it becomes harder for you to lose weight in the future, due to the ill effects of these diets on the health of your bowel and body, which should be keeping you thin, naturally and effortlessly, in the first place.

## A food that helps you lose weight is not necessarily healthy for you

Just because a food helps you lose weight does not mean it is healthy for you, and just because a food does not help you lose weight, or even if you gain weight when you eat it, does not mean it is necessarily unhealthy for you, either.

An enticer on the Internet said, "We always thought applesauce was healthy: 10 things to stop eating now (to lose weight)." No wonder you are confused and frustrated! Applesauce *is* healthy for you.

You need to stop labeling a food as healthy or unhealthy simply by the immediate effect it has on your body.

Along these same lines, your being led to focus on the quantity versus quality of food eaten is dangerous, as it is the quality of a food that affects your health much more than it is the quantity eaten. Stop counting calories, and instead focus on eating foods that are healthy for you. Diet sodas have no calories and may help you lose weight initially, for example, but diet sodas are also very unhealthy for you, and your unhealthy body will cause you to eventually gain back your weight.

## Eating fat does not make you fat

An unhealthy body makes you fat. Some fats improve your health, and some reduce it.

Research shows that people who eat a lot of nuts have a lower body mass index (not a higher one), compared with non-nut eaters. Nuts contain fats that are healthy for your body. When you accept and understand that a healthy body makes you thin, you will move towards eating a diet that makes you healthy.

461

## Societies that are healthier are thinner

We are one of the least healthy societies in this world, and one of the heaviest as well. Health and weight are directly connected to one another.

In other countries, infertility is also less prevalent than it is here. My guess is that children in other countries start out life with healthier bowels than children here do. Most other countries also eat a much less acidic diet than we do.

A vacation to Mexico with my children resulted in their shock by how wonderful the food tasted there. They assumed that because they saw a lot of poverty, the food would be inferior to ours. I explained to them that in poorer countries, food is much less processed than in ours. Food processing is an expensive luxury that results in food that is much more acidic than unprocessed food. In fact, we were leaving to come home on Thanksgiving Day and the resort we were staying in had live turkeys by the restaurant that they were going to kill and cook that day for dinner. The turkey you buy here has usually been frozen for a long time, and it probably has a lot more antibiotics and other harmful chemicals than these did. (I was sorry we missed this rare opportunity.)

The bottom line is that other countries are healthier than we are and they eat more healthfully, too. This is why they are thinner. It is not due to any "magic wine" or "magic olive oil." They are thinner because they are healthier, and health is not created simply by eating a magic food, as is *often* suggested.

## Active and thinner when younger, weight balloons when older and less active

You hear this story often. Many people who were athletic as a youngster and involved in a sport were able to maintain their weight as a result of the exercise involved. Therefore, they never realized that their body was not as healthy as it could be. If you are thin because you exercise, it does not necessarily mean you are healthy.

If you too have had this experience, healing your bowel and body with this program can change it.

## You are not stuck with excess fat cells forever

With many weight loss programs you lose weight and your fat cells shrink, but they still remain, eventually crying out for more calories. This is a story you've heard many times, as an explanation for why you can't effortlessly maintain your weight.

Low carbohydrate, high protein diets do not eliminate fat cells. These only "suck the glucose out of them." Fat cells are made to protect your body from excess acidity; these diets do nothing to reduce this acidity or to heal your bowel so it can eliminate it.

When you heal your bowel and create an organ that can eliminate acids, your body no longer needs to produce fat cells to buffer them. I would be thrilled to have someone do a study on this program and measure the number of fat cells before and after it. This type of study would be worth your hard earned dollars.

## The metabolism myth

Weight problems are not caused by a "faulty metabolism." Blaming excess weight on poor metabolism occurs when one does not know the real reason for it. It is an easy excuse that millions of you have been sold. Unfortunately, no one has taught you the real story about what causes your weight gain (up until you read this book, that is).

All of this metabolism talk is misleading, confusing, and has led many of you in the wrong direction. "Metabolism" describes how fast you burn fat, but it is a frequently misused word. You are told you have a poor metabolism if you are overweight, you are told you have a fast metabolism if you can't gain weight, and you are told you need to eat frequently to keep your metabolism up.

Your liver, adrenal glands, and thyroid are a few of the organs that help regulate your metabolism.

> You can exercise or eat few calories to stimulate the burning of fat, or you can make these organs of metabolism healthy by healing your bowel and body with this program, relying on them to do this for you. It is much easier to rely on your healthier organs, not to mention, much safer, as they will also help you to live much longer.

A 1994 study in *Metabolism* found that vegetarians had an 11% higher resting metabolic rate than non-vegetarians. Your metabolism is controlled by the health of your organs, and many vegetarians are healthier than non-vegetarians.

Also, these organs could be healthy, yet if you have an unhealthy bowel and kidneys, for example, these can lead to weight gain (water weight gain), or underweight conditions (due to mal-absorption of protein in your bowel), but they have nothing to do with "your metabolism."

You have heard that dieting can slow down your metabolism, and this is true of many weight-loss diet crutches, because eventually your body gets "smart" and "slows you down." By doing this there is less need for glucose, and therefore less need to burn fat to get more glucose. Starvation or high-protein diets are dangerous, and eventually your body usually decides to stop the damaging process.

Other diet advice recommends eating often to "keep up your metabolism," which works if you eat frequent protein meals, but this is not due to a better metabolism, as you are led to believe. It works for weight loss because these frequent protein meals stop your body from cleansing, and reduces the fat and water weight that is otherwise created due to this cleansing and incomplete elimination of acids. (Return to the section on high protein diets to understand this concept if you still do not.).

*Just because you lose weight does not mean that your metabolism has improved.*

When it is explained this way, you are falsely and dangerously led to believe that the diet you are on is therefore good for you. If you lose weight on a low carbohydrate, high protein diet, you have actually *reduced* your metabolism, as this diet is harmful to your organs of metabolism.

Finally, if you are thin and can eat all of the time without gaining weight, you are not healthy and you do not have a strong metabolism, as is commonly thought. You have to be just as concerned about your health as the person who struggles to lose weight, and maybe more so, as everyone will wrongly think you are immune to disease due to your thinness, and you too will likely think you can eat unhealthy foods and get away with it.

If you eat a lot and cannot gain weight it is because you have very unhealthy systems of digestion and absorption. See Chapter 2 for more information on how this program helps with needed weight gain.

## More help eliminating fat-causing,
## water-retention-causing acids

Your kidneys, lungs, and skin are organs of elimination that can assist with the elimination of acidity that causes weight problems. Drink more water and lower your refined salt consumption, as this will help flush acids out of your kidneys. Practice deep breathing daily, as this will enhance the elimination of acids by your lungs. Take Epsom salt baths to help eliminate acids through your skin. Saunas, steam rooms, herbal body wraps, "sweaty" yoga (Bikram yoga), and exercise that induce sweating will too. For more information on these approaches refer to Chapter 8 of *Unique Healing*.

## Water weight fluctuations

Whether you follow my program, or use a weight loss crutch, quick, initial weight loss is due to water weight loss. Unfortunately, just as quickly as you can lose this weight, you can put it back on, as well.

During this program your weight may fluctuate, depending on the number of un-eliminated acids in your blood. Keep your stools well formed and these fluctuations will be much less common and noticeable. Keep healing your bowel and body with this program, and one day, they won't occur at all.

When you use weight loss crutches, you are also vulnerable to fluctuations in your weight due to changes in water weight. However, with these programs, this vulnerability never goes away.

## This program does not cause muscle loss, or ketosis

A concern and danger of many weight loss diet crutches is that they can cause you to lose healthy muscle weight. If you starve yourself, or eat a low carbohydrate diet, you limit the amount of life-sustaining glucose that is available (as glucose comes from food, especially carbohydrates and fruit). As a result, your body can eventually turn to your muscles to provide glucose for you. The breakdown of muscle for energy yields a harmful by-product called ketones, and this state is called ketosis.

This program eliminates the acids that cause fat and water retention. It does not rely on starvation or a low carbohydrate diet for this to happen, and therefore, it does not cause you to lose muscle; it does not send you into a state of ketosis.

## Weight gain that occurs as you age is due to poorer health

Most people are healthier when they are younger than when they are older.

If your bowel and body are unhealthy, and then subjected to numerous acids, gradually and cumulatively, they will become less healthy (even if you exercise, take supplements, go to the chiropractor, etc., as these do not prevent the accumulation of acids that harm your bowel and body health). The less healthy you become, the more prone you become to gaining weight.

To blame the difficulties of losing weight as you age on a "slower metabolism" is very un-empowering, and not inevitable.

You can be healthy as you age. You *will* be healthy as you age if you heal your bowel and body with this program. I am significantly healthier now, in my late-forties, than I was in my teens. Maintaining my weight now, as an older woman, is massively easier than it was when I was a teen, and very unhealthy.

## An unhealthy bowel and childhood weight struggles

Childhood obesity is at an all-time high in this country. Additionally, overweight kids are 20%-30% heavier than they were ten years ago. Many other countries are, for the first time ever, seeing alarming increases in childhood weight problems. The most common excuse for this has been a lack of exercise and too many calories, or the same excuses given for adult weight problems.

As with an adult, exercise and diet crutches may work in the short-term for your children, but they will also fail in the long-term as well. More concerning is their future state of health—not because they are overweight, but because their unhealthy bowel and body that causes this condition is not being acknowledged, and these unhealthy bowels and bodies can manifest as even more alarming increases in cancer and heart disease rates later on (and much too early in life).

*Adults who have been obese since childhood have a life expectancy nearly 25 years shorter than those who maintained an average weight.*

If you have a child who struggles with his/her weight, heal his/her bowel and body with this program. I see children all the time who have very unhealthy bowels and bodies. If your child is overweight, I am 100% certain that his/her bowel and body are unhealthy as well. Every concept in this program can be applied (safely) to your child. Nothing pains my heart more than seeing a child who has been put on a high protein diet by a parent who is doing the same to lose weight. While these diets are harmful for everyone, they are most notably damaging to your child. Heal your child's bowel and body so that he/she can live a long, healthy life, free of constant weight obsessions and struggles. Your child has his/

her whole life ahead of him. He/she needs this perhaps even more than you do.

## The genetic component—it can be changed

Overweight problems can be, in part, attributable to poor genetics, but your genetic inheritance can be changed. You can inherit unhealthy organs and bowel bacterial environments from your parents, which is what leaves you vulnerable to weight problems. But unhealthy organs and bowels can be made into healthy ones, by healing them with this program.

In my experience, children with unhealthy bowels and bodies reach for more animal proteins, fewer veggies, and more sugar than children with healthier ones. This less healthy child is more susceptible to weight problems as he/she gets older, unless his/her bowel and body are healed when he/she is young.

On top of this, well-intentioned parents can aggravate an already unhealthy system by forcing their young children to eat more protein than they desire or need. I've seen a one and a half year old, reaching for yogurt and green beans and rejecting the pork chop he was given, being forced to eat it. This very skinny young boy grew into an overweight twelve year old.

When your children are skinny as youngsters you are told not to worry about what they eat. This is unacceptable. A lack of quality food as a youngster contributes to an unhealthy bowel and body in the future, and weight problems later on as a result.

## Diet crutches can increase the levels of toxic pollutants in your blood

The 9/21/10 issue of the *Wall Street Journal* cited a study published in the *International Journal of Obesity* that found that long term weight loss increases the level of pollutants in your bloodstream, especially "persistent organic pollutants," a class of chemicals that includes pesticides and solvents which have been linked to type 2 diabetes and cardiovascular diseases. The participants who had lost weight over the last ten years had "significantly higher" levels of these chemicals than those who had no change in their weight. People who had gained weight had lower than normal levels and those who had lost at least twenty-two pounds had 75% more of an insecticide, beta-hexxachlorocyclohexane, a product of an insecticide that was banned more than 30 years ago, in their blood than people whose weight had not changed!

Fat buffers un-eliminated acids. It protects you from them. When you use a weight-loss crutch, like a high protein, low calorie diet or exercise, fat may be burned/turned into fuel, but the un-eliminated acids, like insecticides, that *caused* the fat production, are then left exposed in your bloodstream, putting you in danger. When you lose weight with this program, fats *and* acids, like dangerous insecticides, are removed from your body, which eliminates this risk.

## Do it for yourself

"Everybody's going to love me" when I'm thin is a thought that leads to trouble in losing and maintaining your weight. If you have these thoughts, your values are wrong. If someone loves you for how you look, they are not a healthy person to have a relationship with. In a healthy relationship you are loved for who you are, and not how you look.

When you embark on this program, do it for yourself. If you feel pressured to lose weight quickly you will fail in the long run.

## Respect yourself

Make your health a priority. You deserve to be healthy and thin. If someone tries to tell you otherwise, tell him or her it is not okay to be spoken to that way. If they try to sabotage your efforts, are jealous or critical, walk away. If needed, find a good therapist to help you with these issues.

## The Quick Fix Versus Long Term, Struggle-Free Weight Loss

Does this weight-loss program sound too good to be true? It really is this good, but yes there is a catch. You may not lose weight nearly as fast as you will on any of the quick-weight-loss programs. You have to accept that it takes time to negatively impact your health and that it takes time to improve it as well. You must decide if you are only interested in a quick, short-term result, or if you are ready to lose weight and keep it off effortlessly in the future, and get healthier and feel better in the process? In the second case, you will need to be patient and persistent, but if you focus on making your bowel and body healthier, then you will *lose weight and keep it off.*

When your organs become unhealthy due to genetics, stress, an acidic diet, and your unhealthy bowel is unable to eliminate acids, you become susceptible to gaining weight. Because it takes a long time, or a lot of acidity, for them to become unhealthy, it will take some time to reverse this. Luckily, healing is quick, relatively speaking.

If your weight has gone up only in the last couple of years, do not be fooled into thinking that it took only a couple of years to put that weight on. There was a long period prior to this in which your bowel and body were becoming unhealthy. It is only when they reach a certain level of ill health that excess weight shows up. (Children can become overweight at a young age because they can inherit very unhealthy bowels, and they can inherit unhealthy bodies, or organs, too.)

Dr. Lee Kaplan says, "Something this complex (i.e. overweight), is not going to be fixed by a quick fix." He believes that we need a different solution for different people. I agree, to the extent that my clients who struggle with their weight all have an unhealthy bowel and body, but the exact supplements, quantity, and length of time needed to heal them are very different.

Be patient and persistent and know that in every way you are healing your bowel and body and becoming healthier. Be grateful that your bowel and body can heal.

Do not weigh yourself everyday. The more often you do, the more likely you will fall for an unhealthy, quick fix with devastating long-term results.

Every day that you follow this program, your bowel and body are becoming healthier. Eventually, excess fat and water weight will leave your body, and it will stay off, naturally and effortlessly. This result is worth waiting for.

For some, this will happen faster than others, but all of you will be rewarded with long-term weight loss and greater physical and mental wellbeing. The end results are remarkable!

## Long-term results are what matter

Weight loss programs that deliver fast results also come with a 95% failure rate in achieving long-term weight loss.

"Diet experts" are experts at helping you achieve short-term weight loss; but their "expert" advice often leads to long-term weight gain, and long-term health loss.

In 2003, three research centers were set up to do a five-year study on the Atkin's diet. Prior to his recommendations this research did not exist, yet millions of you followed his advice anyway. This study was designed to look at weight loss, cholesterol levels, energy levels and the health of the heart; although I could not find if this was going to be measured in a relevant way such as with a heart scan. A five-year study is not nearly long enough to measure the full ill effects of this diet, but it is better than nothing. Most importantly, it needs to measure the *mortality* of people who followed this diet. Finding that cholesterol levels went down and inferring that this diet is healthy as a result is dangerously harmful. The only significant findings of this study will be those that measure mortality and long-term weight loss.

It is now 2012, or nine years later, and the results of this study are something I have never heard of. How come? What happened to this study? I review studies every week, and read the paper and Internet looking for these types of studies. I am pretty sure I would have read about this, or heard about it, had the results been published.

We may never know what happened to this study, but in the meantime, a ten year study in 1997 conducted by a researcher from the American Cancer Society which tracked the dietary habits of a whopping 79,236 healthy adults found that *the more vegetables and less meat* subjects ate the less likely they were to develop a spare tire around their midsection. Also, a moderately high-fat diet with nuts was better than a low-fat plan at helping people lose weight and keep it off.

The most shocking revelation that is certain to be revealed, eventually, is that people who follow low carbohydrate diets have greater weight problems, and a shortened life, in the long-term versus people who use other methods to lose weight.

## Maintaining weight without the struggle

Years ago, during the holiday season, I was deeply reminded, and touched, by how many people lose weight and thereafter find themselves in a daily struggle to maintain it. I was at my daughter's preschool when one of the directors offered me a piece of holiday fudge. I kindly refused, *as the thought of sugary fudge had no appeal to me.* The director proceeded to comment on how strong my willpower was. I responded by saying that it was not willpower; rather I had no interest in eating the fudge. This comment was confusing to her. She couldn't understand how I could not like sugary fudge; she had a strong craving for sweets. I went on to explain that I had been very ill many years ago and that after healing my bowel and body with this program, I wound up with many benefits, among them a sharp reduction in sugar cravings, as well as tremendous ease in maintaining my weight. Now she was completely lost. She told me how she had lost a lot of weight several years ago (she still had the potential to lose another 30 pounds or so) and that she is healthy; however, she struggles with her weight daily. She said that if she eats too much sugar or food one day, she starves herself the next and/or spend hours exercising. I was filled with feelings of sadness, and compassion for her, and for the many of you who are in her shoes. Is this where you want to be? It doesn't have to be this way.

In a 1997 study conducted at the Obesity Nutrition Research Center, National Weight Control Registry, of people who had successfully kept their weight off for at least one year (which is not very long) and who had lost at least thirty pounds, 89% had changed both their eating patterns and physical activity. 88% ate less of certain foods, although exactly which ones were limited was not stated. On average, they reported eating 1,380 calories a day. This is not much! How long can that go on? They reported very high levels of physical activity (about 2,800 calories burned a week, which is equivalent to walking 3-4 miles a day). That's a lot. Half of the participants weighed themselves every day, and 75% weigh themselves at least once a week. That is very obsessive, and a very stressful way to live. What a struggle!

If maintaining your weight is a struggle, you are not healthy.

Maintaining your weight will be effortless after you heal your bowel and body with this program.

You will be healthier, and in this state, you will stop producing extra fat and water weight, even if you eat a higher-calorie, higher-carbohydrate diet, or stop exercising religiously. On this program you can take a vacation from exercising, or eat a lot of food one week, and not gain the weight back, because your healthy body that keeps you thin cannot become unhealthy in only one week.

With this program you will maintain your weight loss results because it would take another 20, 30, 40 or so years of eating a highly acidic diet for your bowel and body to become unhealthy again. It is not until your bowel and body become unhealthy that you become vulnerable to weight gain.

When you finish healing your bowel and body, you will have the health of many teenagers. Many of you have experienced a time in your life when you could eat whatever you wanted, not go to the gym, and still not gain weight. This is because for many of you, your bowel and body were still pretty healthy as teenagers. Unfortunately, because it takes a lot of acidity to damage your bowel and body, you may have thought that all of the unhealthy foods that you ate were okay to eat because you didn't gain weight while eating them. A lot of the foods and beverages you consumed *were* damaging your bowel and body, and now many of you are suffering the consequences.

When your bowel and body are healed, you will neither over-eat nor under-eat. You will not crave sugar, soda, coffee, alcohol, or other foods that stimulate fat and water production.

When you have healed your bowel and body with this program, you will stay thin, even if you are not always eating well. A strong roof can tolerate some rain. A healthy body can tolerate some acidity from your diet, stress, and the environment without gaining weight.

## Unwanted Weight Gain On This Program: What to Blame? And How to Prevent It

There are two reasons why you *might* gain weight while following this program, *neither of which are caused by this program itself.* If the principles behind this program are understood and followed, and you are patient with healing your bowel and body, neither of these will occur. If you occasionally slip up and they do occur, they can be quickly reversed.

## You reduce or stop a weight loss crutch too quickly

If *prior* to starting this program, or *during* this program, you lost or maintained your weight by a program of exercise, low calorie, or high protein consumption, and you change, eliminate or reduce these "crutches" before you have healed your bowel and body so that they are healthy enough to help you maintain your weight easily and naturally (i.e. you reduce your exercise, increase your caloric intake, or eat less protein), your weight may go up. If you get rid of your crutches before your leg is healed, you won't be able to walk.

In other words, any weight loss that you achieved prior to or during this program because you exercised, reduced your calories, or increased your protein intake, is not permanent, and changing these variables before you heal your bowel and body will cause your weight to "go up" even as you are healing your bowel and body. It is only once your bowel and body are healthier that you will achieve permanent weight loss. (Your weight will go up if you stop or reduce these crutches and do *not* do this program, as well. Only with this program, *one day* this will not occur.)

To prevent this from happening, do not change your exercise or diet habits too quickly. If you do, and you gain weight, know that it is caused by these actions, and not by this program. Also know that while you may not like the extra weight, you have not done anything to stop this program from working. Eventually, you will lose weight without these crutches.

## You cleanse too quickly

If you *over*-cleanse your body during this process, you may gain weight. Over-cleansing occurs when you eat fruits, carbohydrates, and other glucose-containing foods that move acids from your organs into your blood and bowel faster than you can eliminate them. Over-cleansing occurs when your stools become too soft, hard, skinny, mushy, or infrequent.

Your body may respond to these un-eliminated acids with extra fat production and/or water storage (water weight).

To prevent this from happening, do not increase your consumption of fruit and/or carbohydrates (i.e. breads, grains, even gluten-free, pastas, cereals, yogurt, etc.), or reduce your intake of protein (i.e. meats, fish, chicken, turkey), too quickly. If you do, and you gain weight, know that it is caused by these actions, and not by this program. And again, know that while you may not like the extra weight, you have not done anything to stop this program from working. Eventually, you will lose weight without these crutches.

### Watch my video "Not Losing Weight?"

This video, and all of my videos, can be found at *www.UniqueHealing.com* or at *www.YouTube.com/UniqueHealing*.

# Success With Weight Loss

"Since following this program for six months, I have lost over 15 pounds. What is most amazing about this however is that I have not increased my exercise, and I find the foods that I am eating are very appealing and easy to stick with. Even when I eat poorly, I don't immediately gain weight, like I used to."

"I went from a size 14 to a size 4. Since doing this program, I do not exercise, and I eat carbohydrates and I do not follow a low calorie diet, and my weight stays at a size 4. It is amazing."

"I used to gain 5-7 pounds on vacation, during the holidays, etc. I have been gradually losing weight on this program, and I love that I have the freedom to travel, enjoy the holidays, and not gain the extra weight that I used to."

"For the first time in my life, I have thrown out my "fat clothes." After doing a zillion diets, I know that this time, the weight is going to stay away for good. (I was led to believe that on all of the other diets, but deep down, I didn't believe it. This feels completely different.)"

"When I started this program I ate nothing but protein and vegetables, but I was still 10 pounds overweight. I was completely frustrated. The main thing I couldn't give up was wine, and Donna explained how the acidity of it was causing me to retain water. She also gave me her vitamin B-12 and it completely stopped my wine cravings. It made it super easy to cut back on it, and doing so has resulted in my losing those stubborn 10 pounds."

"When I came to Donna I exercised all the time but I still had a good 15-20 pounds to lose. I tried to exercise even more but that seemed to backfire. Donna had me reduce my exercise, and with this program, I was finally able to lose my extra weight."

"I didn't come to Donna for weight loss. I came to see her because I suffered from horrible headaches, fatigue, depression, and high cholesterol.

I was focused on getting rid of these. I had given up all hope of ever losing weight as I had tried everything, and I mean everything, to lose it in the past, and I just couldn't ever stick with the programs. So I was amazed when I started losing weight with this program. I was even more amazed when my cholesterol went down and I started feeling a lot better."

"After doing this program for a while I had to have surgery and could not exercise for a while. I was freaked out because I knew I was going to gain weight, because I always did in the past when I stopped working out. This time, my weight remained the same. Yea!"

## My personal struggles to lose weight

When I was in high school I was constantly dieting. At first I could easily lose an extra five pounds simply by eating less. When I went to college, however, it wasn't that easy. It took an even lower calorie diet to lose weight, and this very restrictive diet was extremely hard to follow. I was confused, and really frustrated.

I drank a lot of diet soda (I was addicted to "TAB"), ate low calorie frozen yogurt for lunch, and starved myself, because I was told that you lose weight by reducing calories. (The healthfulness of these foods was never discussed.)

In my early twenties, I added obsessive exercise to my daily routine in order to maintain my weight. My weight remained down because of this, *but I was never happy*. The daily struggle and obsession were all consuming, mentally exhausting, and massively stressful, and left me feeling very weak and vulnerable. Because I was able to manipulate my weight, I was convinced that all of my other abusive behaviors were not harming me. Of course they were, and one day they all caught up with me and I crashed to rock bottom.

Today I eat twice as much food as I used to, I eat a lot of carbohydrates, and my body looks better than it did when I was in high school starving myself. More importantly, my mind is now free from the daily obsession about what I am eating and what my stomach is doing. And if I do not exercise (and I rarely do), or if I eat poorly for a week or so, I do not gain a single pound.

I no longer belong to a gym. I stopped going many years ago. Even though I love to take long walks and be active, I don't follow an exercise program.

I never think or obsess about my weight and I am a million times happier emotionally and physically than I was years ago, when I maintained my weight the average way of starving and exercising. I feel empowered and confident as a result. I never weigh myself.

You can have this too. It takes longer to get here than it does the other way, but look at your options. You can lose weight quickly in the short-term, only to spend your entire life losing and gaining it back and having your entire life controlled by this. With this option, you will also feel less than ideal physically and emotionally, and you have not reduced your odds of dying from a degenerative disease prematurely.

Or, you can spend the time needed to heal your bowel and body with this program. This may take longer to get results, but when you do, they will be effortless and permanent, and you will be free of a weight loss obsession. It's like getting out of jail! Additionally, you will enjoy greater confidence in your life and greater emotional wellbeing, not to mention the fact that you will also likely live much longer to enjoy your new body.

## Watch my video "Why THIS Program Eliminates Weight Problems"

This video, and all of my videos, can be found at *www.UniqueHealing.com* or at *www.YouTube.com/UniqueHealing*.

(For information on difficulty *gaining* weight, see Chapter 2).

# Chapter 5

## How to Look and Feel Better NOW!

Because it takes time to heal your bowel and body, even with the extraordinarily aggressive program that I have developed, it is *highly* recommended that you use dietary and supplement crutches during this process. They will help you look and feel better while you are healing, which will help give you the patience you need to complete this healing process. Additionally, why not look and feel better while you are healing? I wish someone had this information when I was sick; I definitely would have taken advantage of it, as you should do now.

(For more information on this topic, review Chapter 10 of "Unique Healing.")

### Supplement Crutches to Help
### You Look and Feel Better Now

The following supplement crutches are the ones that I have found to be most helpful. They address 95% of the symptoms that clients present themselves with.

These crutches are: *Body Bentonite, Unique Healing Methyl Vitamin B-12, Unique Healing Colloidal Silver, Unique Healing Calcium Citrate*, natural progesterone cream, and melatonin.

When your bowel and body are unhealthy, these crutches can help you look and feel better. There is zero possibility of them making you look or feel worse. Never blame them for these problems.

Make buying and taking *Bowel Strength* or *Unique Healing Probiotics*, and *Body Bentonite* and *Unique Healing Calcium Citrate*, your priority, and then add in as many of the other crutches listed below as desired. Many of your symptoms, weight problems, and illnesses are the result of un-eliminated acids and can be eliminated with *Body Bentonite* alone but not all of them. Some of your problems are the direct result of your unhealthy bowel bacterial environment, and these require different crutches. *Unique Healing Methyl Vitamin B-12, Unique Healing Colloidal Silver, Unique Healing Calcium Citrate*, natural progesterone cream, and melatonin, positively reduce symptoms in ways that *Body Bentonite* cannot, and using these will help you feel even better while you are healing your bowel.

> Yet still remember that these are crutches, and when you rely on crutches to look and feel better, you cannot expect to look and feel great *every* day. That can, and only will, happen when you have spent adequate time healing your bowel and body with this program. Do not expect miracles from crutches; expect miracles from healing your bowel and body.
>
> You must give this program time to heal you. Don't start it until you are ready to commit to it.

Refer to Chapter 3 of this book, and Chapter 5 of *Unique Healing*, for information on diet crutches to use while you heal your bowel and body with this program.

## Is it really this simple?

Yes, it is. You may think it isn't, due to the fact that many of you have been using supplement crutches the wrong way and are not looking and/ or feeling better as a result. You may have been led to believe that it is much more complicated to look and feel better quickly than it really is, due to the numerous different supplements recommended in books and by practitioners. But the majority of these supplements do the same thing. Just as there are thousands of different brands of perfume that you can buy to smell better, there are hundreds of supplements that can make you feel better, but in both cases, this large selection is unnecessary; it is simply the result of many people and companies vying for your money who work hard marketing their products to convince you to buy their product, and not someone else's. It is to their advantage to make supplement usage sound *much* more complicated and individualized than it really is. For example, an adrenal supplement will reduce many more symptoms than adrenal ones, because it buffers acids, and acids trigger many different symptoms. You, however, are led to believe that adrenal supplements are different from liver ones, for example, but they are not.

## How much do I take?

Under the description of each crutch I have made recommendations for the amounts to be taken. I cannot guarantee that these recommended dosages will eliminate 100% of your symptoms. *No* one can do this (although many books certainly try to). But for many of my clients, the amounts suggested are valuable and effective at reducing their symptoms to a noticeable degree.

If the amounts I have recommended do not help you look and/or feel better within the first week of using them, you have three options. One, you can double the recommended dosage and give that a week to see if it works. Two, you can schedule an appointment with me to make sure you are using the right crutch at the right dose, and/or if taking larger amounts concern you for any reason. Three, you can spend more time healing your bowel and body, and then you can re-try these crutches later (when you are healthier, as the healthier your bowel and body are, the less of a crutch you will need to look and feel better. In other words, one day, when your body and bowel are healthier, they will prove helpful. If they do not work now, one day they will.)

*Because most of us are impatient, I highly recommend options one or two, if possible.*

Crutches only work if you take the right ones, and the right amount. Review the sections in Chapter 2 to determine that you are taking the right crutches. If you are, and they are not working, it is likely that your bowel and body are too unhealthy to benefit from these, in which case, most of your time, money, and energy needs to be directed towards the healing of your bowel and body. It is likely that your leg is too weak to use crutches right now. This is a concern, as it can imply that your health is in imminent danger.

The amounts given are my recommendations, but they can be taken in lower amounts (with less noticeable improvements in your symptoms, addictions, weight loss, etc.). Also, if you are very patient and your funds are limited, or your willingness to take a lot of supplements is limited, make taking *Bowel Strength* and *Body Bentonite* your priority.

## Do not expect one crutch to solve all of your problems

When judging the effectiveness of a crutch, do not expect one crutch to improve all of your symptoms. It usually takes several of the ones that I have recommended to do this. So if you take 60,000 mcg of vitamin B-12 and you are less depressed, but still have headaches, this crutch has "worked." To eliminate your headaches, you may need to increase your intake of *Body Bentonite*, instead. Review the sections on crutches later in this chapter as well as in Chapter 2 to better understand the selection of crutches that you may need to eliminate or reduce all of your symptoms, if desired.

## Can too much be harmful?

I have found all of these crutches to be both safe, and often only effective, in dosages higher than the standard recommended amounts. I have had clients take 10,000 mcg of vitamin B-12 a day with no improvements, experience significant reductions in their depression after increasing this to 60,000 mcg a day, for example.

Perhaps the greatest danger of taking a high dosage of these supplements is not the potential for harm, but the risk of "burn out," and the low likelihood that you will continue with this.

In the nineteen years that I have been doing this work, I have never had a client experience harm due to the ingestion of these supplements, even at the very large amounts I recommend.

In my experience, it is *much* more harmful to take too few of these, than it is to take large amounts of them.

## Using these crutches with young children and teenagers (and pets, too!)

When drugs are prescribed, your size/weight is very important when it comes to the right, and safe, amount to take. Medications are acidic/toxic, and the less you weigh, the greater the toxicity or danger of taking too large of a dosage.

The supplement crutches I advise are not acidic/toxic and there is no danger to their use. Your child's size/weight is irrelevant. The best amount to give your child has to do with their need (as discussed earlier). Many of my young clients take larger amounts of crutches than their parents do, as they have less healthy bowels or bodies and need larger amounts to look or feel better. My clients with autism, for example are advised to use, and benefit from, amounts that are often much larger than the amounts that my average adult uses, and needs.

The greatest limitation in giving crutches to young children and teenagers is their ability to swallow pills and/or their willingness to do this. (Note: If you have an infant less than one year old, you must work with me personally.)

These same concepts apply to your "over ten pound" pets as well. These crutches are safe and very valuable for them too. While animals have different dietary needs than we do (dogs are carnivores, for example, and mine are fed a very high protein, grain-free diet), they are similar in that a healthy bowel and body will go a long way in extending their life and eliminating disease and symptoms. My two ten-pound dogs are fed two teaspoons of *Body Bentonite* in their food everyday, and because their bowels are about 2x/day and never more frequent, or green or watery, I have not given them *Unique Healing Colloidal Silver* or *Unique Healing Probiotics,* but if they did have these bowel issues, I would (and I encourage you to do the same.) An average dosage of probiotics for a 10-pound dog would be 50 Billion organisms/day, but refer to the concepts in Chapter 7 of *Unique Healing* to better determine their need.

I do not currently have the time or energy to extend my practice to animals (although I have given advise to a number of clients about theirs, with great results), but they need this program, too. This program is unique for them too, as currently, pets are primarily treated the same way as humans—with medication crutches, or with "alternative" crutches like acupuncture and supplements, which do not heal their bowel and body and do not yield the dramatic, health and life-changing results that this program does.

(Note: If you have a pet that weighs less than 10 pounds and would like to help them, contact me for an appointment.)

## Crutches need to be used daily for best results

Remember that these are crutches. They do not heal your bowel or body. If you had a broken leg and used crutches to get around on Monday, you would still need to use them on Tuesday to be able to move around. There is no lingering, cumulative affect of them.

If you take *Unique Healing Methyl Vitamin B-12* and have more energy on Monday, you will need to take this supplement again on Tuesday to keep having more energy. Surely you have been led to believe differently, as many times you have been advised to use these sporadically. For example, you may have been given weekly or monthly vitamin B-12 injections. This approach is not only wrong, but it does not work. If you get an injection on Wednesday, you will not feel better on Friday. You will only feel better on Wednesday, the day you used this crutch. Because crutches are wrongly touted as healing agents, you have been led to use these wrongly, and ineffectively, as well.

You do not have to take these daily, but do not expect to feel as good off of them as you do on them. It is not until your bowel and body are much healthier that you will be able to reduce and/or stop them and still feel good.

Using these crutches does not make you "addicted" to them. You are using them because you deserve to look and feel better now, and there is no harm, only benefit, in taking advantage of this knowledge and using these crutches. You are healing your bowel and body with this program and as a result, one day, you will look and feel great without them. Your using these daily only helps you be more successful in getting to this precious outcome.

## How did I figure out that using large amounts was safe, and helpful?

I get this question a lot. The recommendations that I give for supplement crutches are high. They are higher than what is recommended by any other practitioner I know or read about. However, I make these recommendations with great confidence. I "figured this out" due to the following.

One, I read a lot of medical nutrition studies. Years ago, I noticed that in some of these, extremely large amounts of supplement crutches were used, with great results. That got me thinking. Two, I have learned a lot about the way our bodies work, and everything I learned pointed to the idea that these larger amounts should be safe and more effective than smaller amounts. Three, in the nineteen years that I have done this work, I have had many clients who were willing to test higher limits of using these. I openly and honestly informed them that I had not previously recommended higher amounts, yet some insisted on trying more, and I supported this (with the very strong belief that it would be safe and effective to do so). In 100% of the cases where a client pushed the previous limits of what I had been recommending, the results were amazingly positive. This prompted me to make similar recommendations to future clients, and cumulatively, this gave me a much larger base of clients following these recommendations, and the observation of 100% positive results by doing so. Four, when clients increase the crutches they take and feel and look a lot better than they did on lower amounts, it confirms the "need" for larger amounts.

You do not have to take advantage of my knowledge and experience in this area. You can be patient and wait to look and feel better (but I don't come across very many patient clients)! Mostly, when I was extremely ill, I would have done anything to feel better quickly (as these large recommendations are capable of achieving for you). I knew it was going to take time to heal my very toxic body, but if someone had the information I now have, I definitely would have taken advantage of it, and I would have been massively appreciative of it. I am offering you the chance to look and feel better, but it is your prerogative to decline this offer.

(Nevertheless, I must state that the amounts I recommend of these supplements have never been *scientifically* tested or proven to be effective or safe.)

## Body Bentonite

*Body Bentonite* helps eliminate acids, toxins, metals, chemicals, pesticides, etc. from your body, and therefore, over time, it heals your body. But *Body Bentonite* is a crutch as well, which can make you quickly feel and look better, and it is one that I *highly* recommend.

### How *Body Bentonite* works/symptoms helped

Bentonite is a natural substance that is largely derived from clay that is found in the earth. It has been ruled G.R.A.S (Generally Regarded as Safe for human consumption.)

It binds to, and eliminates, the acids in your bowel that your bowel is not able to eliminate on its own. Think of it as an extra trashcan for your front yard to handle the trash that your first trashcan cannot, due to the fact that it has holes in it, or is simply too small.

Eliminated acids are not re-absorbed into your blood and body, triggering health and weight problems. Therefore, *Body Bentonite* reduces your health and weight problems. Over the long-term, your use of *Body Bentonite* eliminates your lifetime of stored acidity and damage to your organs, and heals your organs.

> There are *countless* vitamins, herbs, minerals, and other supplements that buffer acids and reduce your symptoms. Buffering the acids that trigger your symptoms is valuable; healing your body so you don't react badly to these acids in the first place is even better. *Body Bentonite* heals your body; most other supplements do not.

While the full effect of healing your body with *Body Bentonite*, and eliminating a lifetime of accumulated acids in your organs takes some time, a more immediate response to its use is an improvement in the frequency and form of your stools, and less gas and bloating. It is especially helpful for loose stools, but it also improves constipation, bloating, gas, stomachaches, and other intestinal discomforts.

> The quicker you improve the form of your stools with *Body Bentonite*, the faster you will feel better, and lose (water) weight.

Your bowel is "at the bottom of your pipe," so bowel symptoms like constipation, loose stools, gas, and bloating, will be the last to become completely eliminated. While you are healing your bowel and body, the daily use of *Body Bentonite* can help reduce (but not completely eliminate) these. On the other hand, if your loose stools, gas, or bloating are caused by an infection, too much fiber, or another variable that is caused by an unhealthy bowel bacterial environment, *Body Bentonite* will not help eliminate these problems. Return to Chapter 2 and re-read the section on "Bowel Problems" for a complete description of the crutches needed to improve your bowel symptoms while you are healing your bowel and body.

Expect to see improvements in your elimination with the daily use of *Body Bentonite*, but do not expect *Body Bentonite* to produce miracles overnight, and keep in mind that, more importantly, every day that you take *Bowel Strength* or *Unique Healing Probiotics*, you are addressing the cause of these problems. The *cause* of your loose stools, gas, bloating, and constipation is an unhealthy bowel and body, and this takes time to fix.

## It is like putting money towards equity in your house not throwing it away on rent

Every day that you use *Body Bentonite*, you are moving towards a healthier body that, one day, won't need crutches to look and feel good. There is a cumulative, healing effect of this product, which you do *not* get with other crutches.

So while you will find that you will need to use this product for a while to look and feel better, there is an end in sight. After a couple of years of using it, you will be healthier, feel and look better, and need fewer crutches. On the other hand, after a couple of years of using crutches like most diets, vitamins, acupuncture, etc., you will *not* have created greater health, and for most of you, you will find that you need *more* crutches to look and feel better.

If you have a mortgage, at the end of a couple of years, you have built equity (think of this as using *Body Bentonite*.) If you pay rent, at the end of a couple of years, you have no equity, but rather you have "lost" some of your money (think of this as using crutches).

*Warning: Body Bentonite* improves the form, and often the frequency, of your elimination—a feat that is extremely valuable, but difficult.

It is very easy to take a laxative and quickly improve the frequency of your stools (which does nothing to eliminate acids, make you healthier, live longer, or help you lose weight and eliminate symptoms or addictions); it is not easy to attain well-formed stools.

For many years, books have commented on the importance of proper elimination, and they have sold products that the authors have claimed will heal it, yet their focus has been entirely on the frequency of your bowels, and not the "all important" form of your stools. Millions of dollars worth of colon cleansing, colon health, and bowel health products have been sold with the *false assurance* to you that they are helping make your bowel healthier, and helping you eliminate acids/toxins/heavy metals.

Because no one ever told you that the form of your stools, not the frequency, determines how many acids are being eliminated, you have bought into these products (that immediately improve your frequency but not the form of your stools), and you have bought into the idea that good form should be just as easy to attain as good frequency.

> It is 100 times more difficult and complicated to have good form to your stools than it is to have good frequency of elimination. Yet good frequency without good form is not healing, or helpful, to your health.

So, if you have had experience with these other colon products—that always contain some type of irritant to your bowel like senna, cascara, aloe, prunes, or psyllium—and noticed an immediate increase in your frequency of elimination, be careful you do not expect the same result (instant results) when you take *Body Bentonite*. (Adding these ingredients sells products, but it is profit for "them" and loss for you.)

In the short run it takes longer to heal your bowel and body and improve the form of your stools, yet in the long run, your health and weight will be 1,000 times better as a result. In other words, while you may like the "quick fix" of immediate and automatic increased frequency of elimination with these other products, you will not like the fact that decades after using these, your health and weight will be the same, or worse.

## Disadvantages/misunderstandings of *Body Bentonite*

> *Body Bentonite* does not eliminate vital nutrients from your body.

While *Body Bentonite* absorbs and eliminates acids from your body—acids that harm you when they are not eliminated—it does not bind to, or eliminate, vital nutrients from your body. You can take it with food and it will not, because it cannot, bind to the nutrients in your diet. Nor does bentonite "stick" to the side of your intestinal walls, causing mal-absorption. Mal-absorption is caused by an unhealthy bowel, which this program heals.

In fact, because it helps eliminate acids, and because un-eliminated acids are the primary cause of nutritional deficiencies, the use of it improves, not reduces, your nutritional status. (For more information on how this product improves your nutrient levels see Chapter 3.)

*Body Bentonite* does not cause dehydration.

Dehydration occurs when your body draws water out of your tissues to buffer un-eliminated acids. Because *Body Bentonite* eliminates acids from your body, its use *improves* the hydration of your body and helps prevent dehydration. If you are dehydrated, increasing the amount of *Body Bentonite* you take will reduce your dehydration. (For more information on how this product reduces dehydration see Chapter 3.)

Constipation which may occur with *Body Bentonite* use is very valuable, and temporary.

Contrary to what many of you have been told, constipation is *not* caused by inadequate water consumption. Un-eliminated acids cause it. If you have poorly formed stools prior to using this product (and the vast majority of you do), and they become less frequent and firmer while taking *Body Bentonite*, this is a very positive, productive occurrence. You will look and feel better if you continue with it. The tendency to reduce or stop this product in this case is high, but do not. Review Chapter 6 of *Unique Healing* for a description of ideal elimination, and watch my video, "Stop Freaking Out About Constipation," available on my website at ***www.UniqueHealing.com*** or at ***www.YouTube.com/UniqueHealing***.

On the other hand, if *Body Bentonite* makes your stools infrequent and very hard, and this makes you uncomfortable, consider taking extra magnesium so that you don't have to stop or reduce taking *Body Bentonite*. You will look and feel better much faster if you do this. (For more advice on this, see Chapter 10 of *Unique Healing*.)

*Body Bentonite* will not make your stools looser.

*Body Bentonite* works very differently from fiber products/ bulking agents, and from numerous colon health products that contain laxatives. *These* products can cause more frequent and looser stools; *Body Bentonite* cannot. Additionally, these products do not eliminate acids from your body, *Body Bentonite* does. If you have had a problem with urgent or loose stools, or cramping, with fiber/bulking agents or other colon health products, you will not have this problem with this product.

## *Body Bentonite* does not cause nausea.

If you become nauseous after taking this product, it is because you either: 1. Are pregnant 2. Have the flu or 3. Have a bacterial infection. The vast majority of the time that a client has this experience it is due to a bacterial infection (which is caused by an unhealthy bowel, not by bentonite). If you experience nausea with this product, stop it for two days and during this time take *Unique Healing Colloidal Silver* (as directed later in this chapter). After you have taken the correct amount for two days, add back *Body Bentonite*, continuing with the colloidal silver for at least another two days while you do so, so that you can see that it was an infection at the root of this reaction, and so that you can be comfortable taking this product.

## *Body Bentonite* does NOT cause "detox" symptoms.

*Body Bentonite* does not detox you, nor can it cause your symptoms to worsen. I am often asked if this product pulls acids (metals, toxins, etc.) out of your organs. It does not. Bentonite does not, and can not, "pull acids out of your organs into your blood and bowel faster than you can eliminate them," which is what happens when you "detox" and feel bad as a result. In order for acids to be released from your organs into your blood and bowel, you need to eat cleansing foods—foods that contain glucose, like fruit, honey, and carbohydrates like breads and pastas and other grains. (Some cleansing also happens monthly during a woman's period, during menopause, during the first trimester of pregnancy, at night while sleeping, and at other times, but your diet has the greatest impact on this.) When acids are not eliminated from your bowel, the consumption of these cleansing foods triggers health and weight problems, leading many of you to avoid them. You end up eating more protein, and this diet reduces the cleansing of acids out of your organs. *Body Bentonite* helps you eliminates acids from your blood, and as a result, you will be more comfortable eating less protein. You will be able to eat cleansing foods and not look or feel bad doing so, and as a result, you will change your diet and consume more of these. You will automatically eat a cleansing, healing diet when you heal your bowel and body with this program, and *this diet* will move the acids out of your organs. So indirectly, *Body Bentonite* helps heal your organs.

To fully understand this concept watch my video "Body Bentonite does NOT Cause "Detox" Symptoms" at ***www.UniqueHealing.com*** or at ***www.YouTube.com/UniqueHealing***

*Body Bentonite* does not eliminate bacterial infections, or the symptoms caused by them.

Apparently there are some claims online that bentonite fights bacterial infections. Not everything that you read online is based on fact. These comments are not true. To the best of my knowledge, I have more experience using extremely large quantities of bentonite with very large quantities of clients than anyone else, and I have never seen bentonite eliminate a bacterial infection, or the symptoms associated with one.

If you are using *Body Bentonite* and you feel sick, have loose stools, are nauseous, have stomach cramping, or experience any other uncomfortable symptoms, do not blame the bentonite. You likely have a bacterial infection, and you will need to use *Unique Healing Colloidal Silver* to eliminate this. See the section later on for information about when and how to use this product.

Likewise, if your stools are green when you take *Body Bentonite*, but brown when you do not, this is not caused by bentonite. Bentonite can accelerate the elimination of infected, green stools, and make it more obvious that you have them, but it does not cause them. Hundreds of my clients take large amounts of *Body Bentonite* and have brown stools.

*Body Bentonite* does not add aluminum to your body or harm you in *any* way.

There *might* be extremely tiny amounts of aluminum in some bentonite products, but it is not in an active form that can harm you.

My experience and testing has revealed that *Body Bentonite does not* add aluminum to your body. On the contrary, it *eliminates* the storage of it in your body (and symptoms and disease associated with excess aluminum stores).

## Fears of bentonite are unfounded

Claims about any concerns of using bentonite are unfounded. They are *not* based on experience or studies. Beware of everything you read and hear. People are allowed to make any claim they want. Before you give these any credibility, ask the questions that you deserve to get the answers to. Where are the studies that show it is dangerous? What experience does the person who is writing these claims, or repeating them, have to make such a statement? *You will find no studies that show it is dangerous, and you will find that the people who make these false claims have zero personal experience using large amounts, and are therefore not qualified to make these claims.* This includes comments about bentonite that may be made by your acupuncturist, naturopath, doctor, or any other practitioner, as he/she is extremely unlikely to be qualified to comment on its use.

Of all the fear-mongering information you will find online or elsewhere about bentonite, none of it that I have seen is credible.

For the last 19 years I have advised the use of bentonite to my clients. I have had hundreds of clients take amounts that are considered "massive" by the alternative and medical field. *Unlike others who might comment about this product, it is I who am qualified to comment about the safety of it.*

I have never seen any harm done by the ingestion of large amounts of bentonite. On the contrary, I have seen people lose weight and keep it off, eliminate polyps, cysts, numerous diseases, congested arteries, high cholesterol, headaches, bloating, blood sugar problems, ADD, alcoholism, etc. I have seen it heal one's organs and greatly extend the quality and quantity of their life.

It is sad that some of you may be led to be afraid of a product that can dramatically improve the quality *and* longevity of your life; something that modern *and* alternative medicine is failing to do.

*Body Bentonite* cannot harm you. Un-eliminated acids do.

## How much *Body Bentonite* do I take?

*Body Bentonite* is food grade bentonite that comes in liquid, powder, and capsule form. Take 3/4 cup of *Body Bentonite* liquid, 10 capsules, or 1 tablespoon of powder, 1-3x/day. If you buy powdered *Body Bentonite*, put it in a bottle with a lid and shake well. Or, for a smoother consistency, blend it in your blender for 30 seconds. Once made, this product can sit on your counter or in the refrigerator for many weeks and it will still retain its blended consistency.

After one week, double this amount if you desire greater improvements in your stools, weight, and/or symptoms. Many of my clients take more than this. If you desire to take more and look and feel better and heal faster, please contact me for an appointment.

Note: If you are taking medications, do not take these at the same time you take *Body Bentonite*, as it absorbs toxins, and drugs are toxic. Wait one hour before or after taking your medications before you take it. Even though I have never personally seen this interfere with someone's medications, it is a standard recommendation that should be followed. You *can* take *Body Bentonite* with other supplements, herbs, vitamins etc. as these are not toxic, and *Body Bentonite* only binds to toxic substances.

## Do not drink bentonite with cleansing or acidic drinks

Take bentonite only with water or unsweetened tea. If desired, to these you can add a slice of lemon, and a non-acidic, non-cleansing sweetener like stevia or erythritol. These two sweeteners can be found as named, or under other names at the health food store.

## Possible negative side effects?

The use of this product may cause constipation. While this is very positive, as has been discussed and explained many times in my books and videos, if it causes you discomfort, try adding 1,000 mg of magnesium citrate (found at health food stores) to relax your colon and make the passage of your stools more comfortable.

If you get constipated with this product, it means you need it, and that if you continue with it, you will look and feel better.

## Where do I purchase *Body Bentonite?*

*Body Bentonite* can be ordered from Unique Healing at ***www. UniqueHealing.com*** on the "Unique Healing Store" page, or by calling 203.286.8932. The source of bentonite in the liquid and powder is a high quality, very fine, food-grade white bentonite powder, which is *greatly* preferred by clients who have tried other products, and by younger clients. No chemicals are used to make this product. Also, while the liquid bentonite is smoother and not as thick as other brands of liquid bentonite, it contains the same amount of bentonite as these products and is equally as effective.

*Body Bentonite* contains 32 ounces/bottle (liquid), 300 capsules/bottle (capsules), or one pound/package, or approximately 50 tablespoons (powder). (See website for a full list of ingredients.)

## Watch my video and read my blog for more information

My videos, "Body Bentonite REDUCES Dehydration" and "Making Bentonite Work for YOU" can be found at ***www.YouTube.com/ UniqueHealing***. My blog post titled "Aluminum in Bentonite?!" can be found at ***www.UniqueHealing.com***.

# Unique Healing Methyl Vitamin B-12

## How *Unique Healing Methyl Vitamin B-12* works/symptoms helped

Vitamin B-12 is a necessary nutrient for numerous functions in your body. It can be especially helpful in cases of persistent fatigue, depression, nervous system disorders like multiple sclerosis, nerve pain or discomfort, addictions to alcohol, drugs, exercise, and other items, and sugar cravings. It can also be extremely helpful for kids and adults with altered brain chemistry and neurological problems, like autism, ADD, Pandas, Tourette's, seizures, etc. It is a great crutch to give you the mental strength to handle a long healing process.

## Disadvantages/misunderstandings of vitamin B-12

If you take a multivitamin, B-complex, or mega-B vitamins, you will not get nearly enough vitamin B-12. The amount of B-12 in most of these products is 100 mcg/day. The amount I recommend is 300x stronger than this. High amounts of vitamin B-12 will not cause the other B-vitamins in your body to go out of balance. Finally, all of the B-vitamins, vitamin B-12 included, are water-soluble. This means that if too much is taken it is urinated out of your body, and not stored. There are no known side effects or harm of using large amounts.

While vitamin B-12 can improve your energy levels, it is not a stimulant like caffeine and will not make you jittery or interfere with your sleep. (Consider the widespread use of Ritalin for A.D.D. Ritalin is a stimulant and it is used to calm down the hyperactive child, just as B-12 calms down hyperactivity, and does not cause it, either.) It also cannot give you energy "immediately," so do not use it this way or expect this reaction.

Meat contains some vitamin B-12, but low levels of vitamin B-12 are not caused by a vegetarian diet, and a meat-based diet won't remedy a level that is too low in your body. An unhealthy bowel causes low levels of vitamin B-12. Your diet—whether you are a meat eater, vegetarian, vegan, or follow any other dietary practice, is irrelevant in regard to your levels of this vitamin. I have found that clients who eat *all* of these diets, yet who have very unhealthy bacterial environments in their bowel, have low levels of this nutrient. (In fact, while meat contains some of this vitamin, the acidity of meat is very destructive to the health of your bowel bacterial environment. If anything, contrary to what you may have been led to believe, if you are a meat eater you are likely to have even *lower* levels of vitamin B-12 than someone who eats a less acidic, more vegetarian-type of diet.)

Finally, it is important that you use a methyl form of vitamin B-12, as found in *Unique Healing Methyl Vitamin B-12.* Do not use a cheap vitamin B-12 product, as these are very difficult to assimilate, and you will receive no value from this crutch if you can't assimilate it. Ironically, the only reason you will find value in this crutch in the first place is because your bowel bacterial environment is unhealthy, and the less healthy it is, the more difficult it is for you to assimilate this vitamin. Once your bowel is healthier you will be better able to assimilate the less expensive form of this nutrient, but then again, at that point, you won't need this crutch anyway!

Twenty years ago when I was very ill, I received weekly B-12 shots. The amount I was given was inadequate to produce results, and because no one knew how to heal my bowel, the results I received from these were minimal and very short-lived. I recommend supplements of vitamin B-12 as a crutch, and find these to be more effective than shots because they can be taken more consistently and for longer periods of time if needed. Not many people will get a shot five days a week for months and years on end.

## How much *Unique Healing Methyl Vitamin B-12* do I take?

I recommend 30,000 mcg/day, or 6 pills/day, of *Unique Healing Methyl Vitamin B-12* (which contains 5,000 mcg/pill). If your symptoms, as described above, do not improve in one week, try 60,000 mcg/day or 12 pills/day. I have worked with many clients who have benefitted from even larger amounts, especially clients with autism, A.D.D., multiple sclerosis, drug and alcohol addictions, etc., and if you have one of these conditions, please contact me to schedule an appointment so we can assess whether a larger amount would be helpful for you, too.

## Possible negative side effects?

None.

## Where do I purchase *Unique Healing Methyl Vitamin B-12?*

*Unique Healing Methyl Vitamin B-12* can be ordered from Unique Healing at ***www.UniqueHealing.com*** on the "Unique Healing Store" page, or ordered by calling 203.286.8932. *Unique Healing Methyl Vitamin B-12* contains 60 capsules/bottle, and each tablet contains 5,000 mcg of B-12. (See website for a full list of ingredients.)

## Watch my video; "Use the Vitamin B-12 Crutch to Look and Feel Better While You Heal."

This video, and all of my videos, can be found at ***www.UniqueHealing.com*** or at ***www.YouTube.com/UniqueHealing***.

# Unique Healing Colloidal Silver

## How *Unique Healing Colloidal Silver* works/symptoms helped

Infections are either viral or bacterial. To generalize, viral infections are prevented by your lymphatic, or immune system. Preventing bacterial infections is the responsibility of the healthy bacteria in your bowel. They are your "army" that kills off these invaders, but while you are healing your bowel with this program, you are vulnerable to these infections.

Sinus infections, some cases of the flu, staph, pneumonia, bronchitis, strep throat, most cases of diarrhea that last more than two days, and e-coli are examples of bacterial infections that can be reduced or eliminated by taking *Unique Healing Colloidal Silver*.

*Unique Healing Colloidal Silver* is also valuable for eliminating fungal, yeast, and parasitic infections. Some cases of acne, psoriasis, itchy skin rashes, toenail fungus, brain fog, autism, PANDAS, fatigue, stomach cramping, bloating, green stools, and bowel movements that are more than 2x/day, can be caused by an excess of fungal growth and can be eliminated with the use of this product.

If you have stools that are green or yellow, or you have bowel movements that are more than twice a day, take *Unique Healing Colloidal Silver* (increasing as described later on, if necessary), until your stools turn brown and/or slow down. These conditions are normally indicative of a fungal, parasitic, or bacterial infection. While you may not care that you have green or too frequent elimination, you *will* care about the other aggravating symptoms that occur as a result of these infections. You may also be wrongly tempted to reduce your *Bowel Strength* or *Body Bentonite* when your elimination is poor and "nothing else" is helping. This is a particularly good reason for you to use this product; it increases your chance of success in healing your bowel and body.

Finally, *Bowel Strength* contains goldenseal, garlic, wormwood and other anti-bacterial crutches, and can be helpful in preventing these infections as well, but *Unique Healing Colloidal Silver* is generally stronger than goldenseal, and many of you will need the extra help this product provides.

(*Unique Healing Probiotics* do not contain anti-bacterial crutches, so if you are taking this product, it is especially advisable that you have colloidal silver on hand in case it is needed.)

## Disadvantages/misunderstandings of
## *Unique Healing Colloidal Silver*

*Unique Healing Colloidal Silver* has natural antibiotic properties, but it is not as strong as a medical antibiotic. If you are very sick, you may need to use a drug instead.

On the other hand, colloidal silver is not toxic, like antibiotics (and therefore it has no side-effects, like antibiotics do), and it does not destroy any beneficial bacteria in your bowel (as antibiotics do).

A few years ago, a man who turned blue, while allegedly using colloidal silver, appeared on *Oprah* and the *Today* show. This created some unfortunate and unnecessary concern about using this product. The man who turned blue took a homemade silver product daily for 15 plus years, and even applied it directly to his skin during this time.

If this man healed his bowel, he would not need to use a natural antibiotic for this many years. He needs to do this program! Even still, it is impressive that he wasn't harmed by this extremely large dosage of silver. If anything, his story confirms the safety of this product.

You will not turn blue, because you are healing your bowel, and therefore you won't need to use very much of this product. Unlike him, you won't need a crutch, like colloidal silver, forever. Secondly, it is said that the form of silver he was using was *not* colloidal silver, anyway, and that the homemade form of the silver he used can have this effect over time, but that no known "turn blue" side-effects of *colloidal silver*, as I recommend, have been reported.

*Unique Healing Colloidal Silver* cannot weaken your immune system or interfere with "immune-suppressant" drugs if you are taking them.

Finally, *Unique Healing Colloidal Silver* is *not* a toxic heavy metal, like lead and mercury, and it will *not* add to the toxic, heavy metal load of your body. This is a fabulous, and extremely safe, product.

## How much *Unique Healing Colloidal Silver* do I take?

Take 12,0000 parts per million (ppm), or two tablespoons, of *Unique Healing Colloidal Silver*/day. Increase this dosage by 6000 ppm/day, or one tablespoon/day, every twenty-four hours until your symptoms have cleared (up to a maximum of 30,000 ppm/day.) Continue with this dosage for five days, even if your symptoms have improved.

(If your partner, a family member, dog, or other living creature in your household has a bacterial or fungal infection (i.e. their stools are more than 2x/day and/or are yellow, green, or they have diarrhea), give them this treatment at the same time that you use it, otherwise it may not work. If you fight your infection but are constantly re-infected by your spouse, for example, you will be fighting a losing battle.)

Bacterial infections can be much more serious than viral ones and much more difficult to treat naturally. If colloidal silver does not work for you soon, or you are very ill, go to your doctor and get antibiotics, if recommended. Don't take chances with bacterial infections, especially if you have frequent vomiting or frequent diarrhea. This is very dehydrating, and very dangerous. It is not one round of antibiotics that made your bowel unhealthy. One round of antibiotics is not going to prevent you from healing it, either. Re-read Chapter 7 of *Unique Healing* for a better explanation of this.

If you get bacterial infections often, or are very bothered by them, consider taking 6000 ppm, or one tablespoon/day, on a daily basis as a preventative, and/or consider healing your bowel faster. I can assist you with this process, if desired.

(Note: the strength of silver is measured by the ppm (parts per million) that it contains (the smaller the stronger). Comparing silver products is very difficult, however, as I have never found a consistency with them. *Unique Healing Colloidal Silver* was developed to fill a need in the marketplace for a silver product that is effective in a relatively small dosage, at a price that is much less than a similar strength product. Again, you cannot simply compare two silver products with the same ppm and determine which is the best buy from that information alone. I have had clients do this with very limited success. I have thousands of bottles manufactured for me directly and cut out the middle man so I can deliver a strong, high quality product at a great price.)

## Possible negative side effects?
None.

## Where do I purchase *Unique Healing Colloidal Silver?*
*Unique Healing Colloidal Silver* can be ordered from Unique Healing at *www.UniqueHealing.com* on the "Unique Healing Store" page, or ordered by calling 203.286.8932. *Unique Healing Colloidal Silver* contains 2,000 ppm/teaspoon, and 30 teaspoons/bottle. (See website for a full list of ingredients.)

**Watch my video; "Use the Colloidal Silver Crutch to Look and Feel Better While You Heal."**

This video, and all of my videos, can be found at ***www. UniqueHealing.com*** or at ***www.YouTube.com/UniqueHealing***, or by calling 203.286.8932.

## Unique Healing Calcium Citrate

### How *Unique Healing Calcium Citrate* works/symptoms helped

*Unique Healing* Calcium Citrate is an alkalinizing mineral. Calcium is highly abundant in your body, particularly in your bones and intra—and extra-cellular fluids. Calcium makes up more than half of the total mineral content of your body.

Calcium buffers un-eliminated acids in your blood. Using calcium is like spraying perfume on the trash leaking out of your trashcan. The perfume does not fix the holes that cause it to leak out, nor does it help eliminate the trash, but it sure makes it smell better.

*Unique Healing Calcium Citrate* can help you look and feel better because when un-eliminated acids are buffered with it, this reduces the irritating and symptom-producing effects of these acids.

U*nique Healing Calcium Citrate* is also helpful if your bowel has been unhealthy a long time, and you have not been absorbing adequate amounts of calcium from your diet. As such, it can be valuable for helping to slow down, and reverse, bone loss. For more information on this, see the section on "Osteoporosis/Osteopenia" in Chapter 2.

While there are many other forms of calcium available, the most widely used are in a form that is very difficult to absorb, and hence of little value. Calcium citrate is a highly absorbable form of this mineral, which is a necessity for it to work. The majority of this product (80%) comes from calcium citrate, and a much smaller amount, 20%, is derived from calcium carbonate.

### Disadvantages/misunderstandings of
### *Unique Healing Calcium Citrate*

Calcium is recommended for women much more often than for men, even though it is highly beneficial for them as well. Men also have too many un-eliminated acids in their bodies. Generally they have a stronger skeletal system than women, so calcium intake is not as important for them as far as reducing their risk of osteoporosis, but all of my male clients benefit, symptom and weight-wise, when they add calcium to their daily intake.

Taking extra calcium in supplement form does not cause calcium deposits; on the contrary, it can help reduce and eliminate these. Calcium deposits, like those that contribute to the clogging of your arteries and deposits that turn into gallstones and kidney stones, are the result of un-eliminated acids.

Medical studies have conclusively shown that when you take extra calcium, you *reduce* these deposits from occurring.

You do not need magnesium for your body to utilize calcium. By increasing your calcium intake to the amount suggested (2,000 mg/day), you reduce the depletion of your magnesium levels, because calcium buffers the acids that would otherwise "use up" some magnesium to do so. I have intentionally made *Unique Healing Calcium Citrate* without added magnesium, as it is known to have a laxative effect. If you take magnesium and your stools become loose you may wrongly blame the bowel-healing supplements and fail to heal your bowel and body. (Magnesium stearate is a filler used in many supplements and is not to be confused with magnesium that can cause loose stools. It cannot do this. It is listed under "other ingredients." Magnesium stearate does not count as a source of magnesium when looking at these products.) Exception: If you currently take calcium with magnesium, do not change this yet, as you may be relying on the laxative effect of magnesium in this product to prevent constipation, and you could wrongly blame the other products for this constipation if you stop this magnesium crutch right away. Additionally, if you experience concerning or uncomfortable constipation during this program, the addition of extra magnesium as a laxative is advisable. See page 323 of *Unique Healing* for advise on using this, and other, crutches for constipation.

Calcium supplements that contain boron or other minerals or vitamins are in no way superior to *Unique Healing Calcium Citrate* (i.e. these additions are not necessary for the effectiveness of this product).

Finally, some calcium citrate products contain large amounts of calcium carbonate, which is difficult to absorb, but inexpensive. Also, beware of products that say "calcium citrate" and not "calcium, as citrate." The former contain a very low percentage of calcium, and you may easily be manipulated to believe that these inexpensive products are a great buy, but they are not. (In other words, if a product lists 1,000 mg of calcium citrate/capsule, the amount of utilizable calcium in each capsule may actually be 250 mg, not 1,000 mg as you are misled to believe.)

## How much *Unique Healing Calcium Citrate* do I take?

*Unique Healing Calcium Citrate* contains 250 mg of calcium/caplet and 100 IU of vitamin D/caplet for added value.

Take 2,000 mg, or 8 caplets/day. If you have had a recent diagnosis of osteoporosis or osteopenia, or are particularly concerned about these issues or have your first bone density scan scheduled in the next three months, I advise that you contact me for an appointment to discuss your special calcium needs.

Note: If you are working with me directly and taking much more aggressive amounts of *Body Bentonite* than is suggested in this book, your "need" for calcium may be much less, and my suggestion is that you take about ½ the amount recommended, or 1,000 mg, or 4 caplets/day (except where you have a diagnosis of osteoporosis or osteopenia, in which case, I advise you take the full amount recommended in this book). *Body Bentonite* eliminates the acids that calcium buffers and is preferable and much more productive than using calcium to reduce the symptoms caused by acids, however, for those of you who are reading this book and not working with me personally, I have intentionally, and with very good reason, kept my *Body Bentonite* recommendations lower, and for you, the addition of the full recommended amount of *Unique Healing Calcium Citrate* to this program is strongly advised.

## Possible negative side effects?
None.

## Where do I purchase *Unique Healing Calcium Citrate?*
*Unique Healing Calcium Citrate* can be ordered from Unique Healing at ***www.UniqueHealing.com*** on the "Unique Healing Store" page, or ordered by calling 203.286.8932.

## Watch my video; "Use the Calcium Citrate Crutch to Look and Feel Better While You Heal."

This video, and all of my videos, can be found at *www. UniqueHealing.com* or at *www.YouTube.com/UniqueHealing*, or by calling 203.286.8932.

# Natural Progesterone Cream

### How natural progesterone cream works/symptoms helped

Natural progesterone is commonly marketed for reducing symptoms of menopause, but this product is not for menopausal women only. Your hormones can be out of balance *at any age*, and this crutch can be valuable to you at any age as well. I have seen it help young girls who show signs of puberty too early, for teens who have uterine or ovarian cysts, and for women in their thirties who have fertility problems and/or PMS.

I have also found natural progesterone very helpful for women who experience uncomfortable periods, heavy periods, irregular periods, fibroids, hot flashes, vaginal dryness or pain, miscarriages, unwanted hair, poor libido, and other symptoms associated with unbalanced hormone levels.

It is a wonderful crutch for any woman who has or has had breast, ovarian, or any other hormonal cancer, or has a family history of these, as these cancers are largely triggered by the re-absorption of excess estrogen. Progesterone helps offset excess estrogen, making it less harmful.

The use of progesterone for men has not been studied enough, but we do know that is vital for sperm motility and male fertility. Progesterone restores an enlarged prostate gland to normal size. It also reduces the effects of "harmful" testosterone, the kind associated with many cases of prostate cancer.

Finally, studies show additional benefits of this product. They show that it improves body temperature. It reduces spasm and relaxes the smooth muscle of the bronchii and is therefore helpful for asthma and sleep apnea. It helps prevent osteoporosis by stimulating osteoblasts, which help bones heal. It is a neuroprotectant, which can be beneficial for multiple sclerosis, memory, brain trauma, epilepsy, and Alzheimer's. It also reduces gallbladder activity, which can have a protective effect on that organ. (These are claims that have been made by others, however, and I have not myself observed them in my clients who use this product.)

## Disadvantages/misunderstandings of natural progesterone

Excess progesterone may be pulled to the site of excess estrogen to buffer its harmful effects, hence its common presence at the breast cancer site. Hence, also, the fear that has been placed into your head, and on the label of these creams, suggesting that it *may* contribute to hormonal cancers. It is appalling to me that this has been allowed to happen. Your fear of *not* using this crutch should be much larger than your fear of using it.

If your house is on fire, hopefully firemen will show up to put it out. Progesterone is the "firemen" called on to put out the fires in your body. The firemen do not cause the fire to happen in the first place, just as progesterone does not cause breast or other hormonal cancers.

The fear of using too much progesterone is very common, both as voiced by my clients and from articles on the Internet. Millions of women have been diagnosed with breast and ovarian cancer that were *not* using this product. Also, I am not aware of any study that has found that giving women extra natural progesterone increases her likelihood of getting or dying from breast, ovarian, or other hormonal cancers. I believe every female would be safer if she used progesterone cream while healing her bowel and body. I *strongly* encourage my female readers to consider this.

> I have never had a female client who was using progesterone cream get breast, ovarian, or uterine cancer.

Natural progesterone and bio-identical hormones and prescription progesterone are *not* the same. I do not recommend bio-identical hormones; I have seen women get breast cancer while using these. My understanding is that these are still toxic to your body, and possibly dangerous. Natural progesterone is not.

Unlike other hormones, there is no chance of water retention and weight gain as a result of using this product. If anything, these can be reduced by using natural progesterone.

Not all of your "hormonal symptoms" are caused by hormonal imbalances; therefore, do not expect all of them to go away with this crutch alone. For more information, review "Female Issues" in Chapter 2.

## Possible negative side effects?

A very small number of you may experience a temporary increase in vaginal bleeding (usually in between your regular period and not accompanied by other menstrual symptoms, pain, or discomforts) when you start using this cream. This can occur as the progesterone "dissolves" fibroids, cysts, and other unwanted and unhealthy growths in your uterus. This is a good thing. If it concerns you, schedule an appointment with me, or with your doctor.

## How much natural progesterone cream do I use?

Apply ½ teaspoon of cream to your body, two times a day. A standard recommendation is made for you to stop the cream, even if your period is irregular, for seven days from the start of menstrual bleeding, however, some of my clients find that they feel bad when they do this, and continue with it during their period. While this goes against the conventional recommendation, I have never found it be harmful, on the contrary.

## Where do I purchase natural progesterone cream?

"Emerita" makes the natural progesterone cream that I recommend, and it can be found at most health food stores as well as online.

## Watch my video; "Use the Natural Progesterone Crutch to Look and Feel Better While You Heal."

This video, and all of my videos, can be found at *www.UniqueHealing. com* or at *www.YouTube.com/UniqueHealing*.

# Melatonin

## How melatonin works/symptoms helped

Melatonin is a very useful crutch for sleep. Specifically, it has been proven very effective in helping clients sleep through the night and/or for helping them fall back to sleep quickly if they wake in the middle of the night.

While some practitioners claim that melatonin has many other uses, I have never found it to be effective for any other use than to improve sleep.

## Disadvantages/misunderstandings of melatonin

The most common concern I hear about the use of melatonin is that large amounts could be dangerous.

Melatonin is *not* a narcotic like sleeping pills. It is used to regulate your sleep cycles; it does not, and cannot, immediately "put you to sleep." Its action is completely different from over-the-counter or prescription sleeping pills. Likewise, do not take this product and expect to fall asleep immediately after taking it. It needs time to get into your system and to be utilized in the pathways that regulate your sleep cycles.

A healthy bowel bacterial environment produces adequate levels of melatonin. Because you are healing your bowel bacterial environment with this program, you will not need this product in the long-term. Likewise, if you find its use helpful, consider that confirmation that your bowel bacterial environment is unhealthy, and use this to further inspire you to heal it with this program.

Melatonin is a crutch that helps sleep problems caused by low levels, and while this is common, sleep problems have other causes as well. If the melatonin crutch does not work for you, review the section on "Sleep Disorders" in Chapter 2.

Melatonin helps regulate your body's circadian rhythm, and it helps you sleep through the night (as this is part of a normal "body clock."). Melatonin is *not* a tranquilizer or narcotic. *If you are fatigued immediately, or soon after taking it, do not blame it for your fatigue.* Likely you are tired because the night before, when you didn't take melatonin, you didn't sleep well, and your fatigue is a result of this! Or perhaps you are fatigued because your blood is overly acidic; you ate too much fruit or sugar or alcohol the day before.

Finally, melatonin is not a dangerous hormone. There are no dangerous side effects of its use that have been scientifically researched. There may be a connection between its use and hormonal problems, but that does not mean one caused the other. If you have an unhealthy bowel bacterial environment, you will have low levels of melatonin. Your unhealthy bowel also makes you more susceptible to breast or prostate cancer, for example, and people in these conditions may also present themselves with low melatonin levels, but that does *not* mean that low levels are the cause of these cancers. It simply means these two variables, the cancer and low levels of melatonin, coexist.

## How much melatonin do I take?

Take 15 mg/day (or three tablets of melatonin that contains 5 mg/tablet). This is best taken a few hours before bed.

## Possible negative side effects?

If you have had difficulty sleeping and the melatonin crutch helps, you may experience a temporary increase in the number of hours of sleep your body requires. It is as though your body is finally getting the rest it needs to heal and be healthy, and it is "catching up" with lost time. On the other hand, you will likely find that during your waking hours you have more energy and are more productive than ever, so the end result is actually very positive.

## Where do I purchase melatonin?

This can be purchased at health food stores, grocery stores and other outlets that carry supplements, and online. Do not purchase time-released melatonin, and buy the strongest strength you can find (which is typically 5 mg/pill).

## Watch my video; "Use the Melatonin Crutch to Look and Feel Better While You Heal."

This video, and all of my videos, can be found at *www. UniqueHealing.com* or at *www.YouTube.com/UniqueHealing*, or by calling 203.286.8932.

Note: I do not, and cannot, stand behind the safety or effectiveness of supplements that are purchased from other companies. I encourage you to consider this when embarking on this program.

Note: If you are pregnant or nursing, consult with your physician before taking any supplements. Although my experience is that all of the crutches recommended in this book are not only extremely safe, but also very helpful while pregnant and nursing, it is my legal responsibility to advise you to consult with your doctor before using these. You must also contact me directly to schedule an appointment if you are pregnant or nursing so that I can guide you through this process.

# Appendix A

## Sequence of Healing

| 1 | • Cells<br>• Heart<br>• Bones |
|---|---|

| 2 | • Esophagus<br>• Liver<br>• Adrenal glands<br>• Stomach<br>• Small intestine<br>• Gallbladder<br>• Pancreas |
|---|---|

| 3 | • Lymphatic<br>• Nervous/brain |
|---|---|

| 4 | • Lungs<br>• Kidneys<br>• Skin |
|---|---|

Bowel

# Order Information

## Book orders

Additional copies of this, and other Unique Healing books, can be purchased at ***www.UniqueHealing.com*** from the "Unique Healing Store" page. You may also order copies from Author House at 1-888-280-7715, or you can request a copy directly from your local bookstore or at www. Amazon.com. Finally, books can be ordered from my office directly by calling 203,286.8932. Have your Visa, MasterCard, or American Express card number and expiration date ready.

## eBook orders

All of the Unique Healing books can also be purchased as ebooks from online ebook distributors, as well as from www.authorhouse.com.

## *Bowel Strength, Unique Healing Probiotics, Body Bentonite,* Unique Healing Calcium Citrate, *Unique Healing Methyl Vitamin B-12, and Unique Healing Colloidal Silver* orders

These products can be purchased at ***www.UniqueHealing.com*** from the "Unique Healing Store" page, or by calling 203.286.8932. Have your Visa, MasterCard or American Express card number and expiration date ready.

Made in the USA
San Bernardino, CA
10 April 2018